Michael A. Angelo
Pharmacist

Pocket Atlas of Pharmacology

Pocket Atlas of Pharmacology

Heinz Lüllmann, Klaus Mohr,
Albrecht Ziegler, and Detlef Bieger

149 color plates by Jürgen Wirth

1993
Georg Thieme Verlag Stuttgart · New York
Thieme Medical Publishers, Inc. New York

Heinz Lüllmann, M. D.
Professor, Dept. of Pharmacology
University of Kiel
Hospitalstrasse 4, 24105 Kiel, Germany

Klaus Mohr, M. D.
Professor, Dept. of Pharmacology
and Toxicology, Institute of Pharmacy,
University of Bonn
An der Immenburg 4, 53121 Bonn, Germany

Albrecht Ziegler, Ph. D.
Professor, Dept. of Pharmacology
University of Kiel
Hospitalstrasse 4, 24105 Kiel, Germany

Detlef Bieger, M. D.
Professor, Division of Basic Medical Sciences
Faculty of Medicine
Memorial University of Newfoundland
St. John's, Newfoundland Canada A1B 3V6

Library of Congress Cataloging-in-Publication Data
    Pocket atlas of pharmacology / Heinz Lüllmann ... [et al.] ; 149 color plates by Jürgen Wirth.
    Rev. and expanded translation of: Taschenatlas der Pharmakologie /
Heinz Lüllmann, Klaus Mohr, Albrecht Ziegler, 1990.
    Includes bibliographical references and indexes.
    1. Pharmacology-Atlases. 2. Pharmacology-Handbooks, manuals.
etc. I. Lüllmann, Heinz. II. Title.
    [DNLM: 1. Pharmacology-atlases. 2. Pharmacology-handbooks. QV
17 T197p 1993]
RM301.12.T3813   1993
615'.1–dc20

Important Note: Medicine is an ever-changing science undergoing continual development. Research and clinical experience are continually expanding our knowledge, in particular our knowledge of proper treatment and drug therapy. Insofar as this book mentions any dosage or application, readers may rest assured that the authors, editors and publishers have made every effort to ensure that such references are in accordance with the state of knowledge at the time of production of the book.

Nevertheless this does not involve, imply, or express any guarantee or responsibility on the part of the publishers in respect of any dosage instructions and forms of application stated in the book. Every user is requested to examine carefully the manufacturers' leaflets accompanying each drug and to check, if necessary in consultation with a physician or specialist, whether the dosage schedules mentioned therein or the contraindications stated by the manufacturers differ from the statements made in the present book. Such examination is particularly important with drugs that are either rarely used or have been newly released on the market. Every dosage schedule or every form of application used is entirely at the user's own risk and responsibility. The authors and publishers request every user to report to the publishers any discrepancies or inaccuracies noticed.

This book is an authorized, revised and expanded translation of the 1st German edition published and copyrighted 1990 by Georg Thieme Verlag, Stuttgart, Germany. Title of the German edition: Taschenatlas der Pharmakologie

1st German edition, 1990
1st French edition, 1991

1st Japanese edition, 1992
1st Spanish edition, 1992

© 1993 Georg Thieme Verlag, Rüdigerstrasse 14, 70469 Stuttgart
Thieme Medical Publishers, Inc., 381 Park Avenue South, New York, N. Y. 10016
Printed in Germany by K. Grammlich, Pliezhausen

ISBN 3-13-781701-3 (Georg Thieme Verlag, Stuttgart)
ISBN 0-86577-455-2 (Thieme Medical Publishers, Inc. New York)   4 5 6

Preface

Pharmacology in the narrow sense is the study of drugs used in medical therapy. The Pocket Atlas of Pharmacology describes in words and pictures this branch of medical science. The first part, General Pharmacology, deals with aspects that can be considered independently of the individual drug, e. g., dosage forms, absorption, distribution, and elimination, as well as concepts of molecular mechanisms of drug action. The second part, Systems Pharmacology, introduces different groups of drugs with an emphasis on functional and therapeutic aspects; the focus is less on the chemical properties of drugs than on the manner in which they affect body functions and on the therapeutic principles derived from such actions. In the final section, on the pharmacotherapy of specific diseases, rational uses of these principles are presented.

In designing the graphics, attempts were made to explain complex concepts with the aid of visual models. The use of diagrammatic illustrations necessarily results in simplified representations of complex structures and systems with minimal anatomical details. Visual representations of chemical substances, organs, and systems are hierarchically organized within the context of each theme. Color and size distinguish important from unimportant parts. Graphics and the facing text page are meant to complement one another in making pharmacological facts and contexts coherent and intelligible. It is hoped that an appealing and mnemonic presentation will help the reader assimilate and retain an abundance of information about the numerous drugs available.

This pocket atlas is intended for readers with different backgrounds. It will serve students of medicine, dentistry, pharmacy, nursing, and other health sciences to quickly acquire the basic pharmacological knowledge that provides a foundation for subsequent in-depth study. The authors' wish is that basic knowledge gained from the atlas may enable students to absorb more effectively the information presented in lectures and standard textbooks. In addition, the pocket atlas will help physicians and pharmacists call back to memory information learned years earlier and to take in at a glance pharmacotherapeutic contexts. Finally, the pocket atlas is also intended to be a readable source of information for those laymen interested in drug therapy.

We thank Dr. L. Matéfi (Basel), Professor Renate Lüllmann-Rauch, J. Mohr, and Dr. H. J. Pfänder (Kiel) for their assistance in designing individual plates and U. Ziegler (Kiel) for his help with the drug index. The Austrian National Library generously provided a facsimile from the Codex Konstantinopolitanus. Several colleagues at Memorial University, Newfoundland, freely contributed advice during the translation of the original text, which has been revised, extended, and updated. Thanks are also due to Dr. David Frost for his cooperation and advice on the style of the translation.

H. Lüllmann	K. Mohr	A. Ziegler	D. Bieger	J. Wirth
Kiel	Bonn	Kiel	St. John's	Darmstadt

April 1993

Table of Contents

General Pharmacology

History of Pharmacology

Since time immemorial, medicaments have been used for treating disease in humans and animals. The herbals of antiquity describe the therapeutic powers of certain plants and minerals. Belief in the curative powers of plants and certain substances rested exclusively upon traditional knowledge, that is, empirical information not subjected to critical examination.

The Idea

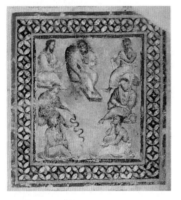

Claudius Galen (129–200 A.D.) first attempted to consider the theoretical background of pharmacology. Both theory and practical experience were to contribute equally to the rational use of medicines through interpretation of the observed and the experienced results.

"The empiricists say that all is found by experience. We, however, maintain that it is found in part by experience, in part by theory. Neither experience nor theory alone is apt to discover all."

The Impetus

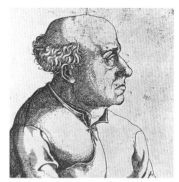

Theophrastus von Hohenheim (1493–1541), called Paracelsus, began to question doctrines handed down from antiquity, demanding knowledge of the active ingredient(s) in prescribed remedies, while rejecting the irrational concoctions and mixtures of medieval medicine. He prescribed chemically defined substances with such success that professional enemies had him prosecuted as a poisoner. He defended himself against such accusations with the thesis that has become an axiom of pharmacology:

"If you want to explain any poison properly, what then isn't a poison? All things are poison, nothing is without poison; the dose alone causes a thing not to be poison."

Early Beginnings

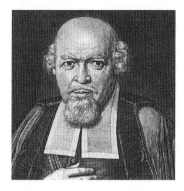

Johann Jakob Wepfer (1620–1695) was the first to verify by animal experimentation assertions about pharmacological or toxicological actions.
"I pondered at length. Finally I resolved to clarify the matter by experiments."

Foundation

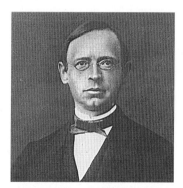

Rudolf Buchheim (1820–1879) founded the first institute of pharmacology at the University of Dorpat (Tartu, Estonia) in 1847, ushering in pharmacology as an independent scientific discipline. In addition to a description of effects, he strove to explain the chemical properties of drugs.
"The science of medicines is a theoretical, i.e., explanatory, one. It is to provide us with knowledge by which our judgement about the utility of medicines can be validated at the bedside."

Consolidation – General Recognition

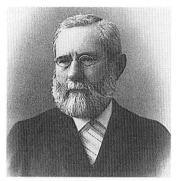

Oswald Schmiedeberg (1838–1921), together with his many disciples (12 of whom were appointed to chairs of pharmacology), helped to establish the high reputation of pharmacology. Fundamental concepts such as structure–activity relationship, drug receptor, and selective toxicity emerged from the work of, respectively, T. Frazer (1841–1920) in Scotland, J. Langley (1852–1925) in England, and P. Ehrlich (1854–1915) in Germany. A. J. Clark (1885–1941) in England first formalized receptor theory in the early 1920s by applying the Law of Mass Action to drug–receptor interactions. Together with the internist Bernhard Naunyn (1839–1925), Schmiedeberg founded the first journal of pharmacology, which has been published ever since without interruption. The "Father of American Pharmacology," John J. Abel (1857–1938), was among the first Americans to train in Schmiedebergs's laboratory and was founder of the *Journal of Pharmacology and Experimental Therapeutics* (published from 1909 until present).

Status Quo
After 1920, pharmacological laboratories sprang up in the pharmaceutical industry, outside established university institutes. After 1960, additional departments of clinical pharmacology were set up at many universities and in industry.

Drug and Active Principle

Until the end of the 19th century, medicines were natural organic or inorganic products, mostly dried, but also fresh, plants or plant parts. These might contain substances possessing healing (therapeutic) properties, but might also contain substances exerting a toxic effect.

In order to secure a supply of medically useful products not merely at the time of harvest but year-round, plants were preserved by drying or by soaking them in vegetable oils or alcohol. Drying of a plant or of a vegetable or animal product yielded a **drug** (from French "drogue"—dried herb). Colloquially, this term nowadays often refers to narcotics and chemical substances with high potential for physical dependence and abuse. Used scientifically, this term implies nothing about the quality of action, if any. In its original wider sense, drug could refer equally well to dried leaves of peppermint, dried lime blossoms, dried flowers and leaves of the female cannabis plant (hashish, marijuana), or the dried milky exudate obtained by slashing the unripe seed capsules of *Papaver somniferum* **(raw opium)**.

Soaking plants or plant parts in alcohol (ethanol) creates a **tincture**. In this process, pharmacologically active constituents of the plant are extracted by the alcohol. Tinctures do not contain the complete spectrum of substances that exist in the plant or crude drug, but only those that are soluble in alcohol. In the case of opium tincture, these ingredients are **alkaloids** (i.e., basic substances of plant origin) including: morphine, codeine, narcotine = noscapine, papaverine, narceine, and others.

Using a natural product or extract to treat a disease thus usually entails the administration of a number of substances possibly possessing very different activities. Moreover, the dose of an individual constituent contained within a given amount of the natural product is subject to large variations, depending upon the product's geographical origin, time of harvesting, or conditions and length of storage. For the same reasons, the relative proportions of individual constituents may vary considerably. Starting with the extraction of morphine from opium in 1804 by F.W. Sertürner (1783–1841) the active principles of many other natural products were subsequently isolated in chemically pure form by pharmaceutical laboratories.

The aims of isolating active principles are:

1. Identification of the active ingredient(s).
2. Analysis of the biological effects (pharmacodynamics) of individual ingredients and of their fate in the body (pharmacokinetics).
3. Ensuring a precise and constant dosage in the therapeutic use of chemically pure constituents.
4. The possibility of chemical synthesis, which would afford independence from limited natural supplies and create conditions for the analysis of structure–activity relationships. Finally, derivatives of the original constituent may be synthesized in an effort to optimize pharmacological properties. Thus, derivatives of the original constituent with improved therapeutic usefulness may be developed.

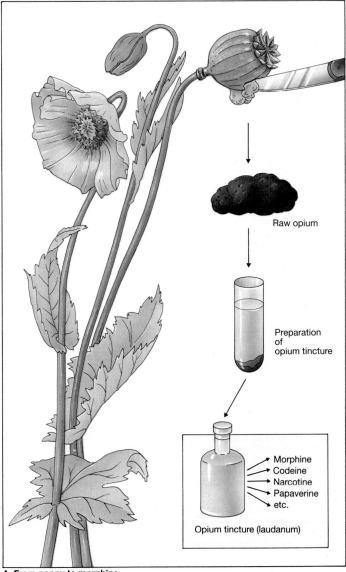

Raw opium

Preparation
of
opium tincture

Morphine
Codeine
Narcotine
Papaverine
etc.

Opium tincture (laudanum)

A. From poppy to morphine

Drug Development

This process starts with the **synthesis** of novel chemical compounds. Substances with complex stuctures may be obtained from various sources, e.g., plants (cardiac glycosides), animal tissues (heparin), cultures of microbes (penicillin G) or of human cells (urokinase), or by means of gene technology (human insulin).

Preclinical testing yields information on the biological effects of new substances. Initial screening may employ biochemical–*pharmacological investigations* (e.g., receptor binding assays, p. 56) or experiments on cell cultures, isolated cells, and isolated organs. Since these models invariably fall short of replicating complex biological processes in the intact organism, any potential drug must be tested in the whole animal. Only animal experiments can reveal whether the desired effects will actually occur at dosages that produce little or no toxicity. Toxicological investigations serve to evaluate the potential for: (1) toxicity associated with acute or chronic administration; (2) genetic damage (genotoxicity, mutagenicity); (3) production of tumors (onco- or carcinogenicity); and (4) causation of birth defects (teratogenicity). In animals, compounds under investigation also have to be studied with respect to their absorption, distribution, metabolism, and elimination (*pharmacokinetics*). Even at the level of preclinical testing, only a very small fraction of new compounds will prove potentially fit for use in humans. *Pharmaceutical technology* provides the methods for drug formulation.

Clinical testing starts with **Phase I** studies on healthy subjects and seeks to determine whether effects observed in animal experiments also occur in humans. Dose–response relationships are determined. In **Phase II** potential drugs are first tested on selected patients for therapeutic efficacy in those disease states for which they are intended. Should a beneficial action be evident and the incidence of adverse effects be acceptably small, **Phase III** is entered, involving a larger group of patients in whom the new drug will be compared with standard treatments in terms of therapeutic outcome. As a form of human experimentation, these clinical trials are subject to review and approval by institutional ethics committees according to international codes of conduct (Declarations of Helsinki, Tokyo, and Venice). During clinical testing, many drugs are revealed to be unusable. Thus, one new drug ultimately remains from approximately 10,000 newly synthesized substances.

The decision to **approve a new drug** is made by a national regulatory body (the Food & Drug Administration in the USA, the Health Protection Branch Drugs Directorate in Canada) to which manufacturers are required to submit their applications. Applicants must document by means of appropriate test data (from preclinical and clinical trials) that the criteria of efficacy and safety have been met and that product formulations (tablet, capsule, etc.) satisfy general standards of quality control.

Following approval, a new drug may be marketed under a trade name and, thus, become available for prescription by physicians and dispensing by pharmacists. As the drug gains more widespread use, regulatory surveillance continues in the form of post-licensing studies (**Phase IV** of clinical trials). Only on the basis of long-term experience will the risk benefit ratio be properly assessed and, thus, the therapeutic value of the new drug be determined.

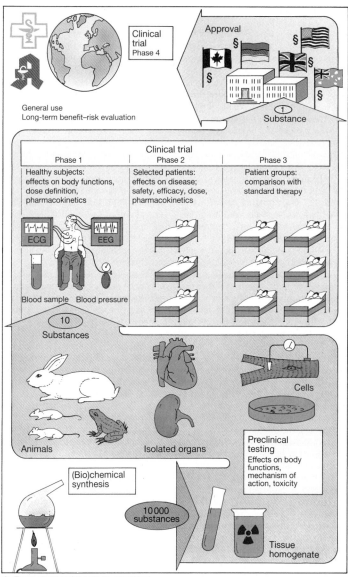

A. From drug synthesis to approval

Dosage Forms for Oral, Ocular, and Nasal Applications

A medicinal agent becomes a medication only after formulation suitable for therapeutic use (i.e., in an appropriate **dosage form**). The dosage form takes into account the intended mode of use and also ensures ease of handling (e.g., stability, precision of dosing) by patients and physicians. *Pharmaceutical technology* is concerned with the design of suitable product formulations and quality control.

Liquid preparations (A) may take the form of **solutions, suspensions** (a sol or mixture consisting of small water-insoluble solid drug particles dispersed in water), or **emulsions** (dispersion of minute droplets of a liquid agent or a drug solution in another fluid, e.g., oil in water). Since storage will cause sedimentation of suspensions and separation of emulsions, solutions are generally preferred. In the case of poorly water-soluble substances, solution is often accomplished by adding ethanol (or other solvents); thus, there are *aqueous* and *alcoholic solutions*. These solutions are made available to patients in specially designed drop bottles, enabling single doses to be measured exactly in terms of a defined number of drops, the size of which depends on the area of the drip opening at the bottle mouth and on the viscosity and surface tension of the solution. The advantage of a drop solution is that the dose, that is, the number of drops, can be precisely adjusted to the patient's need. Its disadvantage lies in the difficulty that some patients, disabled by disease or age, will experience in measuring a prescribed number of drops.

When the drugs are dissolved in a larger volume—as in the case of *syrups* or *mixtures*—the single dose is measured with a measuring spoon. Dosing may also be done with the aid of a tablespoon or teaspoon. However, due to the wide variation in the size of commercially available spoons, dosing will not be very precise. (Standardized medicinal teaspoons and tablespoons are available.)

Eye drops and **nose drops** (A) are designed for application to the mucosal surfaces of the eye (conjunctival sac) and nasal cavity, respectively. In order to prolong contact time, nasal drops are formulated with solutions of increased viscosity.

Solid dosage forms include **tablets, coated tablets,** and **capsules** (B). **Tablets** have a disklike shape, produced by mechanical compression of active drug substance, filler (e.g., lactose, calcium sulfate), binder, and auxiliary material (excipients). The filler provides bulk enough to make the tablet easy to handle and swallow. It is important to consider that the individual dose of many drugs lies in the range of a few milligrams or less. In order to convey the idea of a 10-mg weight, two squares are marked below, the paper mass of each weighing 10 mg. Disintegration of the tablet can be hastened by the use of dried starch, which swells on contact with water, or of $NaHCO_3$, which release CO_2 gas on contact with gastric acid. Auxiliary materials are important with regard to tablet production, shelf-life, palatability, and identifiability (color).

Effervescent tablets (compressed effervescent powders) do not represent a solid dosage form, because they are dissolved in water immediately prior to ingestion and are, thus, taken in solution.

| 10 mg | 10 mg | |

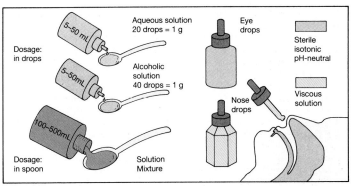

A. Liquid preparations

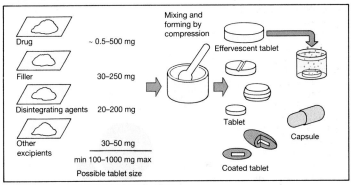

B. Solid preparations for oral application

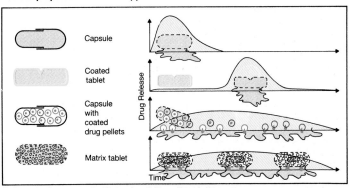

C. Dosage forms controlling rate of drug dissolution

The **coated tablet** contains a drug with a core that is covered by a shell, e.g., a wax coating, that serves to (1) protect perishable drugs from decomposing; (2) mask a disagreeable taste or odor; (3) facilitate passage on swallowing; or (4) permit color coding.

Capsules usually consist of an oblong casing—generally made of gelatin—that contains the drug in powder or granulated form (see p. 9 C).

In the case of the **matrix-type tablet**, the drug is embedded in an inert meshwork, from which it is released by diffusion upon being moistened.

In contrast to *solutions,* which permit direct absorption of drug, the use of solid dosage forms initially requires *tablets* to break up and *capsules* to open (**disintegration**), before the drug can be dissolved (**dissolution**) and pass through the gastrointestinal mucosal lining and into the blood (**absorption**). The **liberation of drug**, hence the site and timecourse of absorption, are subject to modification by appropriate production methods, as illustrated for matrix-type tablets and capsules (p. 9 C).

For acid-labile drugs, a coating of wax or of a cellulose acetate polymer is used to prevent disintegration of solid dosage forms in the stomach. Accordingly, disintegration and dissolution take place in the duodenum at normal speed and drug liberation *per se* is not retarded.

Drug liberation and, hence, absorption can be slowed when the drug is presented in the form of a granulate consisting of pellets coated with a waxy film of graded thickness. As a result, dissolution occurs gradually (p. 9 C) during enteral transit. This kind of **retarded drug release** is employed when a rapid rise in blood level of drug is undesirable, or when absorption is being slowed in order to prolong the action of drug that has a short sojourn in the body. The principle illustrated for a *capsule* (p. 9 C) can also be applied to tablets. In this case, either drug pellets coated with films of various thicknesses are compressed into a tablet or the drug is incorporated into a *matrix-type tablet* (p. 9 C). On contact with water, the drug slowly leaches out of the tablet matrix, the external shape of which remains unaltered. Contrary to timed-release capsules (e.g., Spansules) slow-release tablets have the advantage of being dividable *ad libitum;* thus, fractions of the dose contained within the entire tablet may be administered.

Because disintegration of a tablet and dissolution of the drug in a *tablet* or *capsule* require time, drug absorption will take place largely in the intestine.

When solutions are administered, absorption starts in the stomach. In the case of *coated tablets* (or *pills*), the coating must be detached before disintegration and dissolution can make the drug available for absorption (A).

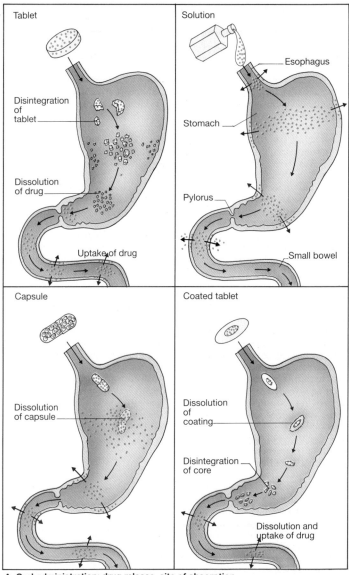

A. Oral administration: drug release, site of absorption

Dosage Forms for Parenteral (1), Pulmonary (2), Rectal or Vaginal (3), and Cutaneous Application

Drugs need not always be administered **orally** (i.e., by swallowing), but may also be given **parenterally**. This route usually refers to an injection, although enteral absorption is also bypassed when drugs are inhaled or applied to the skin.

For intravenous, intramuscular, or subcutaneous injections, drugs are most often given as solutions; less frequently, crystalline suspensions may be used for intramuscular, subcutaneous, or intra-articular injection. An **injectable solution** must be free of infectious agents, pyrogens, or suspended matter. It should have the same osmotic pressure and pH as body fluids in order to avoid tissue damage at the site of injection. Solutions for injection are preserved in airtight glass or plastic sealed containers. From **ampules for multiple or single use**, the solution is aspirated via a needle into a syringe; the **cartridge ampule** is fitted into a special injector that enables its contents to be emptied via a needle. An infusion refers to a solution being administered over an extended period of time. **Solutions for infusion** must meet the same standards as solutions for injection.

Drugs can be sprayed in **aerosol** form onto the mucosa of body cavities accessible from the outside (e.g., the respiratory tract [p. 14]). An aerosol is a dispersion of liquid or solid particles in a gas, such as air. An aerosol results when a drug solution or micronized powder is reduced to a spray on being driven through the nozzle of a pressurized container.

Mucosal application of drug via the rectal or vaginal route is achieved by means of **suppositories and vaginal tablets**, respectively. On rectal application, absorption into the systemic circulation may be intended. With vaginal tablets, the effect is generally confined to the site of application. Usually the drug is incorporated into a fat that solidifies at room temperature, but melts in the rectum or vagina. The resulting oily film spreads over the mucosa and enables drug to pass into the mucosa.

Powders, ointments, and **pastes** (p. 16) are applied to the skin surface. In many cases, these do not contain drugs but are used for skin protection or care. However, drugs may be added if a topical action on the outer skin or, more rarely, a systemic effect is intended.

Transdermal drug delivery systems are pasted to the epidermis. They contain a reservoir from which drugs may diffuse and be absorbed through the skin. They offer the advantage that a drug depot is attached noninvasively to the body, enabling the drug to be administered in a manner similar to an infusion. Drugs amenable to this type of delivery must : (1) be capable of penetrating the cutaneous barrier; (2) be effective in very small doses (restricted capacity of reservoir); and (3) possess a wide therapeutic margin (dosage not adjustable).

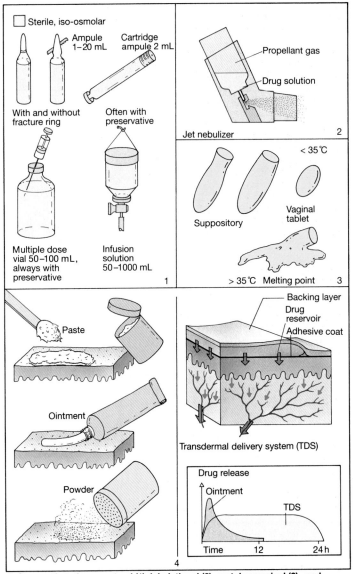

Sterile, iso-osmolar

Ampule 1–20 mL

Cartridge ampule 2 mL

With and without fracture ring

Often with preservative

Multiple dose vial 50–100 mL, always with preservative

Infusion solution 50–1000 mL

1

Propellant gas

Drug solution

Jet nebulizer 2

< 35 °C

Suppository

Vaginal tablet

> 35 °C Melting point 3

Paste

Ointment

Powder

Backing layer
Drug reservoir
Adhesive coat

Transdermal delivery system (TDS)

Drug release

Ointment

TDS

Time 12 24 h

4

A. Preparations for parenteral (1), inhalational (2), rectal or vaginal (3), and percutaneous application

Drug Administration by Inhalation

Inhalation in the form of an aerosol, a gas, or a mist permits drugs to be applied to the bronchial mucosa and, to a lesser extent, to the alveolar membranes. This route is chosen for drugs intended to affect bronchial smooth muscle or the consistency of bronchial mucus. Furthermore, gaseous or volatile agents can be administered by inhalation with the goal of alveolar absorption and systemic effects (e.g., inhalational anesthetics, p. 208). **Aerosols** are formed when a drug solution or micronized powder is converted into a mist or dust, respectively.

In conventional sprays (e.g., nebulizer), the air blast required for the aerosol formation is generated by the stroke of a pump. Alternatively, drug is delivered from a solution or powder packaged in a pressurized canister equipped with a valve through which a metered dose is discharged. During use, the inhaler (spray dispenser) is held directly in front of the mouth and actuated at the start of inspiration. The effectiveness of delivery depends on the position of the device in front of the mouth, the size of aerosol particles, and the coordination of the opening of the spray valve and inspiration. The size of aerosol particles determines the speed at which they are swept along by inhaled air and hence the **depth of penetration into the respiratory tract.** Particles > 100 μm in diameter are trapped in the oropharyngeal cavity, whereas those having diameters between 10 and 60 μm will be deposited on the epithelium of the bronchial tract. Particles < 2 μm in diameter can reach the alveoli, but they will be exhaled again unless they settle out.

Drug deposited on the mucous lining of the bronchial epithelium is partly absorbed and partly transported with bronchial mucus towards the larynx. Bronchial mucus moves as a result of the orally directed undulatory beat of epithelial cilia. Physiologically, this mucociliary transport functions to remove inspired dust particles. Thus, only a portion of the drug aerosol (approx. 10%) gains access to the respiratory tract and just a fraction of this amount penetrates the mucosa, whereas the remainder of the aerosol undergoes mucociliary transport to the laryngopharynx and is swallowed. The advantage of inhalation (i.e., localized application) is fully exploited by using drugs that are poorly absorbed from the intestine (isoproterenol, ipratropium, cromolyn) or are subject to first-pass elimination (p. 42; beclomethasone, budesonide).

Even when the swallowed portion of an inhaled drug is absorbed in unchanged form, administration by this route has the advantage that drug concentrations at the bronchi will be higher than in other organs.

The efficiency of mucociliary transport depends on the force of kinociliary motion and the viscosity of bronchial mucus. Both factors can be altered pathologically (e.g., by smoker's cough, bronchitis) or can be adversely affected by drugs (atropine, antihistamines).

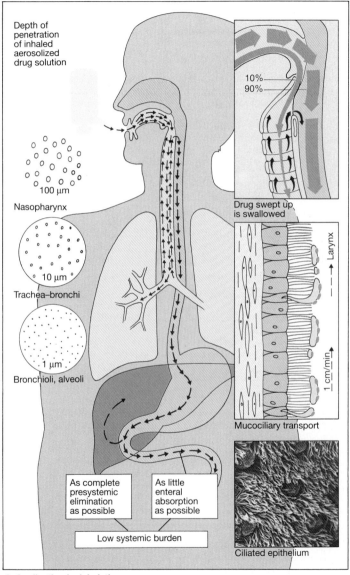

Depth of penetration of inhaled aerosolized drug solution

100 µm

Nasopharynx

10 µm

Trachea–bronchi

1 µm

Bronchioli, alveoli

10%
90%

Drug swept up is swallowed

Larynx

1 cm/min

Mucociliary transport

As complete presystemic elimination as possible

As little enteral absorption as possible

Low systemic burden

Ciliated epithelium

A. Application by inhalation

Dermatologic Agents

Pharmaceutical preparations applied to the outer skin are intended either to provide skin care and protection from noxious influences (A), or to serve as vehicles for drugs that are to be absorbed into the skin or, if appropriate, into the general circulation (B).

Skin Protection (A)

Protective agents are of several kinds to meet different requirements according to skin condition (dry, low in oil, chapped vs. moist, oily, elastic), and the type of noxious stimuli (prolonged exposure to water, regular use of alcohol-containing disinfectants [p. 272], intense solar irradiation). Distinctions among protective agents are based on consistency, physicochemical properties (lipophilic, hydrophilic) and the presence of additives.

Dusting powders are sprinkled onto the intact skin and consist of talc, magnesium stearate, silicon dioxide (silica), or starch. They adhere to the skin, forming a low-friction film that attenuates mechanical irritation. Powders exert a drying (evaporative) effect.

Lipophilic ointment (oil ointment) consists of a lipophilic base (paraffin oil, petroleum jelly, lanolin) and may contain up to 10% powder materials, such as zinc oxide, titanium oxide, starch, or a mixture of these. Emulsifying ointments are made of paraffins and an emulsifying wax, and are miscible with water.

Paste (oil paste) is an ointment containing more than 10% pulverized constituents.

Lipophilic (oily) cream is an emulsion of water in oil, easier to spread than oil paste or oil ointments.

Hydrogel and water-soluble ointment achieve their consistency by means of different gel-forming agents (gelatin, methylcellulose, polyethylene glycol). **Lotions** are aqueous suspensions of water-insoluble and solid constituents.

Hydrophilic (aqueous) cream is an emulsion of an oil in water formed with the aid of an emulsifier; it may also be considered an oil-in-water emulsion of an emulsifying ointment.

All dermatologic agents having a lipophilic base adhere to the skin as a water-repellent coating. They do not wash off and they also prevent (**occlude**) outward passage of water from the skin. The skin is protected from drying and its hydration and elasticity increase.

Diminished evaporation of water results in warming of the occluded skin.

Hydrophilic agents wash off easily and do not impede transcutaneous output of water. Evaporation of water is felt as a cooling effect.

Dermatologic Agents as Vehicles (B)

In order to reach its site of action, a drug (D) must leave its pharmaceutical preparation and enter the skin, if a local effect is desired (e.g., glucocorticoid ointment), or be able to penetrate it, if a systemic action is intended (transdermal delivery system e.g., nitroglycerin patch, p. 12). The tendency for the drug to leave the vehicle (V) is higher the more the drug and the vehicle differ in lipophilicity (high tendency: hydrophilic D and lipophilic V, and vice versa). Because the skin represents a closed lipophilic barrier (p. 22), only lipophilic drugs are absorbed. Hydrophilic drugs fail even to penetrate the outer skin when applied in a lipophilic vehicle. This formulation can be meaningful when high drug concentrations are required at the skin surface (e.g., neomycin ointment for bacterial skin infections).

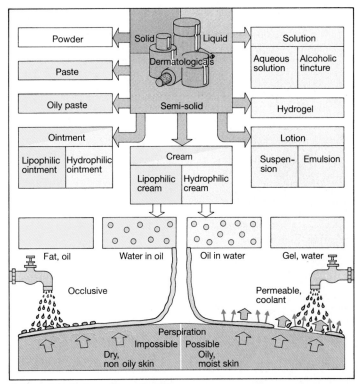

A. Dermatologicals as skin protectants

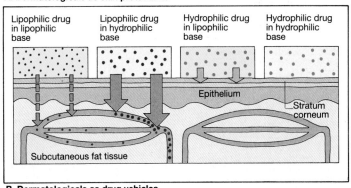

B. Dermatologicals as drug vehicles

From Application to Distribution in the Body

As a rule, drugs reach their target organs via the blood. Therefore, they must first enter the blood, usually the venous limb of the circulation. There are several possible sites of entry.

The drug may be injected or infused *intravenously*, in which case the drug is introduced directly into the bloodstream. In *subcutaneous* or *intramuscular* injection, the drug has to diffuse from the site of application into the blood. Because these procedures entail injury to the outer skin, strict requirements must be met concerning technique. For that reason, the *oral* route (i.e., simple application by mouth) involving subsequent uptake of drug across the gastrointestinal mucosa into the blood is chosen much more frequently. The disadvantage of this route is that the drug must first pass through the liver on its way into the general circulation. This fact assumes practical significance with any drug that may be rapidly transformed or posssibly inactivated in the liver (first-pass hepatic elimination; p. 42). Even with *rectal* administration, at least a fraction of the drug enters the general circulation via the portal vein, because only veins draining the short terminal segment of the rectum communicate directly with the inferior vena cava. Hepatic passage is circumvented when absorption occurs buccally or sublingually, because venous blood from the oral cavity drains directly into the superior vena cava. The same would apply to administration by *inhalation* (p. 14). However, with this route, a local effect is usally intended, and a systemic action is intended only in exceptional cases. Under certain conditions, drug can also be applied percutaneously in the form of a *transdermal* delivery system (p. 12). In this case, drug is slowly released from the reservoir, and then penetrates the epidermis and subepidermal connective tissue where it enters blood capillaries. Only a very few drugs can be applied transdermally. The feasibility of this route is determined by both the physicochemical properties of the drug and the therapeutic requirements (acute vs. long-term effect).

Speed of absorption is determined by the route and method of application. It is fastest with *intravenous* injection, less fast with *intramuscular* injection, and slowest with *subcutaneous* injection. When the drug is applied to the oral mucosa (*buccal, sublingual* route), plasma levels rise faster than with conventional *oral* administration, because the drug preparation is deposited at its actual site of absorption and very high concentrations in the saliva occur upon the dissolution of a single dose. Thus, uptake across the oral epithelium is accelerated. The same does not hold true for poorly water-soluble or poorly absorbable drugs. Such agents should be given orally, because both the volume of fluid for dissolution and the absorbing surface are much larger in the small intestine than in the oral cavity.

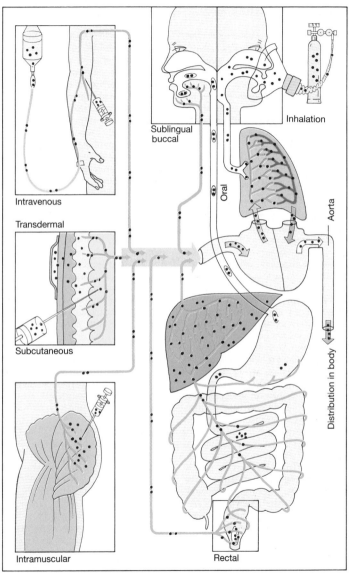

Intravenous

Transdermal

Subcutaneous

Intramuscular

Sublingual
buccal

Inhalation

Oral

Aorta

Distribution in body

Rectal

A. From application to distribution

Potential Targets of Drug Action

Drugs are designed to exert a selective influence on vital processes in order to alleviate or eliminate symptoms of disease. The smallest viable basic unit of an organism is the cell. The outer cell membrane, or plasmalemma, effectively demarcates the cell from its surroundings, thus permitting a large degree of internal autonomy. Embedded in the plasmalemma are **transport proteins** that serve to mediate *controlled metabolic exchange with the cellular environment*. These include energy-consuming pumps (e.g., Na, K-ATPase, p. 130), carriers (e.g., for Na/glucose–co-transport, p. 174), and ion channels e.g., for sodium (p. 136) or calcium (p. 122) (**1**).

Functional coordination between single cells is a prerequisite for the viability of the organism, hence also for the survival of individual cells. Cell functions are regulated by means of messenger substances for the transfer of information. Included among these are "transmitters" released from the nerves, which the cell is able to recognize with the help of specialized membrane binding sites or **receptors.** Hormones secreted by endocrine glands into the blood, then into the extracellular fluid, represent another class of chemical signals. Finally, signalling substances can originate from neighboring cells, e.g., the prostaglandins (p. 188).

The **effect of drugs** frequently results from interference with cellular function. Receptors for the recognition of endogenous transmitters are obvious sites of drug action (receptor agonists and antagonists, p. 60). Altered activity of transport systems affects cell function (e.g., cardiac glycosides, p. 130; loop diuretics, p. 158; calcium antagonists, p. 122). Drugs may also directly interfere with intra-cellular metabolic processes, for instance by inhibiting (phosphodiesterase inhibitors, p. 132) or by activating (organic nitrates, p. 120) an enzyme (**2**).

In contrast to drugs acting from the outside on cell membrane constituents, agents acting on the cell's interior need to penetrate the cell membrane.

The **cell membrane** basically consists of a **phospholipid bilayer** (80Å [8 nm] thickness), embedded in which are proteins (integral membrane proteins, such as receptors and transport molecules). **Phospholipid** molecules contain two long-chain *fatty acids* in ester linkage with two of the three hydroxyl groups of *glycerol*. Bound to the third hydroxyl group is *phosphoric acid* which, in turn, carries a *further residue*, e.g., choline, (phosphatidylcholine = lecithin), the amino acid serine (phosphatidyl-serine) or the cyclic polyhydric alcohol inositol (phosphatidylinositol). In terms of solubility, phospholipids are amphiphilic: the tail region containing the apolar fatty acid chains is lipophilic, the remainder—the polar head—is hydrophilic. By virtue of these properties, phospholipids aggregate spontaneously into a bilayer in an aqueous medium, their polar heads being directed outwards into the aqueous medium, the fatty acid chains facing each other and projecting into the inside of the membrane (**3**).

The **hydrophobic interior** of the phospholipid membrane constitutes a **diffusion barrier** virtually impermeable for charged particles. Apolar particles, however, penetrate the membrane easily. This fact is of major importance with respect to the absorption, distribution, and elimination of drugs.

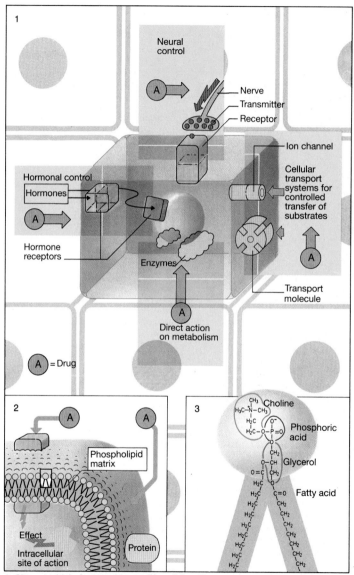

A. Sites at which drugs act to modify cell function

External Barriers of the Body

Prior to its uptake into the blood (i.e., during absorption), the drug has to overcome barriers that demarcate the body from its surroundings, i.e., separate the internal milieu from the external milieu. These boundaries are formed by the skin and mucous membranes.

When absorption takes place in the **gut** (enteral absorption), the intestinal epithelium is the barrier. This single-layered epithelium is made up of enterocytes and mucus-producing goblet cells. On their luminal side, these cells are joined together by *zonulae occludentes* (indicated by black dots in the inset, bottom left). A *zonula occludens* or tight junction is a region in which the phospholipid membranes of two cells establish contact and become fused for a short distance (semicircular inset, left center). The region of fusion surrounds the cell like a ring, so that it is joined to its neighboring cells in a continuous belt. On the whole, an unbroken phospholipid layer is formed (yellow area in the schematic drawing, bottom left) that separates the intestinal lumen (dark blue) from the cell interior and the interstitial space (light blue). This phospholipid bilayer represents the intestinal mucosa–blood barrier that a drug must cross during its enteral absorption. The only drugs to be absorbed enterally are those whose physicochemical properties allow permeation through the lipophilic membrane interior (yellow) or that are subject to a special carrier transport mechanism. Absorption of drugs meeting these conditions proceeds rapidly, because the absorbing surface is greatly enlarged due to the formation of the epithelial brush border (submicroscopic foldings of the plasmalemma).

In the **respiratory tract**, cilia-bearing epithelial cells are also joined on the luminal side by *zonulae occludentes*, so that the bronchial space and the interstitium are separated by a continuous phospholipid bilayer membrane.

With sublingual or buccal application, the drug encounters the non-keratinized, multilayered squamous epithelium of the **oral mucosa**. The cells establish punctate contacts with each other in the form of desmosomes (not shown) that, however, do not seal the intercellular clefts. Instead, the cells have the property of sequestering phospholipid-containing membrane fragments that assemble into layers within the extracellular space (semicircular inset, center right). In this manner, a continuous phospholipid barrier arises also inside squamous epithelia, although at an extracellular location, unlike that of intestinal epithelia. A similar barrier principle operates in the multi-layer keratinized squamous epithelium of the outer **skin**. The presence of a continuous phospholipid layer means that squamous epithelia will permit passage of lipophilic drugs only, i.e., agents capable of diffusing through phospholipid membranes, with the epithelial thickness determining the extent and speed of absorption. In addition, cutaneous absorption is impeded by the keratin layer, the stratum corneum, which is very unevenly developed in various areas of the skin.

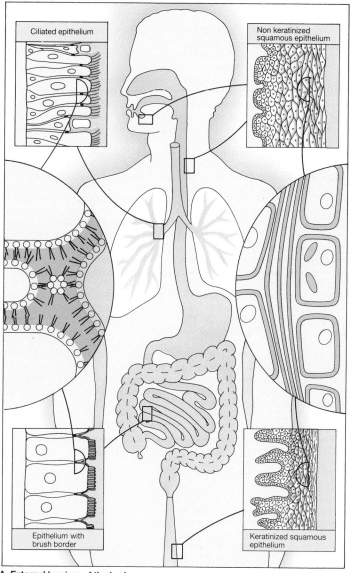

Ciliated epithelium

Non keratinized squamous epithelium

Epithelium with brush border

Keratinized squamous epithelium

A. External barriers of the body

Blood–Tissue Barriers

Drugs are transported in the blood to different tissues of the body. In order to reach their sites of action, they must leave the bloodstream. Drug permeation occurs largely in the capillary bed, where both surface area and time available for exchange are maximal (extensive vascular branching, low velocity of flow). The capillary wall forms the **blood–tissue barrier**. Basically, this consists of an endothelial cell layer and a basement membrane enveloping the latter (black solid line in the schematic drawings). The endothelial cells are "welded" to each other by tight junctions or occluding zonulae (labeled Z in the electron micrograph, top left) such that no clefts, gaps, or pores remain that would permit drugs to pass unimpeded from the blood into the interstitial fluid.

The blood–tissue barrier is developed differently in the various capillary beds. Permeability to drugs of the capillary wall is determined by the structural and functional characteristics of the endothelial cells.

In many capillary beds, e.g., those of **cardiac muscle**, endothelial cells are characterized by pronounced **endo**- and **transcytotic activity**, as evidenced by numerous invaginations and vesicles (arrows in the EM micrograph, top right). Transcytotic activity entails transport of fluid or macromolecules from the blood into the interstitium and vice versa. Any solutes trapped in the fluid, including drugs, may cross the blood–tissue barrier. In this form of transport the physicochemical properties of drugs are of little importance.

In some capillary beds (e.g., in the **pancreas**) endothelial cells exhibit fenestrations. Although the cells are tightly connected by continuous junctions, they possess **pores** (arrows in

EM micrograph, bottom left) that are closed only by diaphragms. Both the diaphragm and basement membrane can be readily penetrated by substances of low molecular weight—the majority of drugs—but less so by macromolecules, e.g., proteins. Penetrability of the latter is determined by molecular size and electrical charge. Fenestrated endothelia are found in the capillaries of the *gut* and the *endocrine glands*.

In the central nervous system **(brain and spinal cord)**, capillary endothelia lack pores and there is little endo- and transcytotic activity. In order to cross the **blood–brain barrier**, drugs must diffuse transcellularly, i.e., penetrate the luminal and basal membrane of endothelial cells. Drug movement along this path requires specific physicochemical properties (p. 26) or the presence of a transport mechanism (e.g., L-dopa, p. 182). Thus, the blood–brain barrier is permeable only to certain types of drugs.

Drugs exchange freely between blood and interstitium in the **liver**, where endothelial cells exhibit large fenestrations (100 nm in diameter) facing Disse's spaces (D) and where neither diaphragms nor basement membrane impede drug movement.

(Vertical bars in the EM micrographs represent 1 μm; E: cross-sectioned erythrocyte; AM: actomyosin; G: insulin-containing granules.)

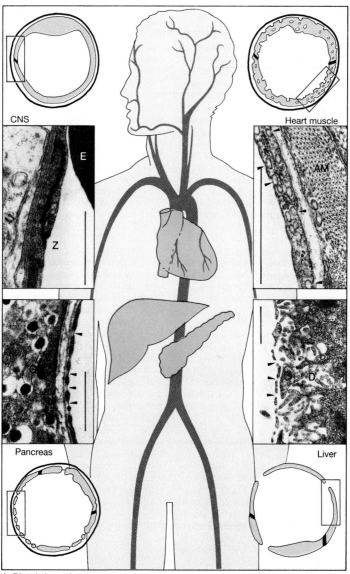

A. Blood-tissue barriers

Membrane Permeation

An ability to penetrate lipid bilayers is a prerequisite for the absorption of drugs, their entry into cells or cellular organelles, and passage across the blood–brain barrier. Due to their amphiphilic nature, phospholipids form bilayers possessing a hydrophilic surface and a hydrophobic interior (p. 20). Substances may traverse this membrane in three different ways.

Diffusion (A). Lipophilic substances (red dots) may enter the membrane from the extracellular space (area shown in ochre), accumulate in the membrane, and exit into the cytosol (blue area). Direction and speed of permeation depend on the relative concentrations in the fluid phases and the membrane. The steeper the gradient (concentration difference), the more drug will be diffusing per unit of time (Fick's Law). The lipid membrane represents an almost insurmountable obstacle for hydrophilic substances (blue triangles).

Transport (B). Some drugs may penetrate membrane barriers with the help of transport systems (carriers), irrespective of their physicochemical properties, especially lipophilicity. As a prerequisite, the drug must have affinity for the carrier (blue triangle matching recess on "transport system") and, when bound to the latter, be capable of being ferried across the membrane. Membrane passage via transport mechanisms is subject to competitive inhibition by another substance possessing similar affinity for the carrier. Substances lacking in affinity (blue circles) are not transported. Drugs utilize carriers for physiological substances, e.g., L-dopa uptake by L-amino acid carrier across the blood–intestine and blood–brain barriers (p. 182) and uptake of aminoglycosides by the carrier transporting basic polypeptides through the luminal membrane of kidney tubular cells (p. 264). Only drugs bearing sufficient resemblance to the physiological substrate of a carrier will exhibit affinity for it.

Finally, membrane penetration may occur in the form of small membrane-covered vesicles. Two different systems are considered.

Endocytosis (vesicular transport, phago- and pinocytosis) (C). When new vesicles are pinched off, substances dissolved in the extracellular fluid are engulfed and then ferried through the cytoplasm, unless the vesicles (phagosomes) undergo fusion with lysosomes to form phagolysosomes and the transported substance is metabolized.

Receptor-mediated endocytosis (C). The drug first binds to membrane surface receptors. Newly formed complexes migrate laterally in the membrane and aggregate in coated pits with other drug-bearing receptors. As soon as a sufficient number has been assembled, the subjacent membrane invaginates and eventually pinches off to form a detached coated vesicle. This vesicle sheds its "bristle coat"; its subsequent maturation into an endosome is still debatable. The endosome delivers its contents to a predetermined destination, e.g., the Golgi complex, the cell nucleus, lysosomes, or the opposite cell membrane (transcytosis). Unlike simple endocytosis, receptor-mediated endocytosis is contingent on affinity for specific receptors and operates independently of concentration gradients.

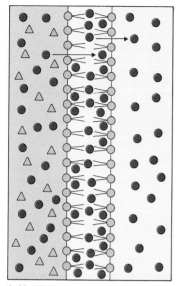

A. Membrane permeation: diffusion

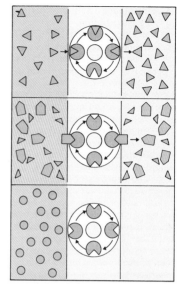

B. Membrane permeation: transport

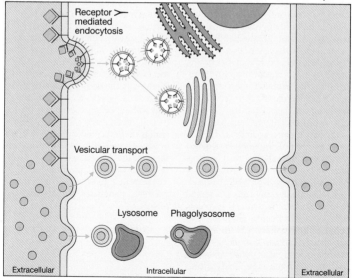

C. Membrane permeation: vesicular uptake and transport

Possible Modes
of Drug Distribution

Following its uptake into the body, the drug is distributed in the blood (1) and through it to the various tissues of the body. Distribution may be restricted to the extracellular space (plasma volume plus interstitial space) (2) or may also extend into the intracellular space (3). Certain drugs may bind strongly to tissue structures, so that plasma concentrations fall significantly even before elimination has begun (4).

After being distributed in blood, macromolecular substances remain largely confined to the vascular space, because they only penetrate the blood–tissue barrier poorly, or the endothelium, even where capillaries are fenestrated. This property is exploited therapeutically when loss of blood necessitates refilling the vascular bed, e.g., by infusion of dextran solutions (p. 150). The vascular space is, moreover, predominantly occupied by substances highly bound to plasma proteins (p. 30; determination of the plasma volume with protein-bound dyes). Unbound, free drug may leave the bloodstream, albeit with varying ease, because the blood–tissue barrier is differently developed in different segments of the vascular tree. These regional differences are not illustrated in the accompanying figures.

Distribution in the body is determined by the ability to penetrate membranous barriers (p. 20). Hydrophilic substances (e.g., inulin) are neither taken up into the cells nor bound to cell surface structures and can, thus, be used to determine the extracellular fluid volume (2). Lipophilic substances diffuse through the cell membrane and, as a result, achieve a uniform distribution in body fluids (3). Assuming an even distribution, the accessible fluid volume amounts to 60% of the total body weight (the remaining body water is structurally bound and unavailable as solvent space). Intracellular water makes up 40% of body weight (65% of total body water) with extracellular fluid, including red blood cells, comprising 20% (35% of total body water). Extracellular fluid consists of interstitial fluid (10.5–11.5 L) and blood volume (4–5 L). About 40% of the blood volume is accounted for by erythrocytes, leaving 2.5–3 L for blood plasma.

The volume ratio interstitial:intracellular water varies with age and body weight. On a percentage basis, interstitial fluid volume is large in premature or normal neonates (up to 50% of body water) and smaller in the obese and the aged.

The concentration (c) of the solution corresponds to the amount (D) of substance dissolved in a volume (V); thus, $c = D/V$. If the amount of drug present in the body (D) and its plasma concentration (c) are known, a volume of distribution (V) can be calculated from $V = D/c$. However, this represents an *apparent* volume of distribution (V_{app}), because an even distribution in the body is assumed in its calculation. Homogeneous distribution will not occur if drugs are bound to cell membranes (5) or to membranes of intracellular organelles (6) or are stored within the latter (7). In these cases, V_{app} can exceed the actual size of the available fluid volume. The significance of V_{app} as a pharmacokinetic parameter is discussed on p. 44.

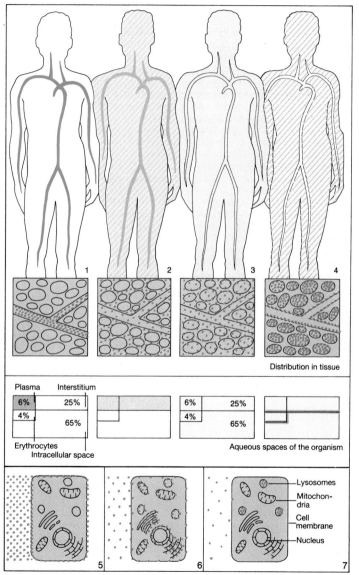

Distribution in tissue

Plasma   Interstitium
6%   25%
4%   65%
Erythrocytes
Intracellular space

6%   25%
4%   65%

Aqueous spaces of the organism

Lysosomes
Mitochondria
Cell membrane
Nucleus

A. Compartments for drug distribution

Binding to Plasma Proteins

Having entered the blood, drugs may bind to the protein molecules that are present in abundance, resulting in the formation of drug–protein complexes.

Protein binding involves primarily albumin and, to a lesser extent, β-globulins and acidic glycoproteins. Other plasma proteins (e.g., transcortin, transferrin, thyroxine-binding globulin) serve specialized functions in connection with specific substances. The degree of binding is governed by the concentrations of the reactants and the affinity of a drug for a given protein. Albumin concentration in plasma amounts to 4.6 g/100 mL or 0.6 mM, and thus provides a very high binding capacity (two sites per molecule). As a rule, drugs exhibit much lower affinity (K_D approx. 10^{-5}–10^{-3} M) for plasma proteins than for their specific binding sites (receptors). In the range of therapeutically relevant concentrations, protein binding of most drugs increases linearly with concentration (exceptions: salicylate and certain sulfonamides).

The albumin molecule has different binding sites for anionic and cationic ligands, but van der Waals' forces also contribute (p. 58). The extent of binding correlates with drug hydrophobicity (repulsion of drug by water).

Binding to plasma proteins is instantaneous and reversible, i.e., any change in the concentration of unbound drug is immediately followed by a corresponding change in the concentration of bound drug. Protein binding is of great importance, because it is the concentration of free drug that determines the intensity of the effect. At an identical total plasma concentration (say, 100 ng/mL) the *effective* concentration will be 90 ng/mL for a drug 10% bound to protein, but 1 ng/mL for a drug 99% bound to protein. The reduction in concentration of free drug resulting from protein binding affects not only the intensity of the effect but also affects biotransformation (e.g., in the liver) and elimination in the kidney, because only free drug will enter hepatic sites of metabolism or undergo glomerular filtration. When concentrations of free drug fall, drug is resupplied from binding sites on plasma proteins. Binding to plasma protein is equivalent to a depot, in prolonging the duration of the effect by retarding elimination, whereas the intensity of the effect is reduced.

If two substances have affinity for the same binding site on the albumin molecule, they may compete for that site. One drug may displace another from its binding site and thereby elevate the free (effective) concentration of the displaced drug (a form of **drug interaction**). Elevation of the free concentration of the displaced drug means increased effectiveness and accelerated elimination.

A decrease in the concentration of albumin (liver disease, nephrotic syndrome, poor general condition) leads to altered pharmacokinetics of drugs that are highly bound to albumin.

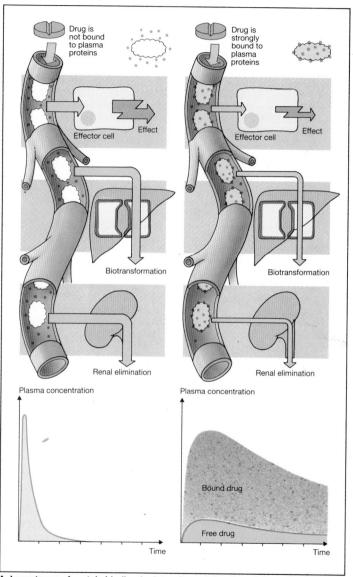

A. Importance of protein binding for intensity and duration of drug effect

The Liver as an Excretory Organ

As the chief organ of drug biotrans-formation, the liver is richly supplied with blood, of which 1100 mL is re-ceived each minute from the intes-tines through the portal vein and 55 mL through the hepatic artery, comprising nearly one-third of cardi-ac output. The blood content of hepat-ic vessels and sinusoids amounts to 500 mL. Due to the widening of the portal lumen, intrahepatic blood flow decelerates (**A**). Moreover, the endo-thelial lining of hepatic sinusoids (p. 24) contains pores large enough to permit rapid exit of plasma proteins. Thus, blood and hepatic parenchyma are able to maintain intimate contact and intensive exchange of substances which is further facilitated by micro-villi covering the hepatocyte surfaces abutting Disse's spaces.

The hepatocyte secretes biliary fluid into the bile canaliculi (dark green), tubular intercellular clefts that are sealed off from the blood spaces by tight junctions. Secretory activity in the hepatocytes results in move-ment of fluid towards the canalicular space (**A**). The hepatocyte has an abundance of enzymes carrying out metabolic functions; these are local-ized in part in mitochondria, in part on the membranes of the rough (rER) or smooth (sER) endoplasmic reticulum.

Enzymes of the sER play a most important role in drug biotransforma-tion. At this site, molecular oxygen is used in oxidative reactions. Because these enzymes can catalyze either hy-droxylation or oxidative cleavage of –N–C– or –O–C– bonds, they are re-ferred to as "mixed-function" oxi-dases or hydroxylases. The essential component of this enzyme system is cytochrome P450, which in its oxi-dized state binds drug substrates (R–H). The Fe^{III}–P450–RH binary

complex is first reduced by NADPH, then forms the ternary complex, O_2–Fe^{II}–P450–RH, which accepts a sec-ond electron and finally disintegrates into Fe^{III}–P450, one equivalent of H_2O and hydroxylated drug (R–OH).

Compared with hydrophilic drugs not undergoing transport, lipo-philic drugs are more rapidly taken up from the blood into hepatocytes and more readily gain access to mixed-function oxidases embedded in sER membranes. For instance, a drug having lipophilicity by virtue of an ar-omatic substituent (phenyl ring) (**B**) can be hydroxylated and, thus, be-come more hydrophilic (Phase I reac-tion, p. 34). Besides oxidases, sER al-so contains reductases and glucuronyl transferases. The latter conjugate glucuronic acid with hydroxyl, car-boxyl, amine, and amide groups (p. 38); hence also phenolic products of Phase I metabolism (Phase II con-jugation). Phase I and Phase II metab-olites can be transported back into the blood—probably via a gradient-de-pendent carrier—or actively secreted into bile.

Prolonged exposure to certain substrates, such as phenobarbital, re-sults in a proliferation of sER mem-branes (cf **C** and **D**). This **enzyme in-duction**, a load-dependent hypertro-phy, affects equally all enzymes localized on **sER** membranes. En-zyme induction leads to accelerated biotransformation, not only of the in-ducing agent but also of other drugs (a form of **drug interaction**). With con-tinued exposure, it develops in a few days, resulting in an increase in reac-tion velocity, maximally 2- or 3-fold, that disappears after removal of the inducing agent.

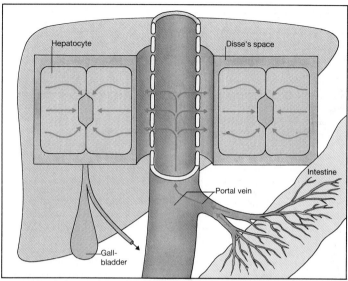

A. Flow patterns in portal vein, Disse's space, and hepatocyte

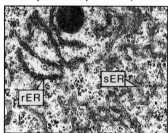

C. Normal hepatocyte

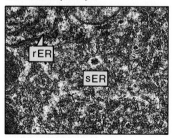

D. Hepatocyte after phenobarbital administration

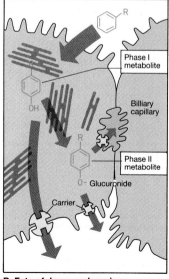

B. Fate of drugs undergoing hepatic hydroxylation

Biotransformation of Drugs

Many drugs undergo chemical modification in the body (**biotransformation**). Most frequently, this process entails a loss of biological activity and an increase in hydrophilicity (water solubility), thereby promoting elimination via the renal route (p. 40). Since rapid drug elimination improves accuracy in titrating the therapeutic concentration, drugs are often designed with built-in weak links. Ester bonds are such a weak link, which is subject to enzymatic attack (hydrolysis) by esterases that are ubiquitous. Along with *oxidations, reductions, alkylations, and dealkylations, hydrolytic cleavages* constitute **Phase I reactions** of drug metabolism. These reactions subsume all metabolic processes apt to alter drug molecules chemically and take place chiefly in the liver. In **Phase II (synthetic) reactions, conjugation products** of either the drug itself or of its Phase I metabolites are formed, for instance, with glucuronic acid or sulfuric acid (p. 38).

The special case of the endogenous transmitter acetylcholine illustrates well the high velocity of ester hydrolysis. Acetylcholine is broken down at its sites of release and action by acetylcholinesterase (pp. 80, 100) so rapidly as to negate its therapeutic use. Hydrolysis of other esters catalyzed by various esterases is slower, though relatively fast in comparison with other biotransformations. The local anesthetic procaine is a case in point; it exerts its action at the site of application while being largely devoid of undesirable effects at other locations because it is inactivated by hydrolysis during absorption from its site of application.

Ester hydrolysis does not invariably lead to inactive metabolites, as exemplified by acetylsalicylic acid.

The cleavage product, salicylic acid, retains pharmacological activity. In certain cases, drugs are administered in the form of esters in order to facilitate absorption (enalapril → enalaprilate; testosterone undecanoate → testosterone) or to reduce irritation of the gastrointestinal mucosa (erythromycin succinate → erythromycin). In these cases, the ester itself is not active, but the cleavage product is. Thus, an inactive precursor or *prodrug* is applied, formation of the active molecule occurring only after hydrolysis in the blood.

Some drugs possessing amide bonds, such as prilocaine and, of course, peptides, can be hydrolyzed by peptidases and inactivated in this manner. Peptidases are also of pharmacological interest because they are responsible for the formation of highly reactive cleavage products (fibrin, p. 146) and potent mediators (angiotensin II, p. 124; enkephalin, p. 200) from biologically inactive peptides.

Peptidases exhibit some substrate selectivity and can be selectively inhibited, as exemplified by the formation of angiotensin II, whose actions *inter alia* include vasoconstriction. Angiotensin II is formed from angiotensin I by cleavage of the C-terminal dipeptide histidylleucine. Hydrolysis is catalyzed by angiotensin-converting enzyme (ACE). Peptide analogs such as captopril (p. 124) block this enzyme. Angiotensin II is degradated by angiotensinase A, which clips off the N-terminal asparagine residue. The product angiotensin III lacks vasoconstrictor activity.

Oxidation reactions can be divided into two kinds: those in which oxygen is incorporated into the drug molecule, and those in which primary oxidation causes part of the original molecule to be lost. The former include **hydroxylations, epoxidations,**

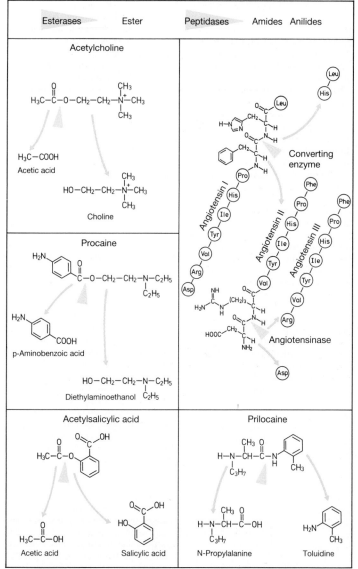

A. Examples of chemical reactions in drug biotransformation (hydrolysis)

and **sulfoxidations**. Hydroxylations may involve alkyl substituents (e.g., pentobarbital) or an aromatic ring system (e.g., propranolol). In both cases, products are formed that are conjugated to an organic acid residue, e.g., glucuronic acid, in a subsequent Phase II reaction. Hydroxylation may also take place at nitrogens, resulting in hydroxylamines (e.g., acetaminophen). Benzene, polycyclic aromatic compounds (e.g., benzopyrene), and unsaturated cyclic carbohydrates can be converted by mono-oxygenases to **epoxides**, highly reactive electrophiles that are hepatotoxic and possibly carcinogenic.

The second type of oxidative biotransformation comprises **dealkylations.** In the case of primary or secondary amines, dealkylation of an alkyl group starts at the carbon adjacent to the nitrogen; in the case of tertiary amines, with hydroxylation of the nitrogen (e.g., lidocaine). The intermediary products are labile and break up into the dealkylated amine and aldehyde of the alkyl group removed. O- and S-dealkylation proceed via a mechanism analogous to that of primary or secondary amine dealkylation (e.g., phenacetin and azathioprine).

$$H{-}\underset{R_2}{\overset{R_1}{N}}{-}CH_2{-}CH_3$$

$$\bigg\downarrow{-}O$$

$$\underset{R_2}{\overset{R_1}{N}}{-}\underset{OH}{\overset{}{C}H}{-}CH_3$$

$$\bigg\downarrow$$

$$\underset{R_2}{\overset{R_1}{N}}H + HC{-}CH_3$$
$$\qquad\qquad \overset{\|}{O}$$

Oxidative **deamination** basically resembles the dealkylation of tertiary amines, beginning with the formation of a hydroxylamine that then decomposes into ammonia and the corresponding aldehyde. The latter is partly reduced to an alcohol and partly oxidized to a carboxylic acid.

$$\underset{H}{\overset{H}{N}}{-}CH_2{-}R \quad\xrightarrow{\overset{O}{\downarrow}}\quad \underset{H}{\overset{H}{N}}H + HC{-}R$$
$$\qquad\qquad\qquad\qquad\qquad \overset{\|}{O}$$

Reduction reactions may occur at oxygen or nitrogen atoms. Keto-oxygens are converted into a hydroxyl group, as in the reduction of the prodrugs cortisone and prednisone to the active glucocorticoids cortisol and prednisolone, respectively. N-reductions occur in azo- or nitro-compounds (e.g., nitrazepam). Nitro groups can be reduced to amine groups via nitroso and hydroxyl-amino-intermediates. Likewise, dehalogenation is a reductive process involving a carbon atom (e.g., halothane, p. 208).

Methylations are catalyzed by a group of relatively specific methyl-transferases involving the transfer of methyl groups to hydroxyl groups (O-methylation as in norepinephrine [noradrenaline]) or to amino groups (N-methylation of norepinephrine, histamine, or serotonin).

In thio compounds, **desulfuration** results from substitution of sulfur by oxygen (e.g., parathion). This example again illustrates that biotransformation is not always to be equated with bioinactivation. Thus, paraoxon formed in the organism from parathion is the actual active agent (p. 102).

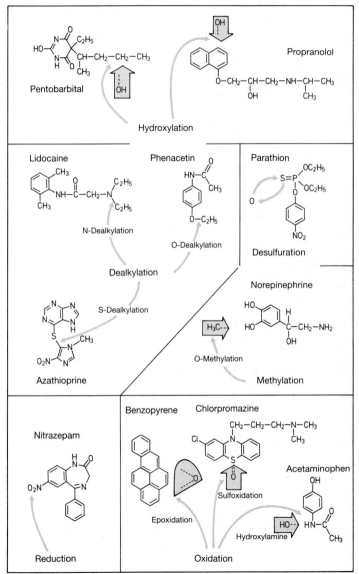

A. Examples of chemical reactions in drug biotransformation

Enterohepatic Cycle (A)

After an orally ingested drug has been absorbed from the gut, it is transported via the portal blood to the liver, where it can be conjugated to glucuronic or sulfuric acid (shown in **B** for salicylic acid and deacetylated bisacodyl, respectively) or to other organic acids. At the pH of body fluids, these acids are predominantly ionized; the negative charge confers high polarity upon the conjugated drug molecule and, hence, low membrane penetrability. The conjugated products may pass from hepatocyte into biliary fluid and from there back into the intestine. O-glucuronides can be cleaved by bacterial β-glucuronidases in the colon, enabling the liberated drug molecule to be **reabsorbed.** The **enterohepatic cycle** acts to trap drugs in the body. However, conjugated products enter not only the bile but also the blood. Glucuronides with a molecular weight (MW) < 300 preferentially pass into the blood, whereas those with MW > 300 enter the bile to a larger extent. Glucuronides circulating in the blood undergo glomerular filtration in the kidney and are excreted in urine because their decreased lipophilicity prevents tubular reabsorption.

Drugs that are subject to enterohepatic cycling are, therefore, excreted slowly. Pertinent examples include digitoxin and acidic nonsteroidal anti-inflammatory agents (NSAIDs) (p. 190).

Conjugations (B)

The most important of Phase II conjugation reactions is *glucuronidation.* This reaction does not proceed spontaneously, but requires the activated form of glucuronic acid, namely, glucuronic acid uridine diphosphate. Microsomal glucuronyl transferases link the activated glucuronic acid with an acceptor molecule. When the latter is a phenol or alcohol, an ether glucuronide will be formed. In the case of carboxyl-bearing molecules, an ester glucuronide is the result. All of these are O-glucuronides. Amines may form N-glucuronides that, unlike O-glucuronides, are resistant to bacterial β-glucuronidases.

Soluble cytoplasmic sulfotransferases conjugate *activated sulfate* (3'- phosphoadenine - 5' - phosphosulfate) with alcohols and phenols. The conjugates are acids, as in the case of glucuronides. In this respect, they differ from conjugates formed by acetyltransferases from *activated acetate* (acetylcoenzyme A) and an alcohol or a phenol.

Acyltransferases are involved in the conjugation of the amino acids *glycine* or *glutamine* with carboxylic acids. In these cases, an amide bond is formed between the carboxyl groups of the acceptor and the amino group of the donor molecule (e.g., formation of salicyluric acid from salicylic acid and glycine). The acidic group of glycine or glutamine remains free.

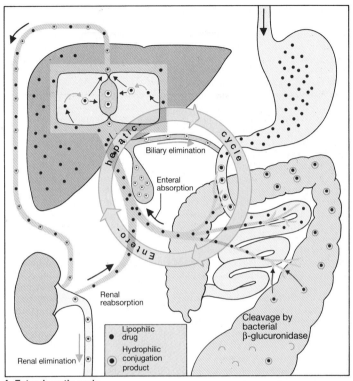

A. Enterohepatic cycle

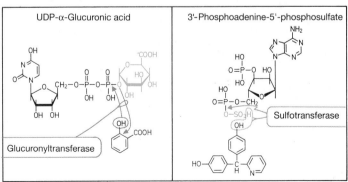

B. Conjugation reactions

The Kidney as Excretory Organ

Most drugs are eliminated in the urine either chemically unchanged or as metabolites. The kidney permits elimination because the vascular wall structure in the region of the glomerular capillaries **(B)** allows unimpeded passage of blood solutes having molecular weights < 5000. Filtration is slowed at molecular weights > 5000 and ceases when they exceed 70,000. With few exceptions, therapeutically used drugs and their metabolites have much smaller molecular weights and can, therefore, undergo **glomerular filtration,** i.e., pass from blood into primary urine. Separating the capillary **endothelium** from the tubular **epithelium,** the **basal membrane** consists of charged glycoproteins and acts as a filtration barrier for high-molecular-weight substances. The relative density of this barrier depends on the electrical charge of the molecules that attempt to permeate it.

Apart from **glomerular filtration (B),** drugs present in blood may pass into urine by **active secretion.** Certain cations and anions are secreted by the epithelium of the proximal tubules into the tubular fluid via special, energy-consuming transport systems. These transport systems have a limited capacity. When several substrates are present simultaneously, competition for the carrier may occur (see p. 290).

During passage down the renal tubule, urinary volume shrinks more than 100-fold; accordingly, there is a corresponding concentration of filtered drug or drug metabolites **(A).** The resulting concentration gradient between urine and interstitial fluid is preserved in the case of drugs incapable of permeating the tubular epithelium. However, with lipophilic drugs the concentration gradient will favor **reabsorption** of the filtered molecules. In this case, reabsorption is not based on an active process but results instead from passive diffusion. Accordingly, for protonated substances, the extent of reabsorption is dependent on urinary pH or the degree of dissociation. In the case of endobiotics (glucose, amino acids, peptides), specific transport processes operate in the proximal tubule that also handle certain drugs (aminoglycosides, p. 264).

The degree of dissociation varies as a function of the urinary pH and the pK_a, which represents the pH value at which half of the substance exists in protonated (or unprotonated) form. This relationship is graphically illustrated **(D)** with the example of a protonated amine having a pKa of 7. In this case, at urinary pH 7, 50% of the amine will be present in the protonated, hydrophilic, membrane-impermeant form (blue dots), whereas the other half, representing the uncharged amine (orange dots), can leave the tubular lumen in accordance with the resulting concentration gradient. If the pK_a of an amine is higher ($pK_a = 7.5$) or lower ($pK_a = 6.5$), a correspondingly smaller or larger proportion of the amine will be present in the uncharged, reabsorbable form. Lowering or raising urinary pH by half a pH unit would result in analogous changes.

The same considerations hold for acidic molecules, with the important difference that alkalinization of the urine (increased pH) will promote the deprotonization of –COOH groups and thus impede reabsorption. Intentional alteration in urinary pH can be used in cases of intoxication with proton-acceptor substances in order to hasten elimination of the toxin (alkalinization → phenobarbital; acidification → amphetamine).

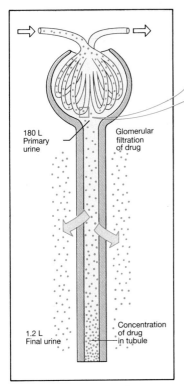

A. Filtration and concentration

180 L Primary urine

Glomerular filtration of drug

1.2 L Final urine

Concentration of drug in tubule

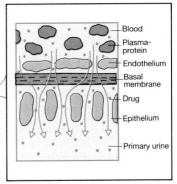

B. Glomerular filtration

Blood
Plasma-protein
Endothelium
Basal membrane
Drug
Epithelium
Primary urine

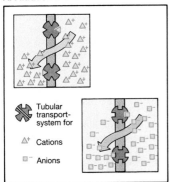

C. Active secretion

Tubular transport-system for

$\triangle^+$ Cations

$\square^-$ Anions

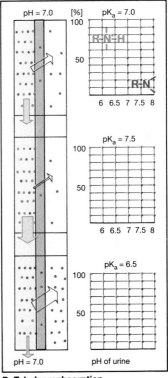

D. Tubular reabsorption

pH = 7.0 [%] pK$_a$ = 7.0

pK$_a$ = 7.5

pK$_a$ = 6.5

pH = 7.0 pH of urine

Elimination of Lipophilic and Hydrophilic Substances

The terms **lipophilic** and **hydrophilic** (or hydro- and lipophobic) refer to solubility of substances in media of low and high polarity, respectively. Blood plasma, interstitial fluid, and cytosol are highly polar aqueous media, whereas lipids—at least in the interior of the lipid bilayer membrane—and fat constitute apolar media. Most polar substances are readily dissolved in aqueous media (i.e., are hydrophilic) and lipophilic ones in apolar media. A **hydrophilic drug**, on reaching the bloodstream, probably after a partial, slow absorption (not illustrated), passes through the liver unchanged, because it either cannot, or will only slowly, permeate the lipid barier of the hepatocyte membrane and thus will fail to gain access to hepatic biotransforming enzymes. The unchanged drug reaches the arterial blood and the kidneys, where it is filtered. With hydrophilic drugs, there is little binding to plasma proteins (protein binding increases as a function of lipophilicity), hence the entire amount present in plasma is available for glomerular filtration. A hydrophilic drug is not subject to tubular reabsorption and appears in the urine. Hydrophilic drugs undergo **rapid elimination.**

If a **lipophilic drug**, because of its chemical nature, cannot be converted into a polar product, despite having access to all cells, including metabolically active liver cells, it is to be retained in the body. The portion filtered during glomerular passage will be reabsorbed from the tubules. Reabsorption will be nearly complete, because the free concentration of a lipophilic drug in plasma is low (usually lipophilic substances are largely protein-bound). The situation portrayed for a lipophilic **nonmetaboliz-able** drug would seem undesirable, because pharmacotherapeutic measures once initiated would be virtually irreversible (poor control over blood concentration).

Lipophilic drugs that are converted in the liver to **hydrophilic metabolites** permit better control, because the lipophilic agent can be eliminated in this manner. The speed of formation of hydrophilic metabolite determines the length of the drug's stay in the body.

If hepatic conversion to a polar metabolite is rapid, only a portion of the absorbed drug enters the systemic circulation in unchanged form, the remainder having undergone **presystemic** (first pass) **elimination**. When biotransformation is rapid, oral administration of the drug is impossible (e.g., lidocaine, p. 134). Parenteral or, alternatively, sublingual, intranasal, or transdermal administration is then required in order to bypass the liver. Irrespective of the route of administration, a portion of administered drug may be taken up into and transiently stored in lung tissue before entering the general circulation. Biotransformation (e.g., liver) and transient storage (e.g., lung) may contribute to presystemic elimination. **Presystemic elimination** refers to the fraction of drug absorbed that is excluded from the general circulation by biotransformation or by first-pass binding.

Bioavailability indicates the fraction of drug *administered* that enters the circulation in unchanged form. Two preparations of a particular drug can be said to have equal bioavailability (or bioequivalence) if the same fraction of the administered dose enters the systemic circulation at the same rate and reaches identical peak blood levels.

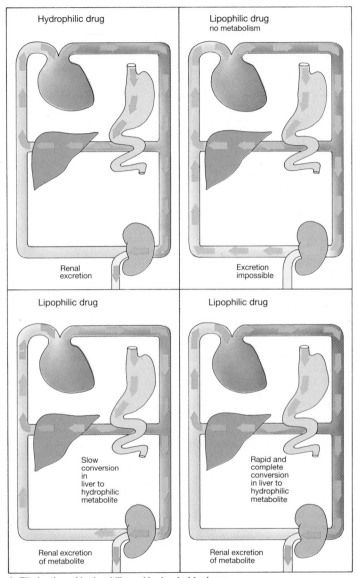

A. Elimination of hydrophilic and hydrophobic drugs

Drug Concentration in the Body as a Function of Time. First-Order (Exponential) Rate Processes

Processes such as drug absorption and elimination display exponential characteristics. As regards the former, this follows from the simple fact that the amount of drug being moved per unit of time depends on the concentration difference (gradient) between two body compartments (Fick's Law). In drug absorption from the alimentary tract, the intestinal contents and the blood would represent the compartments containing an initially high and low concentration, respectively. In drug elimination via the kidney, excretion often depends on glomerular filtration, i.e., the filtered amount of drug present in primary urine. As the blood concentration falls, the amount of drug filtered per unit of time diminishes. The resulting exponential decline is illustrated in (**A**). The exponential time course implies constancy of the interval during which the concentration decreases by one-half. This interval represents the half-life ($t^1/_2$) and is related to the elimination rate constant k by the equation $t^1/_2 = \ln 2/k$. The two parameters, together with the initial concentration c_o, describe a first-order (exponential) rate process.

The constancy of the process permits calculation of the plasma volume that would be cleared of drug, if the remaining drug were not to assume a homogeneous distribution in the total volume (a condition not met in reality). The **notional plasma volume freed of drug per unit of time** is termed the **clearance.** Depending on whether plasma concentration falls as a result of urinary excretion or of metabolic alteration, clearance is considered to be renal or hepatic. Renal and hepatic clearances add up to total clearance (Cl_{tot}) in the case of drugs

that are eliminated unchanged via the kidney and biotransformed in the liver. Cl_{tot} represents the sum of all processes contributing to elimination; it is related to the half-life ($t^1/_2$) and the apparent volume of distribution V_{app} (p. 28) by the equation:

$$t^1/_2 = \ln 2 \cdot \frac{V_{app}}{Cl_{tot}}$$

The smaller the volume of distribution or the larger the total clearance, the shorter is the half-life.

In the case of drugs renally eliminated in unchanged form, the half-life of elimination can be calculated from the cumulative excretion in urine; the final total amount eliminated corresponds to the amount absorbed.

Hepatic elimination obeys exponential kinetics because metabolizing enzymes operate in the quasilinear region of their concentration–activity curve, and hence the amount of drug metabolized per unit of time diminishes with decreasing blood concentration.

The best-known exception to exponential kinetics is the elimination of alcohol (ethanol), which obeys a linear time course (zero-order kinetics), at least at blood concentrations > 0.02%. It does so because the rate-limiting enzyme, alcohol dehydrogenase, achieves half saturation at very low substrate concentrations, i.e., at about 80 mg/L (0.008%). Thus, reaction velocity reaches a plateau at blood ethanol concentrations of about 0.02%, and the amount of drug eliminated per unit of time remains constant at concentrations above this level.

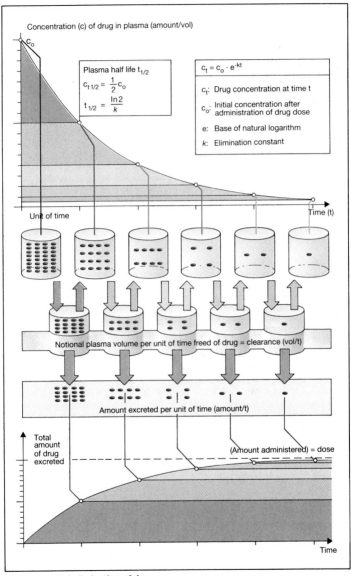

Concentration (c) of drug in plasma (amount/vol)

c_0

Plasma half life $t_{1/2}$

$c_{t\,1/2} = \dfrac{1}{2} c_0$

$t_{1/2} = \dfrac{\ln 2}{k}$

$c_t = c_0 \cdot e^{-kt}$

c_t: Drug concentration at time t

c_0: Initial concentration after administration of drug dose

e: Base of natural logarithm

k: Elimination constant

Unit of time   Time (t)

Notional plasma volume per unit of time freed of drug = clearance (vol/t)

Amount excreted per unit of time (amount/t)

Total amount of drug excreted

(Amount administered) = dose

Time

A. Exponential elimination of drug

Time Course of
Drug Concentration in Plasma

A. Drugs are taken up into and eliminated from the body by various routes. The body thus represents an open system wherein the actual drug concentration reflects the interplay of intake (ingestion) and egress (elimination).

When orally administered drug is absorbed from the stomach and intestine, speed of uptake depends on many factors, including the speed of drug dissolution (in the case of solid dosage forms) and of gastrointestinal transit; the membrane penetrability of the drug; its concentration gradient across the mucosa–blood barrier; and mucosal blood flow. **Absorption** from the intestine causes the drug concentration in blood to increase. Transport in blood conveys the drug to different organs (**distribution**), into which it is taken up to a degree compatible with its chemical properties and rate of blood flow through the organ. For instance, well-perfused organs such as the brain receive a greater proportion than do less well-perfused ones. Uptake into tissue causes the blood concentration to fall. Absorption from the gut diminishes as the mucosa–blood gradient decreases. Plasma concentration reaches a peak when the amount of drug leaving the blood per unit of time equals that being absorbed. Drug entry into hepatic and renal tissue constitutes movement into the **organs of elimination.**

The characteristic phasic time course of drug concentration in plasma represents the sum of the constituent processes of **absorption, distribution,** and **elimination**, which overlap in time. When distribution takes place significantly faster than elimination, there is an initial rapid and then a greatly retarded fall in the plasma level, the former being designated the α-phase (distribution phase), the latter the β-phase (elimination phase). When the drug is distributed more rapidly than it is absorbed, the time course of the plasma level can be described in mathematically simplified form by the Bateman function (k_1 and k_2 represent the rate constants for absorption and elimination, respectively).

B. The velocity of absorption depends on the route of administration. The more rapid the absorption, the shorter will be the time (t_{max}) required to reach the peak plasma level (c_{max}), the higher will be the c_{max}, and the earlier the plasma level will begin to fall again.

The *area under the plasma level time curve* (AUC) is independent of the route of administration, provided the doses and bioavailability are the same (Dost's law of corresponding areas). The AUC can thus be used to determine the extent of **presystemic elimination** or the bioavailability of a drug. The ratio of AUC values determined after oral or intravenous administration of a given dose of a particular drug corresponds to the proportion of drug entering the systemic circulation after oral administration. The determination of plasma levels affords a comparison of different proprietary preparations containing the same drug in the same dosage. Identical plasma level time-curves of different manufacturers' products with reference to a standard preparation indicate **bioequivalence.**

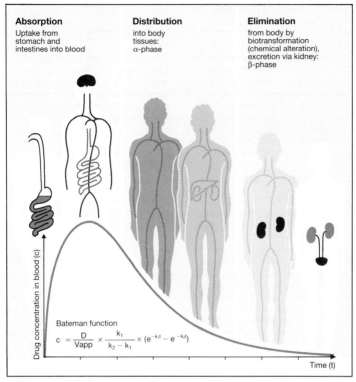

Absorption
Uptake from stomach and intestines into blood

Distribution
into body tissues: α-phase

Elimination
from body by biotransformation (chemical alteration), excretion via kidney: β-phase

Bateman function
$$c = \frac{D}{V_{app}} \times \frac{k_1}{k_2 - k_1} \times (e^{-k_1 t} - e^{-k_2 t})$$

Drug concentration in blood (c)

Time (t)

A. Time course of drug concentration

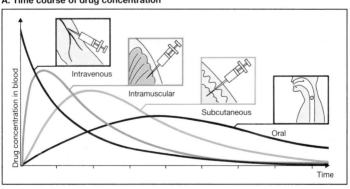

Drug concentration in blood

Intravenous

Intramuscular

Subcutaneous

Oral

Time

B. Mode of application and time course of drug concentration

Time Course of Drug Plasma Levels during Repeated Dosing (A)

When a drug is administered at regular intervals over a prolonged period, the rise and fall of drug concentration in blood will be determined by the relationship between the half-life of elimination and the time interval between doses. If the drug amount administered in each dose has been eliminated before the next dose is applied, repeated intake at constant intervals will result in similar plasma levels. If intake occurs before the preceding dose has been eliminated completely, the next dose will add on to the residual amount still present in the body—i.e., the drug **accumulates.** The shorter the dosing interval relative to the elimination half-life, the larger will be the residual mount of drug to which the next dose is added and the more extensively the drug will accumulate in the body. However, at a given dosing frequency, the drug does not accumulate infinitely and a **steady state** (C_{ss}) or **accumulation equilibrium** is eventually reached. This is so because the activity of elimination processes is concentration-dependent; the higher the drug concentration rises, the greater is the amount eliminated per unit of time. After several doses, the concentration will have climbed to a level at which the amounts eliminated and taken in per unit of time become equal, i.e., a steady state is reached. Within this concentration range, the plasma level will continue to rise (peak) and fall (trough) as dosing is continued at a regular interval. The height of the steady state (C_{ss}) depends upon the amount (D) administered per dosing interval (τ) and the clearance (Cl_{tot}):

$$C_{ss} = \frac{D}{(\tau \cdot Cl_{tot})}$$

The speed at which the steady state is reached corresponds to the speed of elimination of the drug. The time needed to reach 90% of the concentration plateau is about three times the $t \frac{1}{2}$ of elimination.

Time Course of Drug Plasma Levels during Irregular Intake (B)

In practice, it proves difficult to achieve a plasma level that undulates evenly around the desired effective concentration. For instance, if two successive doses are omitted, the plasma level will drop below the therapeutic range and a longer period will be required to regain the desired plasma level. In everyday life, patients will be apt to neglect drug intake at the scheduled time. **Patient compliance** means strict adherence to the prescribed regimen. Apart from poor compliance, the same problem may occur when the daily dose is divided into three individual doses and the first dose is taken at breakfast, the second at lunch, and the third at supper. Under this condition, the nocturnal dosing interval will be twice the diurnal one. Consequently, plasma levels during the early morning hours may have fallen far below the desired or, possibly, urgently needed range.

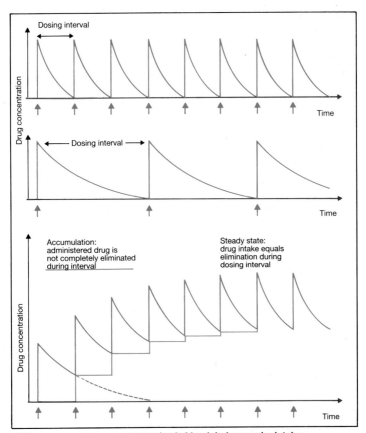

A. Time course of drug concentration in blood during regular intake

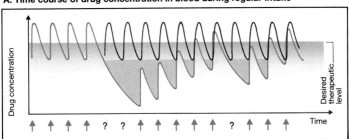

B. Time course of drug concentration with irregular intake

Accumulation: Dose, Dose Interval, and Plasma Level Fluctuation

Successful drug therapy in many illnesses is accomplished only if drug concentration is maintained at a steady high level. This requirement necessitates regular drug intake and a dosage schedule that ensures that the plasma concentration neither falls below the therapeutically effective range nor exceeds the minimal toxic concentration. A constant plasma level would, however, be undesirable if it accelerated a loss of effectiveness (development of tolerance), or if the drug were required to be present at specified times only.

A steady plasma level can be achieved by giving the drug in a constant intravenous infusion, the steady-state plasma level being determined by the infusion rate: dose D per unit of time t:

$$C_{ss} = \frac{D}{t \cdot Cl_{tot}}$$

This procedure is routinely used in hospital settings, but is generally impracticable. With oral administration, dividing the total daily dose into several individual ones, e.g., four, three, or two, offers a practical compromise. When the daily dose is given in several divided doses, the mean plasma level shows little fluctuation. In practice, it is found that a regimen of frequent regular drug ingestion is not well adhered to by patients. The degree of fluctuation in plasma level over a given dosing interval can be reduced by a use of dosage form permitting slow (sustained) release (p. 10).

The time required to reach steady-state accumulation during multiple constant dosing depends on the rate of elimination. As a rule of thumb, a plateau is reached after approximately three elimination half-lives ($t \, ^1/_2$).

For slowly eliminated drugs, which tend to accumulate extensively (phenprocoumon, digitoxin, methadone [p. 204]), the optimal plasma level is attained only after a long period. Here, increasing the initial doses (loading dose) will speed up the attainment of equilibrium, which is subsequently maintained with a lower dose (maintenance dose).

Change in Elimination Characteristics during Drug Therapy (B)

With any drug taken regularly and accumulating to the desired plasma level, it is important to consider that conditions for biotransformation and excretion do not necessarily remain constant. Elimination may be hastened due to enzyme induction (p. 32) or to a change in urinary pH (p. 40). Consequently, the steady-state plasma level declines to a new value corresponding to the new rate of elimination. The drug effect may diminish or disappear. Conversely, when elimination is impaired (e.g., in renal failure), the mean plasma level of renally eliminated drugs rises and may enter a toxic concentration range.

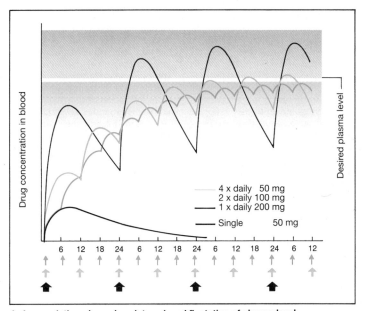

A. Accumulation: dose, dose interval, and fluctation of plasma level

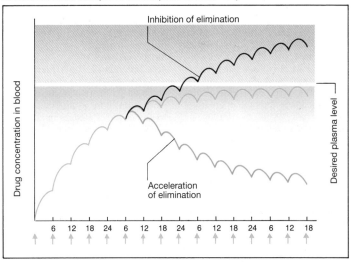

B. Changes in elimination kinetics in the course of drug therapy

Dose–Response Relationship

The effect of a substance depends on the amount administered, i.e., the dose. If the dose chosen is below the critical threshold (subliminal dosing), an effect will be absent. Depending on the nature of the effect to be measured, ascending doses may cause the effect to increase in intensity. Thus, the effect of an antipyretic or hypotensive drug can be quantified in a graded fashion, in that the extent of fall in body temperature or blood pressure is being measured. A dose–effect relationship is then encountered, as discussed on page 54.

The dose–effect relationship may vary depending on the sensitivity of the individual person receiving the drug, i.e., for the same effect, different doses may be required in different individuals. The interindividual variation in sensitivity is especially obvious with effects of the "all-or-none" kind.

To illustrate this point, we consider an experiment in which the subjects individually respond in all-or-none fashion, as in the Straub tail phenomenon (**A**). Mice react to morphine with excitation, evident in the form of an abnormal posture of the tail and limbs. The dose dependence of this phenomenon is observed in groups of animals (e.g., 10 mice per group) injected with increasing doses of morphine. At the low dose, only the most sensitive, at increasing doses a growing proportion, at the highest dose all of the animals are affected (**B**). There is a relationship between the frequency of responding animals and the dose given. At 2 mg/kg, 1 out of 10 animals reacts; at 10 mg/kg, 5 out of 10 respond. The **dose–frequency relationship** results from the different sensitivity of individuals, which as a rule exhibits a log normal distribution

(**C**, graph at right linear scale). If the cumulative frequency (total number of animals responding at a given dose) is plotted against the logarithm of the dose (abscissa), a sigmoidal curve results (**C**, graph at left semi-logarithmic scale). The inflection point of the curve lies at the dose at which one-half of the group has responded. The dose range encompassing the dose–frequency relationship reflects the variation in individual sensitivity to the drug.

Although similar in shape, a dose–frequency relationship has, thus, a different meaning than does a dose–effect relationship. The latter can be evaluated in one individual and results from an (intraindividual) dependency of the effect on drug concentration.

The evaluation of a dose–effect relationship within a group of individuals is compounded by interindividual differences in sensitivity. To account for the biological variation, measurements have to be carried out on a representative sample and the results averaged. Thus, recommended therapeutic doses will be appropriate for the majority of patients, but not necessarily for *each* individual.

The variation in sensitivity may be based on pharmacokinetic differences (same dose → different plasma levels) or on differences in target organ sensitivity (same plasma level → different effects).

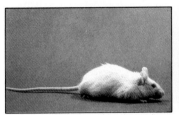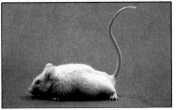

A. Abnormal posture in mouse given morphine

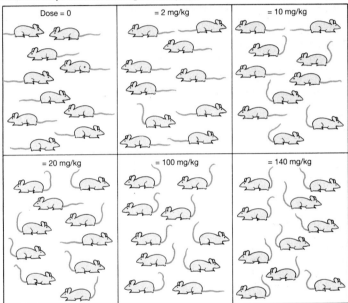

B. Incidence of effect as a function of dose

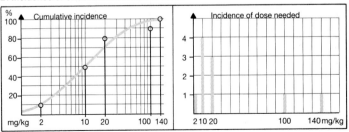

C. Dose–frequency relationship

Concentration–Effect Relationship (A)

The relationship between the concentration of a drug and its effect is determined in order to define the range of active drug concentrations (potency) and the maximum possible effect (efficacy). On the basis of these parameters, differences between drugs can be quantified. As a rule, the therapeutic effect or toxic action depends critically on the response of a single organ or a limited number of organs, e.g., blood flow is affected by a change in vascular luminal width. By isolating critical organs or tissues from a larger functional system, these actions can be studied with more accuracy; for instance, vasoconstrictor agents can be examined in isolated preparations from different regions of the vascular tree, e.g., the portal or saphenous veins, or the mesenteric, coronary, or basilar artery. In many cases, isolated organs or organ parts can be kept viable for hours in an appropriate nutrient medium sufficiently supplied with oxygen and held at a suitable temperature. Responses of the preparation to a physiological or pharmacological stimulus can be determined by a suitable recording apparatus. Thus, narrowing of a blood vessel is recorded with the help of two clamps by which the vessel is suspended under tension.

Experimentation on isolated organs offers several *advantages*:
1. The drug concentration in the tissue is usually known
2. Reduced complexity and ease of relating stimulus and effect
3. It is possible to circumvent compensatory responses that may partially cancel the primary effect in the intact organism—e.g., the heart rate–increasing action of norepinephrine cannot be demonstrated in the intact organism, because a simultaneous rise in blood pressure elicits a counter-regulatory reflex that slows cardiac rate;
4. The ability to examine a drug effect over its full range of intensities—e.g., it would be impossible in the intact organism to follow negative chronotropic effects to the point of cardiac arrest

Disadvantages are:
1. Unavoidable tissue injury during dissection
2. Loss of physiological regulation of function in the isolated tissue
3. The artificial milieu imposed on the tissue

Concentration–Effect Curves (B)

As the concentration is raised by a constant factor, the *increment in effect* diminishes steadily and tends asymptotically toward zero the closer one comes to the maximally effective concentration. The concentration at which a maximal effect occurs cannot be measured accurately; however, that eliciting a half-maximal effect (EC_{50}) is readily determined. It typically corresponds to the inflection point of the concentration–response curve in a semilogarithmic plot (log concentration on abscissa). Full characterization of a concentration–effect relationship requires determination of the EC_{50}, the maximally possible effect (E_{max}), and the slope at the point of inflection.

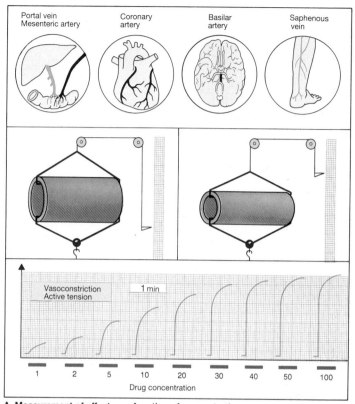

A. Measurement of effect as a function of concentration

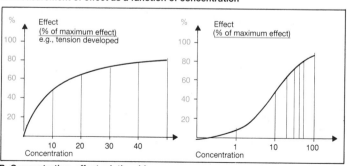

B. Concentration–effect relationship

Concentration–Binding Curves

In order to elicit their effect, drug molecules must be bound to the cells of the effector organ. Binding commonly occurs at specific cell structures, namely the receptors. The analysis of drug binding to receptors aims to determine the affinity of ligands, the kinetics of interaction, and the characteristics of the binding site itself.

In studying the affinity and number of such binding sites, use is made of membrane suspensions of different tissues. This approach is based on the expectation that binding sites will retain their characteristic properties during cell homogenization. Provided that binding sites are freely accessible in the medium in which membrane fragments are suspended, drug concentration at the "site of action" would equal that in the medium. The drug under study is radiolabeled (enabling low concentrations to be measured quantitatively), added to the membrane suspension, and allowed to bind to receptors. Membrane fragments and medium are then separated, e.g., by filtration, and the amount of bound drug is measured. Binding increases in proportion to concentration as long as there is a negligible reduction in the number of *free* binding sites (C=1 and B $\approx$ 10% of maximum binding; C=2 and B $\approx$ 20%). As binding sites approach saturation, the number of free sites decreases and the increment in binding is no longer proportional to the increase in concentration (in the example illustrated, an increase in concentration by 1 is needed to increase binding from 10% to 20%; however, an increase by 20 is needed to raise it from 70% to 80%).

The **law of mass action** describes the hyperbolic relationship between binding (B) and ligand concentration (c). This relationship is characterized by the drug's affinity ($1/K_D$) and the maximum binding (B_{max}), i.e., the total number of binding sites per unit of weight of membrane homogenate.

$$B = B_{max} \cdot \frac{c}{c + K_D}$$

K_D is the equilibrium dissociation constant and corresponds to that ligand concentration at which 50% of binding sites are occupied. The values given in (**A**) and used for plotting the concentration–binding graph (**B**) result when $K_D=10$.

The differing affinity of different ligands for a binding site can be demonstrated elegantly by binding assays. Although simple to perform, these binding assays pose the difficulty of correlating unequivocally the binding sites concerned with the pharmacological effect; this is particularly difficult when more than one population of binding sites is present. Therefore, receptor binding must not be implied until it can be shown that

1. binding is saturable *(saturability)*;
2. the only substances bound are those possessing the same pharmacological mechanism of action *(specificity)*;
3. binding *affinity* of different substances is *correlated with* their pharmacological *potency*.

Binding assays provide information about the affinity of ligands, but they do not give any clue as to whether a ligand is an agonist or antagonist (p. 60).

Radiolabeled drugs bound to their receptors may be of help in purifying and analyzing further the receptor protein.

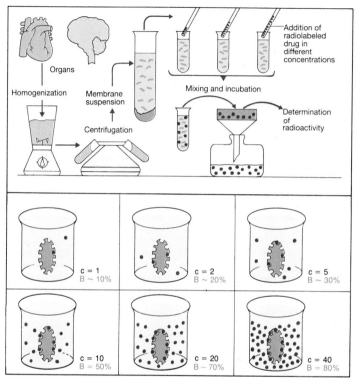

A. Measurement of binding (B) as a function of concentration (c)

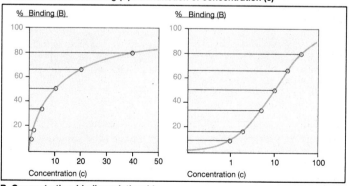

B. Concentration–binding relationship

Types of Binding Forces

Unless a drug comes into contact with intrinsic structures of the body, it cannot affect body function.

Covalent bond. Two atoms enter a covalent bond if each donates an electron to a shared electron pair (cloud). This state is depicted in structural formulas by a dash. The covalent bond is "firm," that is, not reversible or poorly so. Few drugs are covalently bound to biological structures. The bond, and possibly the effect, persist for a long time after intake of a drug has been discontinued, making therapy difficult to control. Examples include alkylating cytostatics (p. 280) or organophosphates (p. 102). Conjugation reactions occurring in biotransformation also represent a covalent linkage (e.g., to glucuronic acid, p. 38).

Noncovalent bond. There is no formation of a shared electron pair. The bond is reversible and typical of most drug–receptor interactions. Since a drug usually attaches to its site of action by multiple contacts, several of the types of bonds described below may participate.

Electrostatic attraction (A). A positive and negative charge attract each other.

Ionic interaction. An ion is a particle charged either positively (cation) or negatively (anion), i.e., the atom lacks or has surplus electrons, respectively. Attraction between ions of opposite charge is inversely proportional to the square of the distance between them; it is the initial force drawing a charged drug to its binding site. Ionic bonds have a relatively high stability.

Dipole–ion interaction. When bond electrons are asymmetrically distributed over both atomic nuclei, one atom will bear a negative (δ^-), and its partner a positive (δ^+) partial charge. The molecule thus presents a positive and a negative pole, i.e., has *polarity* or a *dipole*. A partial charge can interact electrostatically with an ion of opposite charge.

Dipole–dipole interaction. This is the electrostatic attraction between opposite partial charges. When a hydrogen atom bearing a partial positive charge bridges two atoms bearing a partial negative charge, a hydrogen bond is created.

A **van der Waals' bond (B)** is formed between apolar molecular groups that have come into close proximity. Spontaneous transient distortion of electron clouds (momentary faint dipole, $\delta\delta$) may induce an opposite dipole in the neighboring molecule. The van der Waals' bond, therefore, is also a form of electrostatic attraction, albeit of very low strength (inversely proportional to the seventh power of the distance).

Hydrophobic interaction (C). The attraction between water dipoles is strong enough to hinder intercalation of any apolar (uncharged) molecules. By tending toward each other, H_2O molecules squeeze apolar particles from their midst. Accordingly, in the organism, apolar particles have an increased probability of staying in nonaqueous, apolar surroundings, such as fatty acid chains of cell membranes or apolar regions of a receptor.

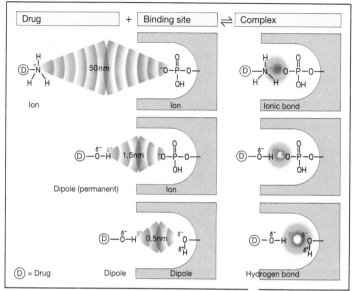

A. Electrostatic attraction

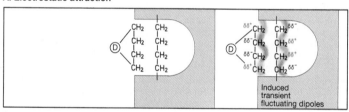

B. van der Waals' bond

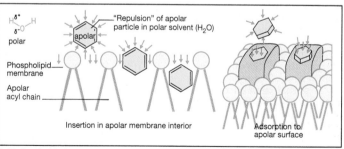

C. Hydrophobic interaction

Agonists–Antagonists (A)

When an agent interacts with a binding site to elicit a specific effect, it does so by virtue of possessing **affinity** and the ability to affect the binding site—the receptor—so that a change occurs in cellular function. This additional property is called **"intrinsic activity."** Affinity and intrinsic activity characterize an **agonist.**

Substances exist in whose presence the effect of an agonist is attenuated; they act therefore anti-agonistically or **antagonistically,** for short.

Competitive antagonists also possess affinity for the receptors; however, their binding does not elicit a change in cell function. In other words, competitive antagonists are devoid of intrinsic activity. When present simultaneously, an agonist and a competitive antagonist vie for occupancy of the receptor. Affinity and the concentrations of both competitors determine whether the agonist or antagonist will be bound and whether or not an effect is evoked. By increasing the concentration of the agonist, blockade induced by an antagonist can be overcome, i.e., the concentration–effect curve of the agonist is shifted right to higher concentrations in the presence of the competitive antagonist.

This type of antagonism implies reversible binding of the antagonist to the receptor. If dissociation from the receptor is slow or impossible (irreversible binding), an existing blockade cannot be overcome by raising the concentration of the agonist.

A **partial agonism** or **antagonism** is present when a drug has an intrinsic activity so low as to generate only a fraction of the maximal effect obtainable with a full agonist, even though all available receptors are occupied. In the presence of the partial agonist, the effect of a full agonist is attenuated because binding of the latter is impeded. Partial agonists, therefore, also display antagonism; however, by themselves they permit a certain level of receptor activation.

Unlike a competitive antagonist, an **allosteric antagonist** is bound outside the receptor area proper. In this type of binding, the receptor is altered so that its affinity for an agonist is decreased. It is also possible that allosteric deformation of the receptor increases affinity for an agonist, resulting in an **allosteric synergism.**

An **inverse agonist** (not illustrated) interacts with the receptor so that cell function is altered in a manner opposite to that of a "normal" agonist. In classic terminology inverse agonists would be assigned a negative intrinsic activity. The effect of an inverse agonist can be abolished by antagonists.

Functional antagonism (B). If two agonists acting by different mechanisms affect the same variable (e.g., bronchial lumen) but in opposite directions (epinephrine: dilation; histamine: constriction), a functional antagonism occurs. Another example is insulin and epinephrine [adrenaline], which behave as functional antagonists in their actions on blood glucose levels. Since different processes are involved in functional antagonism, processes that need not exert similar maximal, albeit opposite, actions, this interaction is not nearly as predictable as is competitive antagonism.

The term **chemical antagonism** is used when a substance reduces the concentration of an agonist by forming a complex (e.g., EDTA with Ca^{2+}; protamine with heparin). A **pharmacokinetic antagonism** is present when one drug accelerates the elimination of another (e.g., enzyme induction by phenobarbital, p. 32).

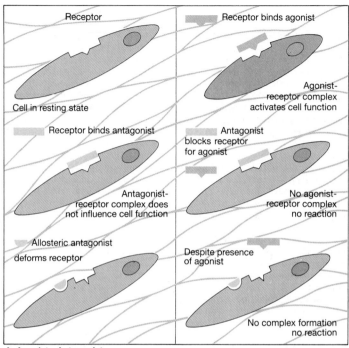

A. Agonist - Antagonist

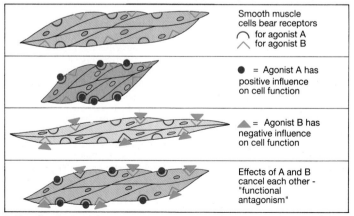

B. Functional antagonism

Enantioselectivity of Drug Action

Many drugs are racemates, including β-blockers, acidic nonsteroidal anti-inflammatory drugs (NSAID), as well as the anticholinergic, *benzetimide* (A). A **racemate** consists of a molecule and its corresponding mirror-image which, like the left and right hand, cannot be superimposed. Such **chiral** ("handed") pairs of molecules are referred to as **enantiomers**. Usually, chirality is due to a carbon atom (C) linked to four different substituents *("asymmetric center")*. Enantio-merism is a special case of stereoiso-merism. Nonchiral stereoisomers are called **diastereomers** (e.g., quinidine/quinine).

Distances between atoms in en-antiomers, but not in diastereomers, are the same. Therefore, enantiomers possess **similar physicochemical properties** (i.e., solubility, melting point) and both forms are usually obtained in equal amounts by chemical synthesis. As a result of enzymatic activity, however, only one of the enantiomers is usually found in nature.

In solution, enantiomers **rotate the wave plane of linearly polarized light in opposite directions**; hence, they are referred to as *"dextro-"* or *"levo-rotatory,"* designated by the prefixes *d* or (+) and *l* or (–), respectively. The direction of rotation gives no clue to the spatial structure of en-antiomers. The absolute configuration, as determined by certain rules, is described by the prefixes s and R. In some compounds, designation as D- and L-form is possible by reference to the structure of D- and L-glyceralde-hyde.

For drugs to exert biological actions, contact with reaction partners in the body is required. When the reaction favors one of the enantiomers, enantioselectivity is observed.

Enantioselectivity of affinity. If a receptor has sites for three of the substituents (symbolized in **B** by a cone, a sphere, and a cube) on the asymmetric carbon to attach to, only one of the enantiomers will have optimal fit. Its affinity will then be higher. Thus, *dexetimide* displays an affinity at the muscarinic ACh receptors (p. 98) almost 10,000 times higher than that of *levetimide*; and at β-adre-noceptors, s(–)-propranolol has an affinity 100 times that of the R(+)-form.

Enantioselectivity of intrinsic activity. The mode of attachment at the receptor also determines whether or not a substance has intrinsic activity, i.e., acts as an agonist or antago-nist. For instance, (–)-dobutamine is an agonist at α-adrenoceptors, where-as the (+)-enantiomer is an antagonist.

Inverse enantioselectivity at another receptor. An enantiomer may possess an unfavorable configu-ration at one receptor that may, how-ever, be optimal for interaction with another receptor. In the case of *do-butamine*, the (+)-enantiomer has an affinity at β-adrenoceptors 10 times higher than that of the (–)-enantiomer, both having agonist activity. Howev-er, the α-adrenoceptor stimulant ac-tion is due to the (–)-form (see above).

As described for receptor interac-tions, **enantioselectivity** may also be manifested in drug interactions **with enzymes and transport proteins**. Enantiomers may display different af-finities and reaction velocities.

Conclusion: The enantiomers of a racemate can differ sufficiently in their pharmacodynamic and pharma-cokinetic properties to constitute two distinct drugs.

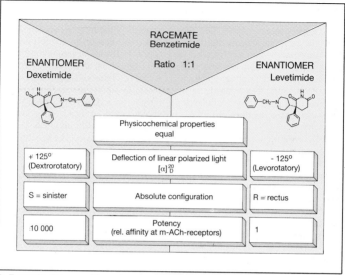

A. Example of an enantiomeric pair with different affinity for a stereoselective receptor

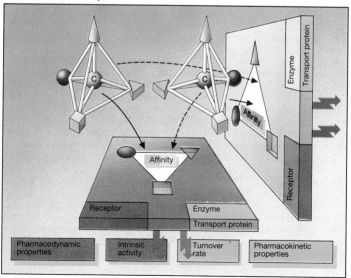

B. Reasons for different pharmacological properties of enantiomers

Receptor Types

Receptors are macromolecules that bind mediator substances and transduce this binding into an effect, i.e., a change in cell function. Receptors differ in terms of their structure and the manner in which they translate occupancy by a ligand into a cellular response (**signal transduction**).

G-Protein-coupled   receptors (A) consist of an amino acid chain that weaves in and out of the membrane in serpentine fashion. The extramembranal loop regions of the molecule may possess sugar residues at different N-glycosylation sites. The seven α-helical membrane-spanning domains probably form a circle around a central pocket that carries the attachment sites for the mediator substance. Binding of the mediator molecule or of a structurally related agonist molecule induces a change in the conformation of the receptor protein, enabling the latter to interact with a G-protein (= guanyl nucleotide–binding protein). G-Proteins lie at the inner leaf of the plasmalemma and consist of three subunits designated α, β, and γ. There are various G-proteins that differ mainly with regard to their α unit. Association with the receptor activates the G-protein, leading in turn to activation of another protein (enzyme, ion channel). A large number of mediator substances act via G-protein-coupled receptors (see p. 66 for more details).

An example of a **ligand-gated ion channel (B)** is the nicotinic cholinoceptor of the motor end plate. The receptor complex consists of five subunits, each of which contains four transmembrane domains. Simultaneous binding of two acetylcholine (ACh) molecules to the two α sub-units results in opening of the ion channel, with entry of Na^+ (and exit of some K^+), membrane depolarization, and triggering of an action potential (pp. 176, 180). The ganglionic N-cholinoceptors apparently consist only of α and β subunits ($\alpha_2 \beta_3$). Some of the receptors for the transmitter γ-aminobutyric acid (GABA) belong to this receptor family; the $GABA_A$ subtype is linked to a chloride channel (and also to a benzodiazepine-binding site, see p. 216). Glutamate and glycine both act via ligand-gated ion channels.

The insulin receptor protein represents a **ligand-regulated enzyme (C),** a catalytic receptor. When insulin binds to the extracellular attachment site, a tyrosine kinase activity is "switched on" at the intracellular portion. Protein phosphorylation leads to altered cell function. Receptors for growth hormones also belong to the catalytic receptor class.

Protein   synthesis–regulating receptors (D) for steroids and thyroid hormone are found in the cytosol and in the cell nucleus, respectively. Binding of hormone exposes a normally hidden domain of the receptor protein, thereby permitting the latter to bind to a particular nucleotide sequence on a gene and to regulate its transcription. Transcription is usually initiated or enhanced, rarely blocked.

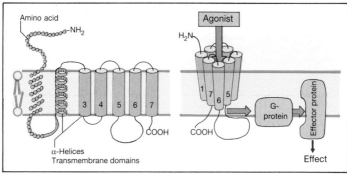

A. G-protein-coupled receptor

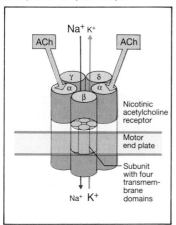

B. Ligand-gated ion channel

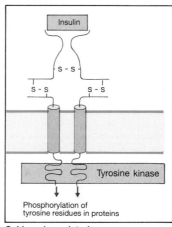

C. Ligand-regulated enzyme

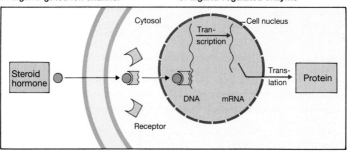

D. Protein synthesis-regulating receptor

Mode of Operation
of G-Protein-coupled Receptors

Signal transduction at G-protein-coupled receptors uses essentially the same basic mechanism (**A**). Agonist binding to the receptor leads to a change in receptor protein conformation. This change propagates to the G-protein; the α subunit exchanges GDP for GTP, then dissociates from the two other subunits, associates with an effector protein, and alters its functional state. The α subunit slowly hydrolyzes bound GTP to GDP. G_{α}-GDP has no affinity for the effector protein and reassociates with the β and γ subunits (**A**). G-Proteins can undergo lateral diffusion in the membrane; they are not assigned to individual receptor proteins. However, a relation exits between receptor types and G-protein types (**B**). Furthermore, the α subunits of individual G-proteins are distinct in terms of their affinity for different effector proteins, as well as the kind of influence exerted on the effector protein. G_{α}-GTP of the G_{s}- protein stimulates adenylate cyclase, whereas G_{α}-GTP of the G_{i}-protein is inhibitory. The G-protein-coupled receptor family includes muscarinic cholinoceptors, adrenoceptors for norepinephrine and epinephrine, receptors for dopamine, histamine, serotonin, morphine, prostaglandins, leukotrienes, and many other mediators and hormones.

Major effector proteins for G-protein-coupled receptors include **adenylate cyclase** (ATP $\rightarrow$ intracellular messenger **cAMP), phospholipase C** (phosphatidyl inositol $\rightarrow$ intracellular messengers **inositol triphosphate** and **diacylglycerol**) as well as ion channel proteins (**D**).

Numerous cell functions are regulated by cellular **cAMP** concentration, because cAMP enhances activi-

ty of protein kinase A, which catalyzes the transfer of phosphate groups onto functional proteins. Elevation of cAMP levels *inter alia* leads to relaxation of smooth muscle tonus, enhanced contractility of cardiac muscle, as well as increased glycogenolysis and lipolysis (p. 84). Phosphorylation of cardiac calcium-channel proteins increases the probability of channel opening during membrane depolarization. It should be noted that cAMP is inactivated by phosphodiesterase. Inhibitors of this enzyme elevate intracellular cAMP concentration and elicit effects resembling those of epinephrine.

The receptor protein itself may undergo phosphorylation, with a resultant loss of its ability to activate the associated G-protein. This is one of the mechanisms that contributes to a decrease in sensitivity of a cell during prolonged receptor stimulation by an agonist ("desensitization").

Activation of phospholipase C leads to cleavage of the membrane phospholipid phosphatidylinositol-4,5-bisphosphate into **inositol triphosphate** (IP$_3$) and **diacylglycerol** (DAG). IP$_3$ promotes release of Ca^{2+} from storage organelles, whereby contraction of smooth muscle cells, breakdown of glycogen, or exocytosis may be initiated. Diacylglycerol stimulates protein kinase C, which phosphorylates certain serine- or threonine-containing enzymes.

The α subunit of some G-proteins may induce opening of a **channel protein.** In this manner, K$^+$ channels can be activated (e.g., ACh effect on sinus node; opioid action on neural impulse transmission).

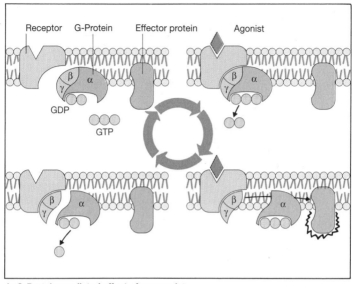

A. G-Protein-mediated effect of an agonist

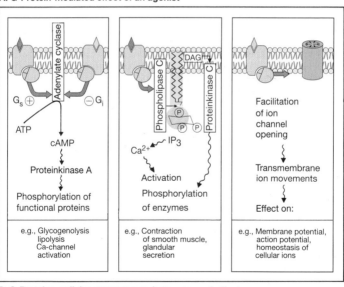

B. G-Proteins, cellular messenger substances, and effects

Time Course of Plasma Concentration and Effect

After the administration of a drug, its concentration in plasma rises, reaches a peak, and then declines gradually to the starting level, due to the processes of distribution and elimination (p. 46). Plasma concentration at a given point in time depends on the dose administered. Many drugs exhibit a linear relationship between plasma concentration and dose within the therapeutic range (**dose–linear kinetics**; (**A**); note different scales on ordinate). However, the same does not apply to drugs whose elimination processes are already sufficiently activated at therapeutic plasma levels so as to preclude further proportional increases in the rate of elimination when the concentration is increased further. Under these conditions, a smaller proportion of the dose administered is eliminated per unit of time.

The time course of the *effect* and of the *concentration* in plasma are not identical, because the **concentration–effect relationship** obeys a hyperbolic function (**B**; cf. also p. 54). This means that the time course of the effect exhibits dose dependence also in the presence of dose–linear kinetics (**C**).

In the lower dose range (example 1), the plasma level passes through a concentration range ($0 \rightarrow 0.9$) in which the concentration–effect relationship is quasilinear. The respective time courses of plasma concentration and effect (**A** and **C**, left graphs) are very similar. However, if a high dose (100) is applied, there is an extended period of time during which the plasma level will remain in a concentration range (between 90 and 20) in which a change in concentration does not cause a change in the size of the effect. Thus, at high doses (100), the time–effect curve exhibits a kind of plateau. The effect declines only when the plasma level has returned (below 20) into the range where a change in plasma level causes a change in the intensity of the effect.

The dose dependence of the time course of the drug effect is exploited when the duration of the effect is to be prolonged by administration of a dose in excess of that required for the effect. This is done in the case of penicillin G (p. 254), when a dosing interval of 8 h is being recommended, although the drug is eliminated with a half-life of 30 min. This procedure is, of course, feasible only if supramaximal dosing is not associated with toxic effects.

Furthermore it follows that a nearly constant effect can be achieved, although the plasma level may fluctuate greatly during the interval between doses.

The hyperbolic relationship between plasma concentration and effect explains why the time course of the effect, unlike that of the plasma concentration, cannot be described in terms of a simple exponential function. A half-life can be given for the processes of drug absorption and elimination, hence for the change in plasma levels, but generally not for the onset or decline of the effect.

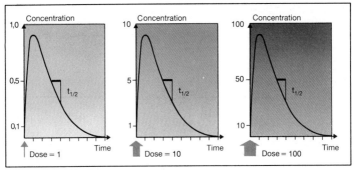

A. Dose–linear kinetics

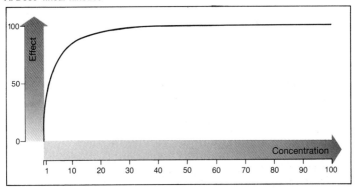

B. Concentration–effect relationship

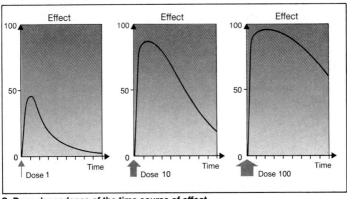

C. Dose dependence of the time course of effect

Adverse Drug Effects

The desired (or intended) principal effect of any drug is to modify body function in such a manner as to alleviate symptoms caused by the patient's illness. In addition, a drug may also cause unwanted effects that can be grouped into minor or side effects and major or adverse effects. These, in turn, may give rise to complaints or illness, or may even cause death.

Causes of adverse effects: overdosage (A). The drug is administered in a higher dose than is required for the principal effect; this directly or indirectly affects other body functions. For instance, morphine (p. 200), given in the appropriate dose, affords excellent pain relief by influencing nociceptive pathways in the CNS. In excessive doses, it inhibits the respiratory center and makes apnea imminent. The dose dependence of both effects can be graphed in the form of dose response curves (DRC). The distance between both DRCs indicates the difference between the therapeutic and toxic doses. This *margin of safety* indicates the risk of toxicity when standard doses are exceeded.

"The dose alone makes the poison" (Paracelsus). This holds true for both medicines and environmental poisons. *No substance as such is toxic!* In order to assess the risk of toxicity, knowledge is required of: 1) the effective dose during exposure; and 2) the dose level at which damage is likely to occur.

Increased sensitivity (B). If certain body functions develop hyperreactivity, unwanted effects can occur even at normal dose levels. Increased sensitivity of the respiratory center to morphine is found in patients with chronic lung disease, in neonates or during concurrent exposure to other respiratory depressant agents. The DRC is shifted to the left and a smaller dose of morphine is sufficient to paralyze respiration. Genetic anomalies of metabolism may also lead to hypersensitivity. Thus, several drugs (aspirin, antimalarials, etc.) can provoke premature breakdown of red blood cells (hemolysis) in subjects with a glucose-6-phosphate dehydrogenase deficiency. The discipline of pharmacogenetics deals with the importance of the genotype for reactions to drugs.

The above forms of hypersensitivity must be distinguished from allergies involving the immune system (p. 72).

Lack of selectivity (C). Despite appropriate dosing and normal sensitivity, undesired effects can occur because the drug does not act specifically on the targeted (diseased) tissue or organ. For instance, the anticholinergic, atropine, is bound only to acetylcholine receptors of the muscarinic type; however, these are present in many different organs. Moreover, the neuroleptic, chlorpromazine, is able to interact with several different receptor types. Thus, its action is neither organ specific nor receptor specific.

The consequences of lack of selectivity can often be avoided if the drug does not require the blood route to reach the target organ, but is, instead, applied locally, as in the administration of parasympatholytics in the form of eye drops or in an aerosol for inhalation.

With every drug use, unwanted effects must be taken into account. Before prescribing a drug, the physician should therefore assess the **risk:benefit ratio;** for this, knowledge of principal and adverse effects is a prerequisite.

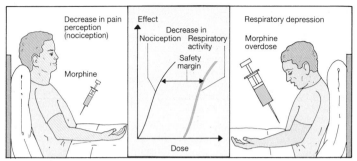

A. Adverse drug effect: overdosing

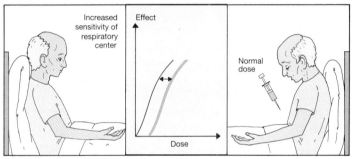

B. Adverse drug effect: increased sensitivity

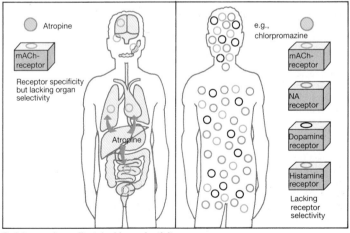

C. Adverse drug effect: lacking selectivity

Drug Allergy

The immune system normally functions to rid the organism of invading foreign particles, such as bacteria. Immune responses can occur without appropriate cause or with exaggerated intensity and may harm the organism, for instance, when allergic reactions are caused by drugs (active ingredient or pharmaceutic excipients). Only a few drugs, e.g. (heterologous) proteins, have a molecular mass ($>$ 10,000) great enough to act as effective **antigens** or immunogens, capable by themselves of initiating an immune response. Most drugs or their metabolites (so-called **haptens**) must first be converted to an antigen by linkage to a body protein. In the case of penicillin G, a cleavage product (penicilloyl residue) probably undergoes covalent binding to protein. During **initial contact** with the drug, the immune system is sensitized; antigen-specific lymphocytes of the T type and B type (antibody formation) proliferate in lymphatic tissue and some of them remain as so-called memory cells. Usually, these processes remain clinically silent. During the **second contact** antibodies are already present and memory cells proliferate rapidly. A detectable immune response, the allergic reaction, occurs. This can be of severe intensity, even at a low dose of the antigen. Four **types of reactions** can be distinguished:

Type 1, anaphylactic reaction. Drug-specific antibodies of the *IgE type* combine via their F_c moiety with receptors on the surface of *mast cells*. Binding of the drug provides the stimulus for the release of histamine and other mediators. In the most severe form, a life-threatening anaphylactic shock develops, accompanied by hypotension, bronchospasm (asthma attack), laryngeal edema, urticaria, stimulation of gut musculature, and spontaneous bowel movements (p. 298).

Type 2, cytotoxic reaction. *Drug-antibody (IgG) complexes* adhere to the *surface of blood cells*, where either circulating drug molecules or complexes already formed in blood accumulate. These complexes mediate the *activation of complement,* a family of proteins that circulate in the blood in an inactive form, but can be activated in a cascade-like succession by an appropriate stimulus. "Activated complement," normally directed against microorganisms, can *destroy the cell membranes* and thereby cause cell death; it also promotes phagocytosis, attracts neutrophil granulocytes (chemotaxis), and stimulates other inflammatory responses. Activation of complement on blood cells results in their destruction, evidenced by hemolytic anemia, agranulocytosis, and thrombocytopenia.

Type 3, immune complex vasculitis (serum sickness, Arthus reaction). *Drug–antibody complexes* precipitate on *vascular walls, complement* is activated, and an *inflammatory reaction* is triggered. Attracted neutrophils, in a futile attempt to phagocytose the complexes, liberate lysosomal enzymes that damage the vascular walls (inflammation, vasculitis). Symptoms may include fever, exanthema, swelling of lymph nodes, arthritis, nephritis, and neuropathy.

Type 4, contact dermatitis. A cutaneously applied drug is bound to the surface of *T-lymphocytes* directed specifically against it. The lymphocytes release signal molecules (*lymphokines*) into their vicinity that activate macrophages and provoke an inflammatory reaction.

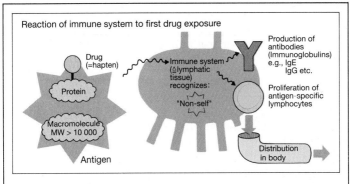

Reaction of immune system to first drug exposure

Drug (=hapten)

Protein

Macromolecule MW > 10 000

Antigen

Immune system (≙lymphatic tissue) recognizes:

"Non-self"

Production of antibodies (Immunoglobulins) e.g., IgE, IgG etc.

Proliferation of antigen-specific lymphocytes

Distribution in body

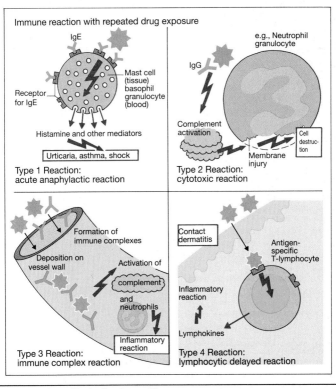

Immune reaction with repeated drug exposure

IgE

Receptor for IgE

Mast cell (tissue) basophil granulocyte (blood)

Histamine and other mediators

Urticaria, asthma, shock

Type 1 Reaction: acute anaphylactic reaction

e.g., Neutrophil granulocyte

IgG

Complement activation

Membrane injury

Cell destruction

Type 2 Reaction: cytotoxic reaction

Formation of immune complexes

Deposition on vessel wall

Activation of complement and neutrophils

Inflammatory reaction

Type 3 Reaction: immune complex reaction

Contact dermatitis

Antigen-specific T-lymphocyte

Inflammatory reaction

Lymphokines

Type 4 Reaction: lymphocytic delayed reaction

A. Adverse drug effect: allergic reaction

Drug Toxicity in Pregnancy and Lactation

Drugs taken by the mother can be passed on transplacentally or via breast milk and adversely affect the unborn or the neonate.

Pregnancy (A)

Limb malformations induced by the hypnotic, thalidomide, first focused attention on the potential of drugs to cause malformations *(teratogenicity)*. Drug effects on the unborn fall into two basic categories:

1. Predictable effects that derive from the known pharmacological properties. Examples are: masculinization of the female fetus by androgenic hormones; brain hemorrhage due to oral anticoagulants; bradycardia due to β-blockers.

2. Effects that specifically affect the developing organism and that cannot be predicted on the basis of the known pharmacological activity profile.

In assessing the risks attending drug use during pregnancy, the following points have to be considered:

a) *Time of drug use.* The possible sequelae of exposure to a drug depend on the stage of fetal development, as shown in **A**. Thus, the hazard posed by a drug with a specific action is limited in time, as illustrated by the tetracyclines, which produce effects on teeth and bones only after the third month of gestation, when mineralization begins.

b) *Transplacental passage.* Most drugs can pass in the placenta from the maternal into the fetal circulation. The fused cells of the syncytiotrophoblast form the major diffusion barrier. They possess a higher permeability to drugs than is suggested by the term "placental barrier."

c) *Teratogenicity.* Statistical risk estimates are available for familiar, frequently used drugs. For many drugs, teratogenic potency cannot be demonstrated; however, in the case of novel drugs it is usually not yet possible to define their teratogenic hazard.

Drugs with established human teratogenicity include derivatives of Vitamin A (etretinate, isotretinoic acid [used internally in skin diseases]), and oral anticoagulants. A peculiar type of damage results from the synthetic estrogenic agent, diethylstilbestrol (DES), following its use during pregnancy: daughters of treated mothers have an increased incidence of cervical and vaginal carcinoma at the age of approx. 20 years.

In assessing the risk:benefit ratio, it is also necessary to consider the benefit for the child resulting from adequate therapeutic treatment of its mother. For instance, therapy with antiepileptic drugs is indispensable, because untreated epilepsy endangers the infant at least as much as does administration of anticonvulsants.

Lactation (B)

Drugs present in the maternal organism can be secreted in breast milk and thus be ingested by the infant. Evaluation of risks should be based on factors listed in **B**. In case of doubt, potential danger to the infant can be averted only by weaning.

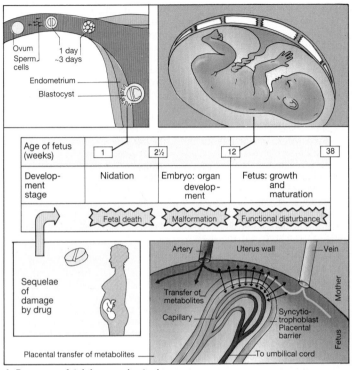

A. Pregnancy: fetal damage due to drugs

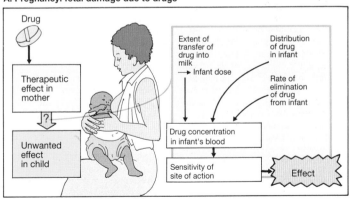

B. Lactation: maternal intake of drug

Placebo (A)

A placebo is a dosage form devoid of an active ingredient, a dummy medication. Administration of a placebo may elicit desired (relief of symptoms) or undesired effects that reflect a change in the patient's psychological situation brought about by the therapeutic setting.

Physicians may consciously or unconsciously communicate to the patient whether or not they are concerned about the patient's problem, or certain about the diagnosis and about the value of prescribed therapeutic measures. In the care of a physician who projects personal warmth, competence, and confidence, the patient in turn feels comfort and less anxiety, and optimistically anticipates recovery.

The physical condition determines the psychic disposition and vice versa. Consider gravely wounded combatants in war, oblivious to their injuries while fighting to survive, only to experience severe pain in the safety of the field hospital, or the patient with a peptic ulcer caused by emotional stress.

Clinical trials. In the individual case, it may be impossible to decide whether therapeutic success is attributable to the drug or to the therapeutic situation. What is therefore required is a comparison of the effects of a drug and of a placebo in matched groups of patients by means of statistical procedures, i.e., a *placebo-controlled trial*. A *prospective trial* is planned in advance, a retrospective (case–control) study follows patients backwards in time. Patients are *randomly allotted* to two groups, namely the *placebo* and the *active* or test drug group. In a *double-blind* trial, neither the patients nor the treating physicians know which patient is given drug and which placebo. Finally, a switch from drug to placebo and vice versa can be made in a successive phase of treatment, the *cross-over trial*. In this fashion, drug vs. placebo comparisons can be made not only between two patient groups, but also within either group itself.

Homeopathy (B) is an alternative method of therapy, developed in the 1800s by Samuel Hahnemann. His idea was this: when given in normal (allopathic) dosage, a drug (in the sense of medicament) will produce a constellation of symptoms; however, in a patient whose disease symptoms resemble just this mosaic of symptoms, the same drug (simile principle) would effect a cure when given in a very low dosage ("potentiation"). The body's self-healing powers were to be properly activated only by minimal doses of the medicinal substance.

The homeopath's task is not to diagnose the causes of morbidity, but to find the drug with a "symptom profile" most closely resembling that of the patient's illness. This drug is then applied in very high dilution.

A direct action or effect on body functions cannot be demonstrated for homeopathic medicines. Therapeutic success is due to the suggestive powers of the homeopath and the expectations of the patient. When an illness cannot be treated well by allopathic means, a case can be made in favor of exploiting suggestion as a therapeutic tool; homeopathy is one of several possible methods of doing so.

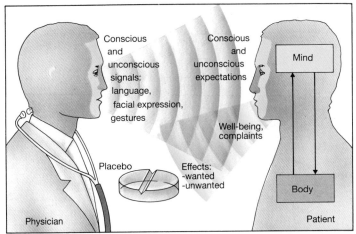

A. Therapeutic effects resulting from physician's power of suggestion

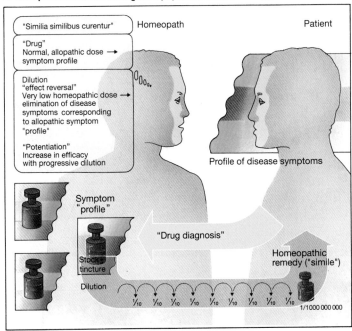

B. Homeopathy: concepts and procedure

Systems Pharmacology

Sympathetic Nervous System

In the course of phylogeny an efficient control system evolved that enabled the functions of individual organs to be orchestrated in increasingly complex life forms and permitted rapid adaptation to changing environmental conditions. This regulatory system consists of the CNS (brain plus spinal cord) and two separate pathways for two-way communication with peripheral organs, viz., the somatic and the autonomic nervous systems. The **somatic nervous system**, comprising extero- and interoceptive afferents, special sense organs, and motor efferents, to perceive *external* states and to target appropriate body movement (sensory perception: threat → response: flight or attack). The **autonomic (vegetative) nervous system** (ANS), together with the endocrine system, controls the *milieu interieur*. It adjusts internal organ functions to the changing needs of the organism. Neural control permits very quick adaptation, whereas the endocrine system provides for a long-term regulation of functional states. The ANS operates largely beyond voluntary control; it functions autonomously. Its central components reside in the hypothalamus, brain stem and spinal cord.

The ANS has **sympathetic** and **parasympathetic** branches. Both are made up of centrifugal (efferent) and centripetal (afferent) nerves. In organs innervated by both branches, respective activation of the sympathetic and parasympathetic input evokes opposing responses.

In various disease states (organ malfunctions), drugs are employed with the intention of normalizing susceptible organ functions. To understand the biological effects of substances capable of inhibiting or exciting sympathetic or parasympathetic nerves, one must first envisage the functions subserved by the sympathetic and parasympathetic divisions (**A, Responses to sympathetic activation**). In simplistic terms, activation of the sympathetic division can be considered a means by which the body quickly achieves a state of maximal work capacity as required in fight or flight situations.

In both cases there is a need for vigorous activity of skeletal musculature. To ensure adequate supply of oxygen and nutrients, blood flow in skeletal muscle is increased; cardiac rate and contractility are enhanced, resulting in a larger blood volume being pumped into the circulation. Narrowing of splanchnic blood vessels, moreover, diverts blood into vascular beds in muscle.

Because digestion of food in the intestinal tract is dispensable and only counterproductive, the propulsion of intestinal contents is slowed to the extent that peristalsis diminishes and sphincters are narrowed. However, in order to increase nutrient supply to heart and musculature, glucose from the liver and free fatty acids from adipose tissue must be released into the blood. The bronchi are dilated, enabling tidal volume and alveolar oxygen uptake to be increased.

Sweat glands are also innervated by sympathetic fibers (wet palms due to excitement); however, these are exceptional as regards their neurotransmitter (ACh) (p. 106).

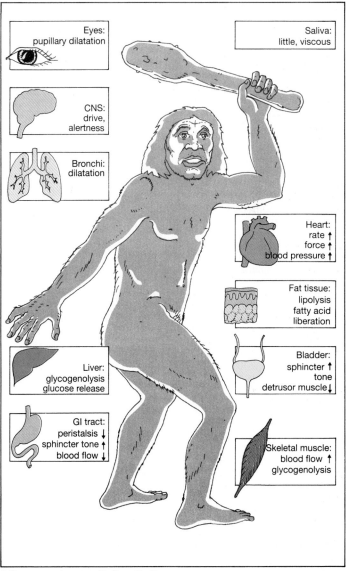

A. Responses to sympathetic activation

Structure of the Sympathetic Nervous System

The sympathetic preganglionic neurons (first neurons) project from the intermediolateral column of the spinal gray matter to the paired paravertebral ganglionic chain lying alongside the vertebral column and to unpaired prevertebral ganglia. These **ganglia** represent sites of synaptic contact between **preganglionic axons** and nerve cells (second neurons or sympathocytes) that emit **postganglionic axons** terminating on cells in various end-organs. In addition, there are preganglionic neurons that project either to peripheral ganglia in end-organs or to the adrenal medulla.

Sympathetic Transmitter Substances

Whereas **acetylcholine** (see p. 100) serves as the chemical transmitter at ganglionic synapses between **neurons (first and second)**, **norepinephrine [noradrenaline]** is the mediator of synapses of the second neuron (**B**). This second neuron does not synapse with only a single cell in the effector organ; rather, it branches out, each branch making *en passant* contacts with several cells. At these junctions the nerve axons form enlargements (**varicosities**) resembling beads on a string. Thus, excitation of the neuron leads to activation of a larger aggregate of effector cells, although the action of released norepinephrine may be confined to the region of each junction. Excitation of preganglionic neurons innervating the adrenal medulla causes a liberation of acetylcholine. This, in turn, elicits a secretion of **epinephrine [adrenaline]** into the blood, by which it is distributed to body tissues as a **hormone (A)**.

Adrenergic Synapse

Within the varicosities, norepinephrine is stored in small membrane-enclosed vesicles (granules, 0.05 to 0.2 μm in diameter). In the axoplasm, L-tyrosine is converted via two intermediate steps to dopamine, which is taken up into the vesicles and there converted to norepinephrine by dopamine-β-hydroxylase. When stimulated electrically, the sympathetic nerve discharges the contents of part of its vesicles, including norepinephrine into the extracellular space. Liberated **norepinephrine** reacts with **adrenoceptors** located postjunctionally on the membrane of effector cells or prejunctionally on the membrane of varicosities. Activation of presynaptic α_2-receptors inhibits norepinephrine release. By this negative feedback, release can be regulated.

The effect of released norepinephrine wanes quickly, because approx. 90% is actively transported back into the axoplasm, then into storage vesicles (**neuronal re-uptake**). Small portions of norepinephrine are inactivated by the enzyme **c**atechol-amine **O**-**m**ethyl **t**ransferase (COMT, present in the cytoplasm of postjunctional cells), and **m**ono**a**mine **o**xidase (MAO, present in the mitochondria of nerve cells and postjunctional cells).

The liver is richly endowed with COMT and MAO; it therefore contributes significantly to the degradation of circulating norepinephrine and epinephrine. The end product of the combined actions of MAO and COMT is vanillylmandelic acid.

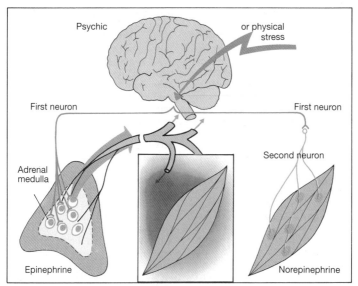

A. Epinephrine as hormone, norepinephrine as transmitter

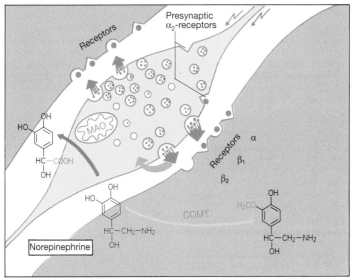

B. Second neuron of sympathetic system, varicosity, norepinephrine release

Adrenoceptor Subtypes and Catecholamine Actions

Adrenoceptors fall into three major groups, designated α_1, α_2 and β, within each of which further subtypes can be distinguished pharmacologically. The different adrenoceptors are differentially distributed according to region and tissue. Agonists at adrenoceptors (**direct sympathomimetics**) are used for various therapeutic effects.

Smooth muscle effects. The opposing effects on smooth muscle (**A**) of α- and β-adrenoceptor activation are due to differences in signal transduction (p. 64, 66). This is exemplified by vascular smooth muscle (**A**). In concert with the protein calmodulin, Ca^{2+} can activate myosin kinase, leading to a rise in tonus via phosphorylation of the contractile protein myosin. cAMP inhibits activation of myosin kinase. Via the former effector pathway, stimulation of α-receptors results in vasoconstriction; via the latter, β_2-receptors mediate vasodilation, particularly in skeletal muscle, an effect that has little therapeutic use.

Vasoconstriction. Local application of α-sympathomimetics can be employed in infiltration anesthesia (p. 196) or for nasal decongestion (naphazoline, tetrahydrozoline, xylometazoline; pp. 90, 296, 298). Systemically administered epinephrine is important in the treatment of anaphylactic shock for combating hypotension (288).

Bronchodilatation. β_2-Adrenoceptor-mediated *bronchodilatation* (e.g., with terbutaline or albuterol) plays an essential part in the treatment of bronchial asthma (p. 298).

Tocolysis. The uterine relaxant effect of β_2-adrenoceptor agonists, such as terbutaline or fenoterol, can be used to prevent *premature labor*.

Cardiostimulation. By stimulating β_1-receptors, hence **cAMP** production, catecholamines augment all heart functions, including systolic force (positive inotropism), velocity of shortening (positive clinotropism), sinoatrial rate (positive chronotropism), conduction velocity (positive dromotropism), and excitability (positive bathmotropism). In pacemaker fibers, diastolic depolarization is hastened, so that the firing threshold for the action potential is reached sooner (positive chronotropic effect, **B**). The cardiostimulant effect of β-sympathomimetics such as epinephrine is exploited in the treatment of cardiac arrest. Use of β-sympathomimetics in heart failure carries the risk of cardiac arrhythmias. Vasodilation with a resultant drop in systemic blood pressure results in reflex tachycardia which is augmented by direct activation of atrial β_1- (and β_2-) receptors.

Metabolic effects (C). β_2-**Receptors** mediate increased conversion of glycogen to glucose (*glycogenolysis*) in both the liver and skeletal muscle. From the liver, glucose is released into the blood. In adipose tissue, triglycerides are hydrolyzed to fatty acids (*lipolysis*, mediated by β_3-receptors?), which then enter the blood. The metabolic effects of catecholamines are not amenable to therapeutic use.

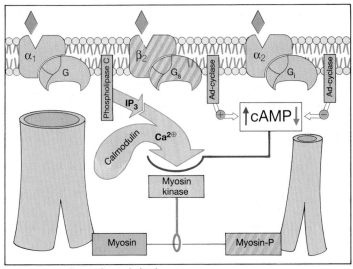

A. Vasomotor effects of catecholamines

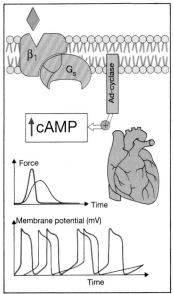

B. Cardiac effects of catecholamines

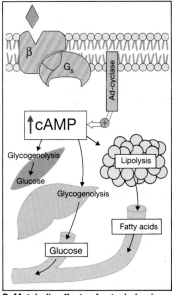

C. Metabolic effects of catecholamines

Structure–Activity Relationships of Sympathomimetics

Due to its equally high affinity for all α- and β-receptors, epinephrine does not permit selective activation of a particular receptor subtype. Like most catecholamines, it is also unsuitable for oral administration (catechole is a trivial name for o-hydroxyphenol). Norepinephrine differs from epinephrine by its low affinity for $β_2$-receptors. In contrast, synthetic isoproterenol has high affinity for β-receptors, but virtually none for α-receptors (**A**). Knowledge of **structure–activity relationships** has permitted the synthesis of sympathomimetics that display a high degree of selectivity at adrenoceptor subtypes.

Direct-acting sympathomimetics (i.e., adrenoceptor agonists) typically share a *phenylethylamine* structure. The *side chain β-hydroxyl group* confers affinity for α- and β-receptors. *Substitution on the amino group* reduces affinity for α-receptors, but increases it for β-receptors, with optimal affinity seen after the introduction of only one isopropyl group. Increasing the bulk of amino substituents favors affinity for $β_2$-receptors. Both *hydroxyl groups on the aromatic nucleus* contribute to affinity; high activity at α-receptors is associated with hydroxyl groups at the 3 and 4 positions. Affinity for β-receptors is preserved in congeners bearing hydroxyl groups at positions 3 and 5 (metaproterenol, terbutaline, fenoterol).

The hydroxyl groups of catecholamines are responsible for the very low lipophilicity of these substances. Polarity is increased at physiological pH due to protonation of the amino group. Deletion of one or all hydroxyl groups improves membrane penetrability at the intestinal mucosa–blood and the blood–brain barriers.

Accordingly, these noncatecholamine congeners can be given orally and can exert CNS actions; however, this structural change entails a loss in affinity.

Absence of one or both aromatic hydroxyl groups is associated with an increase in **indirect sympathomimetic activity**, denoting the ability of a substance to release norepinephrine from its neuronal stores without exerting an agonist action at the adrenoceptor (p. 88).

An altered position of aromatic hydroxyl groups (e.g., in metaproterenol or terbutaline) or their substitution (e.g., salbutamol) protects against *inactivation by COMT* (p. 82). Introduction of a small alkyl residue at the carbon atom adjacent to the amino group (pholedrine, ephedrine, methamphetamine) confers resistance to *degradation by MAO* (p. 82), as does replacement on the amino groups of the methyl residue with larger substituents (e.g., ethyl in etilefrine). Accordingly, the congeners are less subject to presystemic inactivation.

Since structural requirements for high affinity, on the one hand, and for oral applicability, on the other, do not match, choosing a sympathomimetic is a matter of compromise. If the high affinity of epinephrine is to be exploited, absorbability from the intestine must be foregone (epinephrine, isoproterenol). If good bioavailability with oral administration is desired, losses in receptor affinity must be accepted (etilefrine).

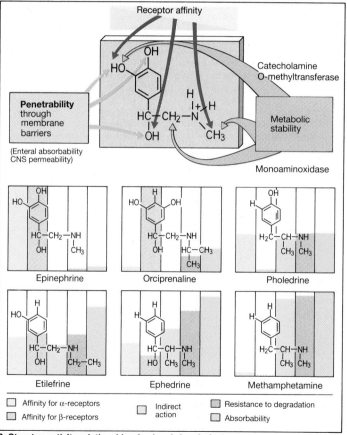

A. Chemical structure of catecholamines and affinity for α- and β-receptors

B. Structur-activity relationship of epinephrine derivates

Indirect Sympathomimetics

Apart from **receptors**, adrenergic neurotransmission involves mechanisms for the **active re-uptake** and **re-storage** of released amine, as well as enzymatic breakdown by **monoamine oxidase (MAO)**. Norepinephrine (NE) displays affinity for receptors, transport systems, and degradative enzymes. Chemical alterations of the catecholamine differentially affect these properties and result in substances with selective actions.

Inhibitors of MAO (A). The enzyme is located predominantly on mitochondria, and serves to scavenge axoplasmic free norepinephrine. Inhibition of the enzyme causes free norepinephrine concentrations to rise. Likewise, dopamine catabolism is impaired, making more of it available for norepinephrine synthesis. Consequently, the amount of norepinephrine stored in granular vesicles will increase, and with it the amount of amine released per nerve impulse.

In the CNS, inhibition of MAO affects neuronal storage not only of norepinephrine but also of dopamine and serotonin. These mediators probably play significant roles in CNS functions (see p. 114, 116) consistent with the stimulant effects of MAO inhibitors on mood and psychomotor drive and their use as antidepressants (e.g., *tranylcypromine*) in the treatment of depression (**A**). Tranylcypromine is an irreversible inhibitor of both MAO subtypes (p. 182). *Moclobemide* affects only MAO_A; the action is reversible.

Indirect sympathomimetics (B) are agents that elevate the concentration of NE at neuroeffector junctions, because they either inhibit re-uptake (*cocaine*), facilitate release, or slow breakdown by MAO, or exert all three of these effects (*amphetamine, meth-*

amphetamine). The effectiveness of such indirect sympathomimetics diminishes or disappears (**tachyphylaxis**) when vesicular stores of norepinephrine close to the axolemma are depleted.

Indirect sympathomimetics can penetrate the blood–brain barrier and evoke such CNS effects as a feeling of well-being, enhanced physical activity and mood (**euphoria**), and decreased sense of hunger or fatigue. Subsequently, the user may feel tired and depressed. These aftereffects are partly responsible for the urge to readminister the drug (high abuse potential). To prevent their misuse, these substances are subject to governmental regulations (e.g., Food and Drugs Act: Canada; Controlled Substances Act: USA) restricting their prescription and distribution.

When amphetamine-like substances are misused to enhance athletic performance (*doping*), there is a risk of dangerous physical overexertion. Because of the absence of a sense of fatigue, a drugged athlete may be able to mobilize ultimate energy reserves. In extreme situations, cardiovascular failure may result (**B**).

Closely related chemically to amphetamine are the so-called appetite suppressants or anorexiants, such as fenfluramine and mazindole. These may also cause dependence and their therapeutic value is questionable.

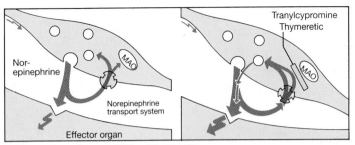

A. Monoamine oxidase inhibitor; Thymeretics

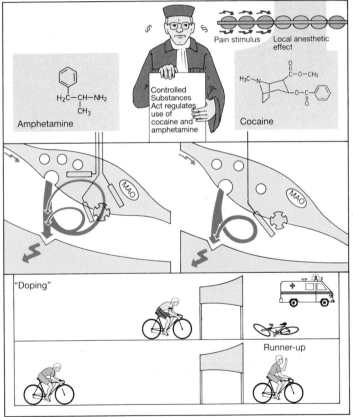

B. Indirect sympathomimetics with central stimulant activity and abuse potential

α-Sympathomimetics, α-Sympatholytics

α-Sympathomimetics can be used systemically in certain types of hypotension (p. 288) and locally for nasal or conjunctival decongestion (pp. 296, 298) or as adjuncts in infiltration anesthesia (p. 196) for the purpose of delaying the removal of local anesthetic. With local use, underperfusion of the vasoconstricted area results in a lack of oxygen (**A**). In the extreme case, local hypoxia can lead to tissue necrosis. The appendages (e.g., digits, toes, ears) are particularly vulnerable in this regard, thus precluding the use of vasoconstrictor adjuncts in infiltration anesthesia at these sites.

Vasoconstriction induced by an α-sympathomimetic is followed by a phase of enhanced blood flow (**reactive hyperemia, A**). This reaction can be observed after the application of α-sympathomimetics (naphazoline, tetrahydrozoline, xylometazoline) to the nasal mucosa. Initially, vasoconstriction reduces mucosal blood flow and, hence, capillary pressure. Fluid exuded into the interstitial space is drained through the veins, thus shrinking the nasal mucosa. Due to the reduced supply of fluid, secretion of nasal mucus decreases. In coryza, nasal patency is restored. However, after vasoconstriction subsides, reactive hyperemia causes renewed exudation of plasma fluid into the interstitial space, the nose is "stuffy" again and the patient feels a need to reapply decongestant. In this way, a vicious cycle threatens. Besides rebound congestion, persistent use of a decongestant entails the risk of atrophic damage caused by prolonged hypoxia of the nasal mucosa.

α-Sympatholytics (B). The interaction of norepinephrine with α-adrenoceptors can be inhibited by α-sympatholytics (α-adrenoceptor antagonists, α-blockers). This inhibition can be put to therapeutic use in antihypertensive treatment (vasodilation → peripheral resistance ↓, blood pressure ↓, p. 118). The first α-sympatholytics blocked the action of norepinephrine at both *post- and prejunctional* α-adrenoceptors (**nonselective α-blockers**, e.g., phenoxybenzamine, phentolamine).

Presynaptic α_2-adrenoceptors function like sensors that enable norepinephrine concentration outside the axolemma to be monitored, thus regulating its release via a local feedback mechanism. When presynaptic α_2-receptors are stimulated, further release of norepinephrine is inhibited. Conversely, their blockade leads to uncontrolled release of norephinephrine with an overt enhancement of sympathetic effects at β_1-adrenoceptor-mediated myocardial neuroeffector junctions, resulting in tachycardia and tachyarrhythmia.

Selective α-Sympatholytics

α-Blockers, such as prazosin, lack affinity for prejunctional α_2-adrenoceptors. They suppress activation of α_1-receptors without a concomitant enhancement of norepinephrine release.

α_1-Blockers may be used in hypertension (p. 286). Because they prevent reflex vasoconstriction, they are likely to cause postural hypotension with pooling of blood in lower limb capacitance veins during change from the supine to the erect position (orthostatic collapse: ↓ venous return, ↓ cardiac output, fall in systemic pressure, ↓ blood supply to CNS, fainting and syncope, p. 288).

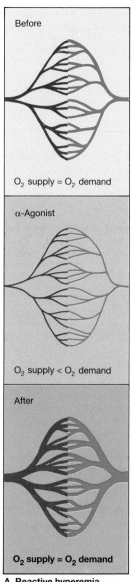

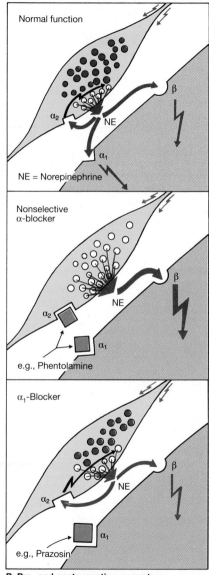

A. Reactive hyperemia due to α-sympathomimetics

B. Pre- and postsynaptic α-receptors and α-sympatholytics

β-Sympatholytics (β-Blockers)

β-Sympatholytics are antagonists of norepinephrine and epinephrine at β-adrenoceptors; they lack affinity for α- receptors.

Therapeutic effects. β-Blockers protect the heart from the oxygen-wasting effect of sympathetic inotropism (p. 282) by blocking cardiac β-receptors; thus, cardiac work can no longer be augmented above basal levels (the heart is "coasting"). This effect is utilized prophylactically in *angina pectoris* in order to prevent myocardial stress that could trigger an ischemic attack (p. 284). β-Blockers also serve to *lower cardiac rate* (sinus tachycardia, p. 134) and elevated blood pressure due to high cardiac output. The mechanism underlying their *antihypertensive action* via reduction of peripheral resistance is unclear.

Applied topically to the eye, β-blockers lower production of aqueous humor (→ glaucoma treatment).

Angina pectoris and hypertension are very common disorders in which β-blockers are now widely used as drugs of first choice.

Undesired effects. The hazards of treatment with β-blockers become apparent particularly when continuous activation of β-receptors is needed in order to maintain the function of an organ.

Congestive heart failure. In myocardial insufficiency, the heart depends on a tonic sympathetic drive in order to maintain adequate cardiac output. Sympathetic activation gives rise to an increase in heart rate and systolic muscle tension, enabling cardiac output to be restored to a level comparable with that in a healthy subject. When sympathetic drive is eliminated during β-receptor-blockade, stroke volume and heart rate decline, a latent myocardial insufficiency is unmasked, and overt insufficiency is exacerbated (**A**).

Bradycardia, AV block. Elimination of sympathetic drive can lead to a marked fall in cardiac rate, as well as to disorders of impulse conduction from the atria to the ventricles.

Bronchial asthma. Increased sympathetic activity prevents bronchospasm in patients disposed to paroxysmal constriction of the bronchial tree (bronchial asthma, bronchitis in smokers). In this condition, β_2-receptor blockade will precipitate acute respiratory distress (**B**).

Hypoglycemia in diabetes mellitus. When treatment with insulin or oral hypoglycemics in the diabetic patient lowers blood glucose below a critical level, epinephrine is released, which then stimulates hepatic glucose release via activation of β_2-receptors. β-Blockers suppress this counter-regulation; in addition, they mask other epinephrine-mediated warning signs of imminent hypoglycemia, such as tachycardia and anxiety, thereby enhancing the risk of hypoglycemic shock.

Altered vascular responses. When β_2-receptors are blocked, the vasodilating effect of epinephrine is abolished, leaving the α-receptor-mediated vasoconstriction unaffected: peripheral blood flow ↓ —"cold hands and feet."

β-Blockers exert an **"anxiolytic"** action that may be due to the suppression of somatic responses (palpitations; trembling) to epinephrine release that is induced by emotional stress; in turn, these responses would exacerbate "anxiety" or "stage fright."

Because alertness is not impaired by β-blockers, these agents are occasionally taken by orators and musicians before a major performance (**C**).

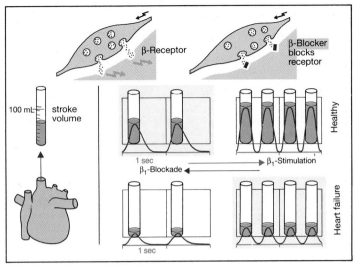

A. β-Sympatholytics: effect on cardiac function

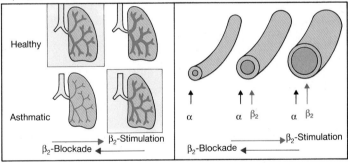

B. β-Sympatholytics: effect on bronchial and vascular tone

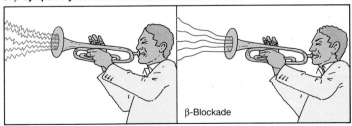

C. "Anxiolytic" effect of β-sympatholytics

Types of β-Blockers

The **basic structure** shared by most β-sympatholytics is the side chain of β-sympathomimetics (cf. isoproterenol with the β-blockers pindolol, propranolol, and atenolol). As a rule, this basic structure is linked to an aromatic nucleus by a methylene and oxygen bridge. The side chain C-atom bearing the hydroxyl group forms the chiral center. With some exceptions (e.g., penbutolol, timolol), all β-sympatholytics exist as racemates (p. 62).

Compared with the dextrorotatory form, the levorotatory enantiomer possesses a greater than 100-fold higher affinity for the β-receptor, and is, therefore, practically alone in contributing to the β-blocking effect of the racemate. The side chain and substituents on the amino group critically affect affinity for β-receptors, whereas the aromatic nucleus determines whether the compound possesses **intrinsic sympathomimetic activity (ISA)**, that is, acts as a *partial* agonist or partial antagonist (p. 60). However, the β-receptor at which such partial agonism can be shown appears to be atypical (β_3 subtype). Whether ISA confers a therapeutic advantage on a β-blocker remains an open question.

As cationic amphiphilic drugs, β-blockers can exert a **membrane–stabilizing effect**, as evidenced by the ability of the more lipophilic congeners to inhibit Na^+-channel function and impulse conduction in cardiac tissues. At the usual therapeutic dosage, the high concentration required for these effects will not be reached.

Some β-sympatholytics possess higher affinity for cardiac β_1-receptors than for β_2-receptors and thus display **cardioselectivity** (e.g., metoprolol, acebutolol, bisoprolol). None of these blockers is sufficiently selective to permit their use in patients with bronchial asthma or diabetes mellitus (p. 92).

The chemical structure of β-blockers also determines their **pharmacokinetic properties**. Except for hydrophilic representatives (atenolol), β-sympatholytics are completely absorbed from the intestines and subsequently undergo **presystemic elimination** to a major extent (**A**).

All the above differences are of little clinical importance. The **abundance of** commercially available **congeners** would thus appear all the more curious (**B**). Propranolol was the first β-blocker to be introduced into therapy in 1965. Twenty-five years later, about 20 different congeners are being marketed in different countries. This questionable development unfortunately is typical of any drug group that has major therapeutic relevance, in addition to a relatively fixed active structure. Variation of the molecule will create a new *patentable* chemical, not necessarily a drug with a novel action. Moreover, a drug no longer protected by patent is offered as a *generic* by different manufacturers under dozens of different proprietary names.

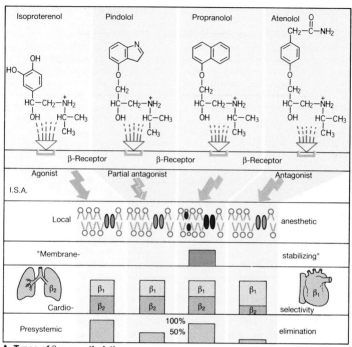

A. Types of β-sympatholytics

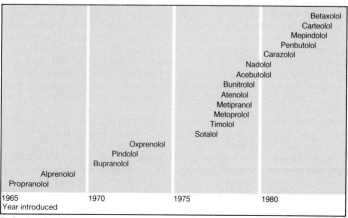

B. Avalanche-like increase in commercially available β-sympatholytics

Antiadrenergics

Antiadrenergics are drugs capable of lowering transmitter output from sympathetic neurons, i. e. the "sympathetic tone." Their action is hypotensive (indication: hypertension, p. 286); however, being poorly tolerated, they enjoy only limited therapeutic use.

Clonidine is an α_2-agonist whose high lipophilicity (dichlorophenyl ring) permits rapid penetration through the blood–brain barrier. The activation of *postsynaptic* α_2-receptors dampens the activity of central vasomotor neurons, resulting in a resetting of systemic arterial pressure at a lower level. In addition, activation of presynaptic α_2-receptors in the periphery (pp. 82, 90) leads to a decreased release of both norepinephrine (NE) and acetylcholine.

Side effects. Lassitude, dry mouth; rebound hypertension after abrupt cessation of clonidine therapy.

Methyldopa (dopa = **d**ihydrox**y**phenyl**a**lanine), as an amino acid, is transported across the blood–brain barrier, decarboxylated in the brain to α-methyldopamine and then hydroxylated to α-methylnorepinephrine. The decarboxylation of α-methyldopa competes for a portion of the available enzymatic activity, so that the rate of conversion of L-dopa to norepinephrine (via dopamine) is decreased. The *false transmitter* α-methylnorepinephrine can be stored; however, unlike the endogenous mediator, it has a higher affinity for α_2- than for α_1-receptors and therefore produces effects similar to those of clonidine. The same events take place in peripheral adrenergic neurons.

Adverse effects. Fatigue, orthostatic hypotension, extrapyramidal Parkinson-like symptoms (p. 182), cutaneous reactions, hepatic damage, immune-hemolytic anemia.

Reserpine, an alkaloid from the Rauwolfia plant, abolishes the vesicular storage of biogenic amines (NE, dopamine = DA, serotonin = 5-HT) by inhibiting an ATPase required for the vesicular amine pump. The amount of NE released per nerve impulse is decreased. To a lesser degree, release of epinephrine from the adrenal medulla is also impaired. At higher doses, there is irreversible damage to storage vesicles ("pharmacological sympathectomy"), days to weeks being required for their resynthesis. Reserpine readily enters the brain, where it also impairs vesicular storage of biogenic amines.

Adverse effects. Disorders of extrapyramidal motor function with development of pseudo-Parkinsonism (p. 182), sedation, depression, stuffy nose, impaired libido, and impotence; increased appetite.

Guanethidine possesses high affinity for the axolemmal and vesicular amine transporters. It is stored instead of NE, but is unable to mimic the functions of the latter. In addition, it stabilizes the axonal membrane, thereby impeding the propagation of impulses into the sympathetic nerve terminals. Storage and release of epinephrine from the adrenal medulla are not affected, owing to the absence of a re-uptake process. The drug does not cross the blood–brain barrier.

Adverse effects. Cardiovascular crises are a possible risk: emotional stress of the patient may cause sympathoadrenal activation with epinephrine release. The resulting rise in blood pressure can be all the more marked because persistent depression of sympathetic nerve activity induces supersensitivity of effector organs to circulating catecholamines.

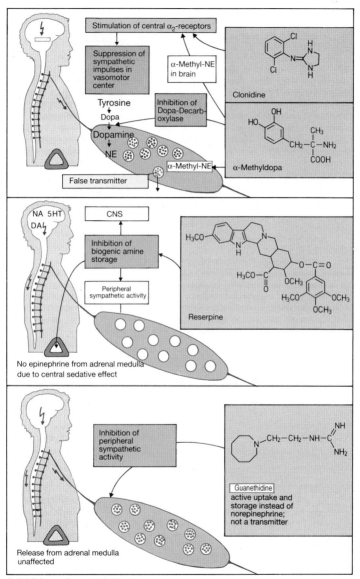

Stimulation of central α_2-receptors

Suppression of sympathetic impulses in vasomotor center

α-Methyl-NE in brain

Clonidine

Tyrosine
Dopa
Dopamine
NE

Inhibition of Dopa-Decarboxylase

α-Methyldopa

α-Methyl-NE

False transmitter

NA 5HT DA

CNS

Inhibition of biogenic amine storage

Peripheral sympathetic activity

Reserpine

No epinephrine from adrenal medulla due to central sedative effect

Inhibition of peripheral sympathetic activity

Guanethidine
active uptake and storage instead of norepinephrine; not a transmitter

Release from adrenal medulla unaffected

A. Inhibitors of sympathetic tone

Parasympathetic Nervous System

Responses to activation of the parasympathetic system. Parasympathetic nerves regulate processes connected with energy assimilation (food intake, digestion, absorption) and storage. These processes operate when the body is at rest, allowing a decreased tidal volume (increased bronchomotor tone) and decreased cardiac activity. Secretion of saliva and intestinal fluids promotes the digestion of foodstuffs; transport of intestinal contents is speeded up because of enhanced peristaltic activity and lowered tone of sphincteric muscles. To empty the urinary bladder (micturition), wall tension is increased by detrusor activation with a concurrent relaxation of sphincter tonus.

Activation of ocular parasympathetic fibers (see below) results in narrowing of the pupil and increased curvature of the lens, enabling near objects to be brought into focus (accommodation).

Anatomy of the parasympathetic system. The cell bodies of parasympathetic preganglionic neurons are located in the brain stem and the sacral spinal cord. Parasympathetic outflow is channelled from the brain stem (1) through the third cranial nerve (oculomotor n.) via the ciliary ganglion to the eye (2); through the seventh cranial nerve (facial n.) via the pterygopalatine and submaxillary ganglia to lachrymal glands and salivary glands (sublingual, submandibular), respectively (3); through the ninth cranial nerve (glossopharyngeal n.) via the otic ganglion to the parotid gland; and (4) via the tenth cranial nerve (vagus n.) to thoracic and abdominal viscera. Approximately 75% of all parasympathetic fibers are contained within the vagus nerve. The neurons of the sacral division innervate the distal colon, rectum, bladder, the distal ureters, and the external genitalia.

Acetylcholine (ACh) as a transmitter. ACh serves as the mediator at terminals of all postganglionic parasympathetic fibers, in addition to fulfilling its transmitter role at ganglionic synapses within both the sympathetic and parasympathetic divisions and the motor end plates on striated muscle. However, different types of receptors are present at these synaptic junctions:

Localization	Agonist	Antagonist	Receptor-Type
Target tissue of the 2. parasympathetic nerve	ACh Muscarine	Atropine	Muscarinic (M) cholinoceptor M-AChR G-protein-coupled receptor protein with 7 transmembrane domains
Sympathetic and parasympathetic ganglia	ACh Nicotine	Trimethaphan	Nicotinic (N) cholinoceptor N-AChR 5 transmembrane subunit receptor protein forming a cation channel
Motor end plate	ACh Nicotine	d-Tubocurarine	

The existence of distinct cholinoceptors at different cholinergic synapses allows selective pharmacological interventions.

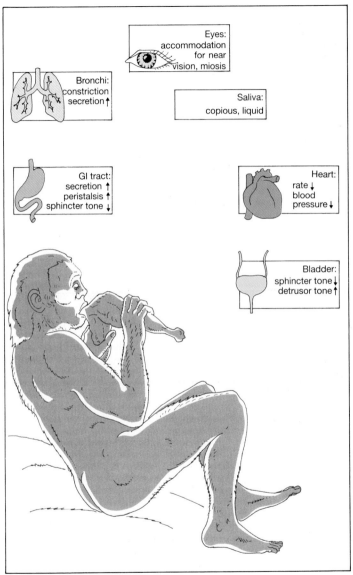

A. Responses to parasympathetic activation

Cholinergic Synapse

Acetylcholine (ACh) is the transmitter at postganglionic synapses of parasympathetic nerve endings. It is highly concentrated in synaptic storage vesicles densely present in the axoplasm of the terminal. ACh is formed from **choline** and activated acetate (**acetylcoenzyme A**), a reaction catalyzed by the enzyme **choline acetyltransferase**. The highly polar choline is actively transported into the axoplasm. The specific choline- transporter is localized exclusively to membranes of cholinergic axons and terminals. The storage vesicles carry negative charges that prevent them from fusing with each other or with the axolemma. During activation of the nerve membrane, Ca^{2+} is thought to enter the axoplasm and to activate contractile proteins (synapsin I) that pull the vesicles towards the presynaptic membrane. The elevated subplasmalemmal Ca^{2+}-concentration may facilitate fusion of vesicle and presynaptic membrane by neutralizing negative surface charges. As a result, the vesicles can fuse with the presynaptic membrane and, in the process, discharge their contents into the synaptic cleft. ACh quickly diffuses through the synaptic gap. At the postsynaptic effector cell membrane, ACh reacts with its **receptors**. Because these receptors can also be activated by the alkaloid muscarine, they are referred to as **muscarinic (M-) cholinoceptors**. In contrast, at ganglionic (p. 98,108) and motor end plate (p. 176) cholinoceptors, the action of ACh is mimicked by nicotine and, hence, mediated by **nicotinic cholinoceptors**.

Released ACh is rapidly hydrolyzed and inactivated by a specific **acetylcholinesterase**, present on pre- and postjunctional membranes, or by a less specific serum cholinesterase (butyryl cholinesterase), a soluble enzyme present in serum and interstitial fluid.

M-cholinoceptors can be classified into subtypes according to their molecular structure, signal transduction, and ligand affinity. M_3-receptors play a role in smooth muscle stimulation involving activation of phospholipase C., membrane depolarisation [mV] and increase in smooth muscle tone [mN]. M_2-receptors mediate the cardiac action of ACh in pacemaker tissues; opening of K^+-channels leads to slowing of diastolic depolarization and a decrease in heart rate. M_3-receptor activation appears to be important in glandular secretion. M_1-receptors occur in neuronal tissue. In ganglia, they facilitate impulse transmission. In the CNS, where all subtypes are present, cholinoceptors serve diverse functions that include regulation of cortical excitability, memory and learning, pain processing, and brain stem motor control. The assignment of specific receptor subtypes to these functions has yet to be achieved.

In blood vessels, the relaxant action of ACh on muscle tone is indirect, because it involves stimulation of M-cholinoceptors on endothelial cells that respond by liberating NO (= endothelium-derived relaxing factor). The latter diffuses into the subjacent smooth musculature, where it causes a relaxation of active tonus (p. 120).

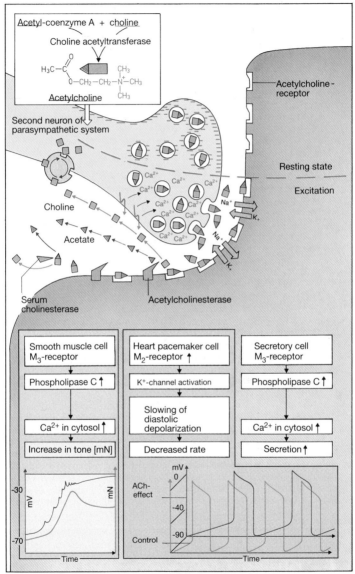

A. Responses of effector organs to acetylcholine release from parasympathetic nerve endings

Parasympathomimetics

Acetylcholine (ACh) is too rapidly hydrolyzed and inactivated by acetylcholinesterase (AChE) to be of any therapeutic use; however, its action can be replicated by other substances, namely direct or indirect parasympathomimetics.

Direct parasympathomimetics. The choline ester, *carbachol*, activates the M-cholinoceptor, but is not hydrolyzed by AChE. Carbachol can thus be effectively employed for local application to the eye (glaucoma, p. 104) and for systemic administration (bowel atonia, bladder atonia). The alkaloids *pilocarpine* (from *Pilocarpus jaborandi*) and *arecoline* (from *Areca catechu*; betelnut) also act as direct parasympathomimetics. As tertiary amines, they moreover exert central effects. The central effect of muscarine-like substances consists of an enlivening, mild stimulation that is probably the effect desired in betel chewing, a widespread habit in South Asia. Of this group, only pilocarpine enjoys therapeutic use, which is limited to local application to the eye in glaucoma.

Indirect parasympathomimetics. AChE can be inhibited selectively, with the result that ACh released by nerve impulses will accumulate at the receptors of cholinergic synapses, with the endogenously released mediator remaining available longer. Inhibitors of AChE are therefore indirect parasympathomimetics. Their action is evident at all cholinergic synapses. Chemically, these agents include esters of carbamic acid (**carbamates** such as *physostigmine, neostigmine*) and of phosphoric acid (**organophosphates** such as *paraoxon* = E600 and *nitrostigmine* = parathion = E605, its prodrug).

Members of both groups react like ACh with AChE and can be considered false substrates. The esters are hydrolyzed upon formation of a complex with the enzyme. The rate-limiting step in ACh hydrolysis is **deacetylation** of the enzyme, which takes only milliseconds, thus permitting a high turnover rate and activity of AChE. **Decarbaminoylation** following hydrolysis of a carbamate takes hours to days, the enzyme remaining inhibited as long as it is carbaminoylated. Cleavage of the phosphate residue, i.e., **dephosphorylation**, is practically impossible; enzyme inhibition is irreversible.

Uses. The quaternary carbamate neostigmine is employed as an indirect parasympathomimetic in postoperative atonia of the bowel or bladder. Furthermore, it is needed to overcome the relative ACh-deficiency at the motor end plate in myasthenia gravis or to reverse the neuromuscular blockade (p. 178) caused by nondepolarizing muscle relaxants (decurarization before discontinuation of anesthesia). The tertiary carbamate physostigmine can be used as an antidote in poisoning with parasympatholytic drugs, because it has access to AChE in the brain. Carbamates (neostigmine, pyridostigmine, physostigmine) and organophosphates (paraoxon, ecothiopate) can also be applied locally to the eye in the treatment of glaucoma. Agents from both classes also serve as insecticides. Although they possess high acute toxicity in humans, they are more rapidly degraded than is DDT following their emission into the environment.

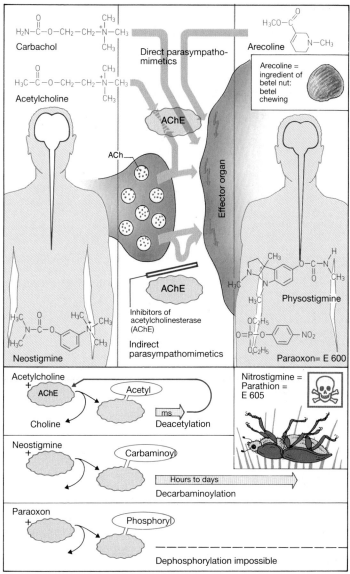

A. Direct and indirect parasympathomimetics

Parasympathomimetics

Therapeutic uses of direct or indirect parasympathomimetics involve mainly **stimulation of smooth musculature**. In *postoperative atonia of the bowel and bladder,* contractility can be restored, e.g., with the help of carbachol.

In *narrow-angle glaucoma,* carbachol or pilocarpine can be employed to constrict the pupil, thereby facilitating drainage of aqueous humor from the anterior chamber, as a result of which intraocular pressure is lowered.

Parasympatholytics
Substances acting antagonistically at the M-cholinoceptor are designated **parasympatholytics** (prototype: the alkaloid **atropine**; actions shown in red in the panels). Therapeutic use of these agents is complicated by their low organ selectivity. Possibilities for a targeted action include:
– local application,
– selection of drugs with either good or poor membrane penetrability, as the situation demands,
– administration of drugs possessing receptor subtype selectivity.
Parasympatholytics are employed for the following purposes:

1. Inhibition of exocrine glands
Bronchial secretion. Premedication with atropine before inhalation anesthesia prevents a possible hypersecretion of bronchial mucus, which cannot be expectorated by coughing during anesthesia.

Gastric secretion. Stimulation of gastric acid production by ACh involves an M-cholinoceptor subtype (M_1-receptor) that has a preferential affinity for *pirenzepine* (p. 107). M_1-receptors have also been demon-

strated in the brain; however, these cannot be reached by pirenzepine because its lipophilicity is too low to permit penetration of the blood–brain barrier. Pirenzepine is used in the treatment of **gastric and duodenal ulcers** (p. 162).

2. Relaxation of smooth musculature
Bronchodilatation. This can be achieved by the use of ipratropium in conditions of increased airway resistance (bronchial asthma, **spastic bronchitis**). When administered by inhalation, this quaternary compound has little effect on other organs because of its low rate of systemic absorption.

Spasmolysis by N-butylscopolamine in **biliary** or **renal colic** (p. 126). Because of its quaternary nitrogen, this drug does not enter the CNS, but requires parenteral administration. Its spasmolytic action is especially marked because of additional ganglionic blocking and direct muscle-relaxant actions.

Lowering of pupillary sphincter tonus and pupillary dilatation by local administration of homatropine or tropicamide (**mydriatics**) allows observation of the ocular fundus. For diagnostic uses, only short-term pupillary dilatation is needed. The effect of both agents subsides quickly in comparison with that of atropine.

3. Cardioacceleration
Ipratropium is used in bradycardia and AV-block to raise **heart rate** and to facilitate cardiac *impulse conduction*. As a quaternary substance, it does not penetrate into the brain, which greatly reduces the risk of CNS disturbances (see below). Relatively high oral doses are required because of an inefficient intestinal absorption.

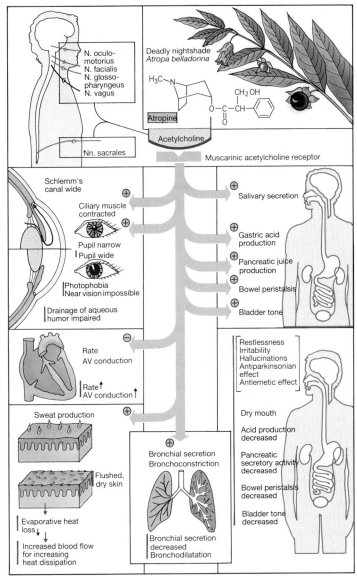

N. oculo-
motorius
N. facialis
N. glosso-
pharyngeus
N. vagus

Deadly nightshade
Atropa belladonna

H_3C-N

CH_2OH

Atropine

Acetylcholine

Nn. sacrales

Muscarinic acetylcholine receptor

Schlemm's
canal wide

⊕

Salivary secretion

Ciliary muscle
contracted

⊕

⊕

Gastric acid
production

Pupil narrow
|Pupil wide

⊕

Pancreatic juice
production

|Photophobia
|Near vision impossible

⊕

Bowel peristalsis

|Drainage of aqueous
|humor impaired

⊕

Bladder tone

⊖

Rate
AV conduction

Restlessness
Irritability
Hallucinations
Antiparkinsonian
effect
Antiemetic effect

|Rate↑
|AV conduction↑

Dry mouth

Sweat production

⊕

Acid production
decreased

⊕

Pancreatic
secretory activity
decreased

|Flushed,
dry skin

Bronchial secretion
Bronchoconstriction

Bowel peristalsis
decreased

|Evaporative heat
loss↓

Bladder tone
decreased

|Increased blood flow
for increasing
heat dissipation

|Bronchial secretion
decreased
Bronchodilatation

A. Effects of parasympathetic stimulation and blockade

Atropine may be given to prevent **cardiac arrest** resulting from vagal reflex activation, incident to anesthetic induction, gastric lavage, or endoscopic procedures.

4. CNS-attenuating effects

Scopolamine is effective in the *prophylaxis of kinetosis* (motion sickness, **sea sickness**, see p. 300); it is well absorbed transcutaneously. Scopolamine ($pK_a = 7.2$) penetrates the blood–brain barrier faster than does atropine ($pK_a = 9$), because at physiologic pH a larger proportion is present in the neutral, membrane-permeating form.

In **psychotic excitement** (agitation), *sedation* can be achieved with scopolamine. Unlike atropine, scopolamine exerts a calming and amnestic action that can also be used to advantage in anesthetic premedication.

Symptomatic treatment in **parkinsonism** for the purpose of restoring a dopaminergic-cholinergic balance in the corpus striatum. Antiparkinsonian agents, such as benztropine (p. 182), readily penetrate the blood–brain barrier. At centrally equieffective dosage, their peripheral effects are less marked than are those of atropine.

Contraindications for Parasympatholytics

Glaucoma. Since drainage of aqueous humor is impeded during relaxation of the pupillary sphincter, intraocular pressure rises.

Prostatic hypertrophy with impaired micturition. Loss of parasympathetic control of the detrusor muscle exacerbates difficulties in voiding urine.

Atropine Poisoning

Parasympatholytics have a wide therapeutic margin. Rarely life-threatening, poisoning with atropine is characterized by the following peripheral and central effects:

Peripheral. **Tachycardia**; **dry mouth**; **hyperthermia** secondary to the inhibition of sweating. Although sweat glands are innervated by sympathetic fibers, these are cholinergic in nature. When sweat secretion is inhibited, the body loses the ability to dissipate metabolic heat by evaporation of sweat (p. 192). There is a compensatory vasodilation in the skin allowing increased heat exchange through increased cutaneous blood flow. Decreased peristaltic activity of the intestines leads to **constipation**.

Central. Motor restlessness, progressing to maniacal agitation, psychic disturbances, **disorientation** and **hallucinations**. Elderly subjects are more sensitive to such central effects. In this context, the diversity of drugs producing atropine-like side effects should be borne in mind, e.g., tricyclic antidepressants, neuroleptics, antihistaminics, antiparkinsonian agents.

Apart from symptomatic, general measures (gastric lavage, cooling with ice water), therapy of severe **atropine intoxication** includes the administration of the indirect parasympathomimetic, physostigmine (p. 102). The most common instances of atropine intoxication occur after ingestion of the berry-like fruits of belladonna by children or intentional overdosage with tricyclic antidepressants.

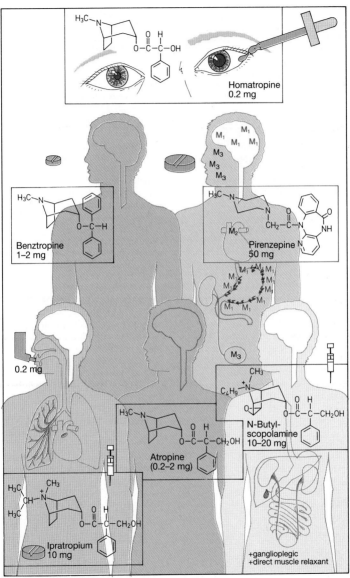

A. Parasympatholytics

Homatropine
0.2 mg

Benztropine
1–2 mg

Pirenzepine
50 mg

0.2 mg

Atropine
(0.2–2 mg)

N-Butyl-scopolamine
10–20 mg

Ipratropium
10 mg

+ganglioplegic
+direct muscle relaxant

Ganglionic Transmission

Whether sympathetic or parasympathetic, all efferent visceromotor nerves are made up of two serially connected neurons. The point of contact (synapse) between the first and second neurons occurs mainly in **ganglia**; therefore, the first neuron is referred to as *preganglionic* and efferents of the second as *postganglionic*.

Electrical excitation (action potential) of the first neuron causes the release of acetylcholine (ACh) within the ganglia. ACh stimulates receptors located on the subsynaptic membrane of the second neuron. Activation of these receptors causes membrane cation conductance to increase, particularly for Na^+, resulting in membrane depolarization (p. 64, 176). If a sufficient number of receptors is activated simultaneously, a threshold potential is reached at which the membrane undergoes rapid depolarization in the form of a propagated action potential. Normally, not all preganglionic impulses elicit a propagated response in the second neuron. The ganglionic synapse acts like a frequency filter (**A**). The effect of ACh elicited at receptors on the ganglionic neuronal membrane can be replicated by nicotine; i.e., it involves **nicotinic cholinoceptors**.

Ganglionic Action of Nicotine

If a small dose of nicotine is given, the ganglionic cholinoceptors are activated. The membrane depolarizes partially, but fails to reach the firing threshold. However, at this point an amount of released ACh smaller than that normally required will be sufficient to elicit a propagated action potential. *At a low concentration*, nicotine acts as a ganglionic stimulant; it alters the filter function of the ganglionic synapse, allowing action potential frequency in the second neuron to approach that of the first (**B**). *At higher concentrations*, nicotine acts to block ganglionic transmission. Simultaneous activation of many nicotinic cholinoceptors depolarizes the ganglionic cell membrane to such an extent that generation of action potentials is no longer possible, even in the face of an intensive and synchronized release of ACh (**C**).

Although nicotine mimics the action of ACh at the receptors, it cannot duplicate the time course of intrasynaptic agonist concentration required for appropriate high-frequency ganglionic activation. The concentration of nicotine in the synaptic cleft cannot build up as rapidly as that of ACh released from nerve terminals nor can nicotine be eliminated from the synaptic cleft as quickly as ACh.

The ganglionic effects of ACh can be blocked by tetraethylammonium, hexamethonium, and other substances (**ganglionic blockers**). None of these has intrinsic activity, that is, they fail to stimulate ganglia even at low concentration, some of them (e.g., hexamethonium) actually block the cholinoceptor-linked ion channel (cf. p. 64, 98), but others (mecamylamine, trimethaphan) are typical receptor antagonists.

Certain sympathetic preganglionic neurons project without interruption to the chromaffin cells of the adrenal medulla. The latter are embryologic homologues of ganglionic sympathocytes. Excitation of preganglionic fibers leads to release of ACh in the adrenal medulla, whose chromaffin cells then respond with a release of epinephrine into the blood (**D**). Small doses of nicotine, by inducing a partial depolarization of adrenomedullary cells, are effective in liberating epinephrine (pp. 110, 112).

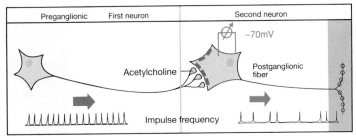

A. Ganglionic transmission: normal state

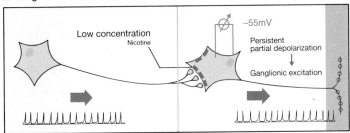

B. Ganglionic transmission: excitation by nicotine

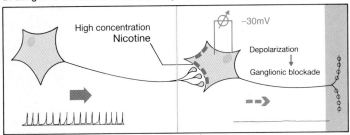

C. Ganglionic transmission: blockade by nicotine

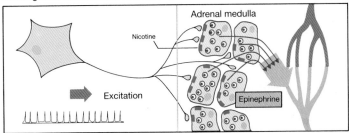

D. Adrenal medulla: epinephrine release by nicotine

Effects of Nicotine on Body Functions

At a low concentration, the tobacco alkaloid **nicotine** acts as a ganglionic stimulant by causing a partial depolarization via activation of ganglionic cholinoceptors (p. 108). A similar action is evident at many other neural sites, considered below in more detail.

Autonomic ganglia. Ganglionic stimulation occurs in both the sympathetic and parasympathetic divisions of the autonomic nervous system. Parasympathetic activation results in increased *production of gastric juice* (smoking ban in peptic ulcer), and enhanced *bowel motility* ("laxative" effect of the first morning cigarette: defecation; diarrhea in the novice).

Although stimulation of parasympathetic cardioinhibitory neurons would tend to lower *heart rate*, this response is overridden by the simultaneous stimulation of sympathetic cardioaccelerant neurons and the adrenal medulla. Stimulation of sympathetic nerves resulting in release of norepinephrine gives rise to *vasoconstriction*; peripheral resistance rises.

Adrenal medulla. On the one hand, release of epinephrine elicits cardiovascular effects, such as increases in *heart rate* and *peripheral vascular resistance*. On the other, it evokes metabolic responses, such as glycogenolysis and lipolysis, that generate energy-rich substrates. The sensation of hunger is suppressed. The metabolic state corresponds to that associated with physical exercise—"silent stress."

Baroreceptors. Partial depolarization of baroreceptors enables activation of the reflex to occur at a relatively smaller rise in blood pressure, leading to decreased sympathetic vasoconstrictor activity.

Neurohypophysis. Release of vasopressin (antidiuretic hormone) results in lowered urinary output (p. 160); in normovolemic subjects, vasoconstriction occurs only at high concentrations of the hormone.

Carotid body. Sensitivity to arterial pCO_2 increases; increased afferent input augments *respiratory rate and depth*.

Receptors for pressure, temperature, and pain. Sensitivity to the corresponding stimuli is enhanced.

Area postrema. Sensitization of chemoceptors leads to *excitation of the medullary emetic center*.

For the sake of completeness, it is worth noting that, at a low concentration, nicotine is also able to augment the excitability of the **motor end plate**. This effect can be manifested in heavy smokers in the form of muscle cramps (calf musculature) and soreness.

The multiplicity of its effects makes nicotine ill-suited for therapeutic use.

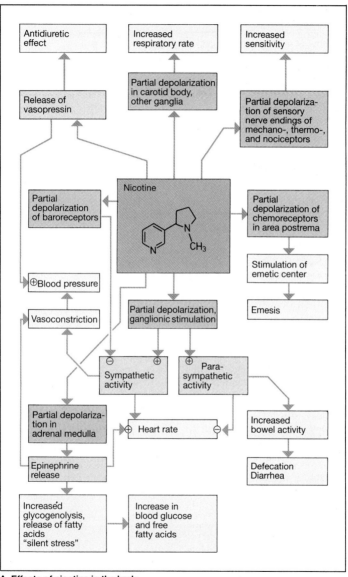

A. Effects of nicotine in the body

Consequences of Tobacco Smoking

The dried and cured leaves of the nightshade plant *Nicotiana tabacum* are known as tobacco. Tobacco is mostly smoked, less frequently chewed or taken as dry snuff. Combustion of tobacco generates approx. 4000 chemical compounds in detectable quantities. The xenobiotic burden on the smoker depends on a range of parameters, including tobacco quality, presence of a filter, rate and temperature of combustion, depth of inhalation, and duration of breath holding.

Tobacco contains 0.2%-5% nicotine. In tobacco smoke, nicotine is present as a constituent of small tar particles. It is rapidly absorbed through bronchi and lung alveoli, and is detectable in the brain only 8 seconds after the first inhalation. Smoking of a single cigarette yields peak plasma levels in the range of 25–50 ng/mL. The effects described on p. 110 become evident. When intake stops, nicotine concentration in plasma shows an initial rapid fall, reflecting distribution into tissues, and a terminal elimination phase with a half-life of 2 h. Nicotine is degradated by oxidation.

The enhanced **risk of vascular disease** (coronary stenosis, myocardial infarction, and central and peripheral ischemic disorders, such as stroke and intermittent claudication) is likely to be a consequence of chronic exposure to nicotine. At the least, nicotine is under discussion as a factor favoring the progression of arteriosclerosis. By releasing epinephrine, it elevates plasma levels of glucose and free fatty acids in the absence of an immediate physiological need for these energy-rich metabolites. Furthermore, it promotes platelet aggregability, lowers fibrinolytic activity of blood, and enhances coagulability.

The health risks of tobacco smoking are, however, attributable not only to nicotine, but also to various other ingredients of tobacco smoke, some of which possess demonstrable **carcinogenic** properties.

Dust particles inhaled in tobacco smoke, together with bronchial mucus, must be removed by the ciliated epithelium from the airways. Cilial activity, however, is depressed by tobacco smoke: mucociliary transport is impaired. This favors bacterial infection and contributes to the chronic bronchitis associated with regular smoking. Chronic injury to the bronchial mucosa could be an important causative factor in increasing the risk in smokers of death from bronchial carcinoma.

Statistical surveys provide an impressive correlation between the number of cigarettes smoked a day and the risk of death from coronary disease or lung cancer. On the other hand, statistics also show that, on cessation of smoking, the increased risk of death from coronary infarction or other cardiovascular disease declines over 5–10 years almost to the level of nonsmokers. Similarly, the risk of developing bronchial carcinoma is reduced.

Abrupt cessation of regular smoking is not associated with severe physical withdrawal symptoms. In general, subjects complain of increased nervousness, lack of concentration, and weight gain.

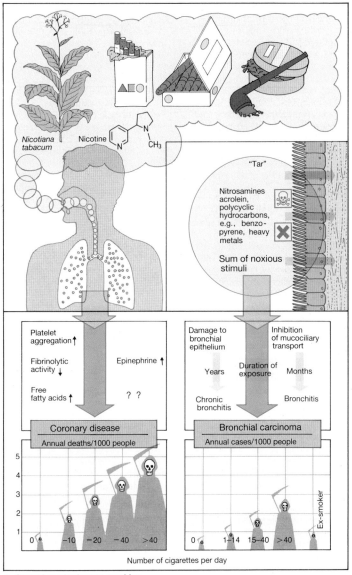

A. Sequelae of tobacco smoking

Biogenic Amines—Actions and Pharmacological Implications

Dopamine (A). *Occurrence and actions.* As the precursor of norepinephrine and epinephrine (p. 82), dopamine is found in sympathetic (adrenergic) neurons and adrenomedullary cells. In the CNS, dopamine itself serves as a messenger substance and is implicated in neostriatal motor programming (p. 182), the elicitation of emesis at the level of the area postrema (p. 300), and inhibition of prolactin release from the anterior pituitary (p. 228).

There are two major receptor subtypes, designated D_1 and D_2. The aforementioned actions are mediated by D_2-receptors. When given by infusion, dopamine causes a dilatation of renal and splanchnic arteries. This effect is mediated by D_1-receptors and is utilized in the treatment of cardiovascular shock. At higher doses, β_1-adrenoceptors and, finally, α-receptors are activated, as evidenced by cardiac stimulation and vasoconstriction, respectively.

Dopamine is not to be confused with dobutamine, which stimulates α- and β-adrenoceptors but *not* dopamine receptors (p. 62).

Dopamine-mimetics. Administration of the precursor L-dopa enables endogenous dopamine synthesis to be enhanced (indication: parkinsonian syndrome, p. 182). The ergot derivatives bromocriptine, pergolide, and lisuride are nonselective D-receptor agonists whose therapeutic effects are probably due to stimulation of D_2-receptors (indications: parkinsonism, suppression of lactation, infertility, acromegaly, p. 228). Typical adverse effects of these substances are nausea and vomiting.

Dopamine antagonists. Classic neuroleptics (p. 224) typically produce a nonselective blockade of D-receptors. The antiemetic effect of metoclopramide involves blockade of D_2-receptors (p. 300). The antihypertensive agents, reserpine and α-methyldopa, exert antidopaminergic effects because they deplete neuronal stores of the amine. A common adverse effect of dopamine antagonists or depletors is parkinsonism.

Histamine (B). *Occurrence and actions.* Histamine is stored in basophils and tissue mast cells. It plays a role in inflammatory and allergic reactions (p. 298) and produces bronchoconstriction, increased intestinal peristalsis, and dilatation and increased permeability of small blood vessels. In the parietal cells of the gastric mucosa, it stimulates the secretion of acid. Two receptor subtypes, H_1 and H_2, can be distinguished; both are involved in vascular responses. Prejunctional H_3-receptors demonstrated in both brain and on peripheral neurons presumably regulate transmitter release.

Antagonists. Most of the so-called *H_1-antihistaminics* also block other receptors, including M-cholinoceptors and D-receptors. H_1-antihistaminics are used for the symptomatic relief of allergies (e.g., chlorpheniramine, clemastine, dimethindine, mebhydroline, pheniramine); as antiemetics (meclizine, dimenhydrinate, p. 300), as over-the-counter hypnotics (e.g., diphenhydramine, p. 212). Promethazine represents the transition to psychopharmacologicals of the phenothiazine-neuroleptic type. Unwanted effects of most H_1-antihistaminics are lassitude (impaired driving skills) and atropine-like reactions (e.g., dry mouth, constipation). Terfenadine and astemizole are thus practically devoid of sedative effects; they also lack anticholinergic properties. *H_2-Antihistaminics* (cimetidine, ranitidine, famotidine, nizatidine) inhibit gastric acid secretion and are used in the treatment of peptic ulcers.

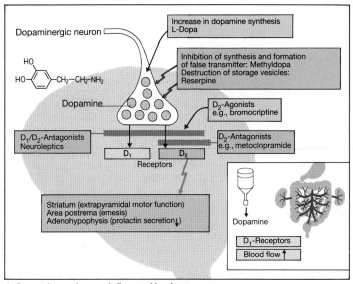

A. Dopamine actions as influenced by drugs

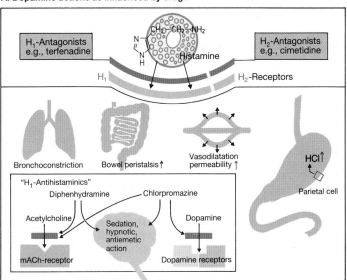

B. Histamine actions as influenced by drugs

Serotonin

Occurrence. Serotonin (5-hydroxy-tryptamine, 5-HT) is synthesized from L-tryptophan in enterochromaffin cells of the intestinal mucosa. 5HT-synthesizing neurons occur in the enteric nerve plexus and the CNS, where the amine fulfills a transmitter function. Blood platelets are unable to synthesize 5-HT, but are capable of taking up, storing, and releasing it.

Serotonin receptors. Based on biochemical and pharmacological criteria, different receptors can be distinguished at present: 5-HT_1, which comprises three subtypes, 5-HT_2, 5-HT_3, and 5-HT_4. Most of these are G-protein linked. The 5-HT_3 subtype is directly coupled to a nonselective cation channel.

Cardiovascular system. The circulatory effects of 5-HT are complex because multiple, in part opposing, effects are exerted via the different receptor subtypes. 5-HT_2 receptors on vascular smooth muscle mediate direct vasoconstriction. Vasodilation and lowering of blood pressure can occur by several indirect mechanisms: 5-HT_{1A} receptors mediate sympatho-inhibition ($\rightarrow$ decrease in neurogenic vasoconstrictor tonus) both centrally and peripherally; 5-HT_1-like receptors on vascular endothelium promote release of vasorelaxant mediators (EDRF, p. 100, 120; prostacyclin, p. 188). 5-HT released from platelets plays a role in thrombogenesis, hemostasis, and the pathogenesis of preeclamptic hypertension. *Ketanserin* is an antihypertensive that acts as an antagonist at 5-HT_2 (and 5-HT_{1C}) receptors. Whether this action accounts for its antihypertensive effect remains questionable, because ketanserin also blocks α-adrenoceptors.

Sumatriptan is an antimigraine drug that possesses agonist activity at 5-HT_{1D} receptors and may thereby exert a favorable effect on this type of headache.

Gastrointestinal tract. Serotonin released from myenteric neurons or enterochromaffin cells acts on 5-HT_3 and 5-HT_4 receptors to enhance bowel motility and enteral fluid secretion. *Cisapride* is a prokinetic agent that promotes propulsive motor activity in the stomach and in the small and large intestines. It is used in motility disorders. Its mechanism of action is unclear; conceivably stimulation of 5-HT_4 receptors is important.

Central nervous system. Serotonergic neurons play a part in various brain functions, as evidenced by the effects of drugs likely to interfere with serotonin. *Fluoxetine* is an antidepressant that, by blocking re-uptake, inhibits inactivation of released serotonin. It produces significant psychomotor stimulation and is considered a second-line antidepressant. Its activity spectrum includes depression of appetite.

Buspirone is an anxiolytic drug whose mode of action is thought to involve central 5-HT_{1A} receptors.

Ondansetron, an antagonist of the 5-HT_3 receptor, possesses striking effectiveness against cytotoxic drug-induced emesis, evident both at the start of and during cytostatic therapy.

Psychedelics (LSD) and other psychotomimetics, such as *mescaline* and *psilocybin,* can induce states of altered awareness, or induce hallucinations and anxiety, probably mediated by 5-HT_2 receptors.

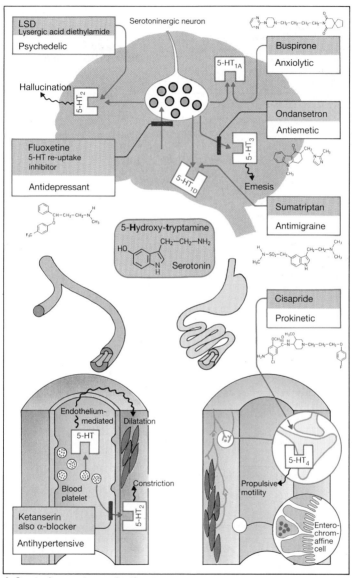

A. Serotonin receptors and actions

Vasodilators—an Overview

The distribution of blood within the circulation is a function of vascular caliber. Venous tone regulates the volume of blood returned to the heart; hence, stroke volume and cardiac output. The luminal diameter of the arterial vasculature determines peripheral resistance. Cardiac output and peripheral resistance are prime determinants of arterial blood pressure (p. 288).

In **A**, the clinically most important vasodilators are presented in the order of approximate frequency of their therapeutic use. Some of these agents possess different efficacies in affecting the venous and arterial limbs of the circulation (width of beam).

Possible uses. *Arteriolar vasodilators* are given to lower blood pressure in cases of hypertension (p. 286), to reduce cardiac work in angina pectoris (p. 284), and to reduce ventricular afterload (pressure load) in cardiac failure (p. 132). *Venous vasodilators* are used to reduce venous filling pressure (preload) in angina pectoris (p. 284) or cardiac failure (p. 132). Practical uses are indicated for each drug group.

Counter-regulation in Acute Hypotension Due to Vasodilators (B). Increased *sympathetic* drive raises heart rate (reflex tachycardia) and cardiac output and thus helps to elevate blood pressure. The patients experience palpitations. Activation of the *renin–angiotensin–aldosterone (RAA) system* (p. 124) serves to increase blood volume, hence cardiac output. Fluid retention leads to an increase in body weight and, possibly, edema. These counter-regulatory processes are susceptible to pharmacological inhibition (β-blockers, ACE inhibitors, diuretics).

Mechanism of Action. ACE inhibitors and α-blockers protect against excitatory mediators such as angiotensin II and norepinephrine, respectively. Prostacyclin analogues, such as iloprost, or prostaglandin E_1 analogues, such as alprostadil, mimic the actions of relaxant mediators. Ca^{2+} antagonists reduce depolarizing inward Ca^{2+} currents, whereas K^+ channel activators promote outward (hyperpolarizing) K^+ currents. Organic nitrovasodilators give rise to NO, an endogenous activator of guanylate cyclase.

Individual vasodilators. Nitrates (p. 120), Ca^{2+} antagonists (p. 122), ACE inhibitors (p. 124) α_1-antagonists (p. 90), and sodium nitroprusside (p. 120) are dealt with elsewhere.

Dihydralazine and **minoxidil** (via its sulfate-conjugated metabolite) dilate arterioles and are used in antihypertensive therapy. They are, however, unsuitable for monotherapy because of compensatory circulatory reflexes. The mechanism of action of dihydralazine is unclear. Minoxidil probably activates K^+ channels, leading to hyperpolarization of smooth muscle cells.

Particular adverse reactions are: lupus erythematosus with dihydralazine; hirsutism with minoxidil—used topically, it is promoted for the treatment of baldness (androgenetic alopecia).

Diazoxide given intravenously causes arteriolar dilation; it can be employed in hypertensive crises. After its oral administration, insulin secretion is inhibited; diazoxide can be used in the management of insulin-secreting pancreas tumors. Both effects are probably due to activation of (ATP-gated) K^+ channels.

The methylxanthine theophylline (p. 298), the phosphodiesterase inhibitor amrinone (p. 132), and nicotinic acid derivatives (p. 152) also possess vasodilating activity.

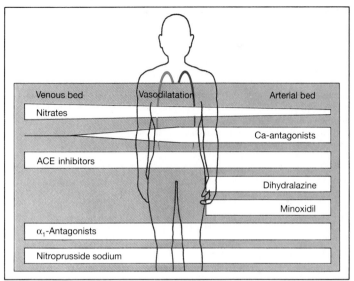

A. Vasodilators

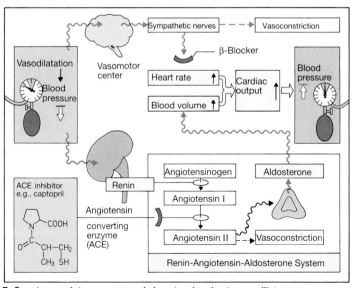

B. Counter-regulatory responses in hypotension due to vasodilators

Organic Nitrates

Various esters of nitric acid (HNO_3) and polyvalent alcohols relax vascular smooth muscle, e.g., nitroglycerin (glyceryl trinitrate) and isosorbide dinitrate. *The effect is more pronounced in venous than in arterial beds.*

These vasodilator effects produce hemodynamic consequences that can be put to therapeutic use. Due to a decrease in both venous return (preload) and arterial afterload, cardiac work is decreased (p. 284). As a result, the cardiac oxygen balance improves. Spasmodic constriction of larger coronary vessels (coronary spasm) is prevented.

Uses. Organic nitrates are used chiefly in *angina pectoris* (p. 282), less frequently in severe forms of chronic or acute congestive heart failure. Continuous intake of higher doses with maintenance of steady plasma levels leads to loss of efficacy, inasmuch as the organism becomes refractory (tachyphylactic). This "nitrate tolerance" can be avoided if a daily nitrate-free interval is maintained, e.g., overnight.

At the start of therapy, **unwanted reactions** occur most often in the form of a throbbing headache, probably caused by dilatation of cephalic vessels. This effect also exhibits tolerance, even when daily "nitrate pauses" are kept. Excessive dosages give rise to hypotension, reflex tachycardia, and circulatory collapse.

Mechanism of action. The reduction in vascular smooth muscle tone is presumably due to activation of guanylate cyclase and elevation of cyclic GMP levels. The causative agent is most likely **NO** generated from the organic nitrate. NO is a physiological messenger molecule that endothelial cells release onto subjacent smooth muscle cells ("endothelium-derived relaxing factor," EDRF). Organic nitrates would thus utilize a preexisting pathway, hence their high efficacy. The generation of NO within the smooth muscle cell depends on a supply of free sulfhydryl (–SH) groups; "nitrate-tolerance" is attributed to a cellular exhaustion of SH-donors.

Nitroglycerin (NTG, glyceryl trinitrate) is distinguished by a high membrane penetrability and very low stability. It is the drug of choice in the treatment of angina pectoris attacks. For this purpose, it is administered as a spray, or in sublingual or buccal tablets for transmucosal delivery. The onset of action is between 1 and 3 minutes. Due to a nearly complete presystemic elimination, it is poorly suited for oral administration. Transdermal delivery (nitroglycerin patch) also avoids presystemic elimination. **Isosorbide dinitrate (ISDN)** penetrates well through membranes, is more stable than NTG, and is partly degraded into the weaker, but much longer-acting, 5-isosorbide mononitrate (ISMN). ISDN can also be applied sublingually; however, it is mainly administered orally in order to achieve a prolonged effect. **ISMN** is not suitable for sublingual use because of its higher polarity and slower rate of absorption. Taken orally, it is absorbed and is not subject to first-pass elimination.

Molsidomine itself is inactive. After oral intake, it is slowly converted into an active metabolite. Apparently, there is little likelihood of "nitrate tolerance."

Sodium nitroprusside contains a nitroso (–NO) group, but is not an ester. It dilates venous and arterial beds equally. It is administered by infusion to achieve controlled hypotension under continuous close monitoring.

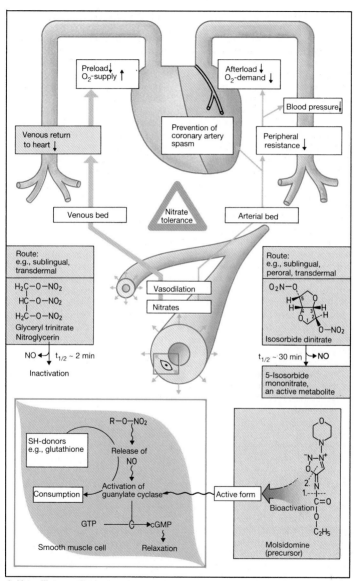

A. Vasodilators: nitrates

Calcium Antagonists

During electrical excitation of the cell membrane of heart or smooth muscle, different ionic currents are activated, including an inward Ca^{2+} current. The term Ca^{2+} antagonist is applied to drugs that inhibit the influx of Ca^{2+} ions without affecting inward Na^+ or outward K^+ currents to a significant degree. Other labels are *calcium-entry blocker* or *calcium-channel blocker*. Therapeutically used Ca^{2+} antagonists can be divided into two groups according to their effects on heart and vasculature.

I. Dihydropyridine derivatives. The dihydropyridines, e.g., nifedipine, are uncharged hydrophobic substances. They induce a *relaxation* of vascular smooth muscle in *arterial beds*. An effect on cardiac function is practically absent at therapeutic dosage. (In pharmacological experiments on isolated cardiac muscle preparations a clear negative inotropic effect is, however, demonstrable.) They are thus regarded as *vasoselective Ca antagonists*. Because of the dilatation of resistance vessels, blood pressure falls. Cardiac afterload is diminished (p. 284) and, therefore, also oxygen demand. Spasms of coronary arteries are prevented.

Indications for nifedipine include *angina pectoris* (p. 284) and *hypertension* (p. 286). In angina pectoris, it is effective when given either prophylactically or during acute attacks. **Adverse effects** are palpitation (reflex tachycardia due to hypotension), headache, and pretibial edema.

Nitrendipine and *felodipine* are used in the treatment of hypertension. *Nimodipine* is given prophylactically after subarachnoid hemorrhage to prevent vasospasms due to depolarization caused by excess K^+ liberated from disintegrating erythrocytes or blockade of NO (EDRF) by free hemoglobin.

II. Verapamil and related catamphiphilic Ca^{2+} antagonists. Verapamil contains a nitrogen atom bearing a positive charge at physiological pH and thus represents a *cationic amphiphilic molecule*. It exerts inhibitory effects not only on *arterial smooth muscle*, but also on *heart muscle*. In the heart, Ca^{2+} inward currents are important in generating depolarization of sinoatrial node cells (impulse generation), in impulse propagation through the AV-junction (atrioventricular conduction), and in electromechanical coupling in the ventricular cardiomyocytes. Verapamil thus produces negative chrono-, dromo-, and inotropic effects.

Indications. Verapamil is used as an *antiarrhythmic* drug in supraventricular tachyarrhythmias. In atrial flutter or fibrillation, it is effective in reducing ventricular rate by virtue of inhibiting AV-conduction. Verapamil is also employed in the prophylaxis of *angina pectoris attacks* (p. 284) and the treatment of *hypertension* (p. 286).

Adverse effects. Because of verapamil's effects on the sinus node, a drop in blood pressure fails to evoke a reflex tachycardia. Heart rate changes; bradycardia may even develop; AV-block and myocardial insufficiency can occur. Patients frequently complain of constipation.

Gallopamil (= methoxyverapamil) is closely related to verapamil in terms of both structure and biological activity.

Diltiazem is a catamphiphilic benzothiazepine derivative with an activity profile resembling that of verapamil.

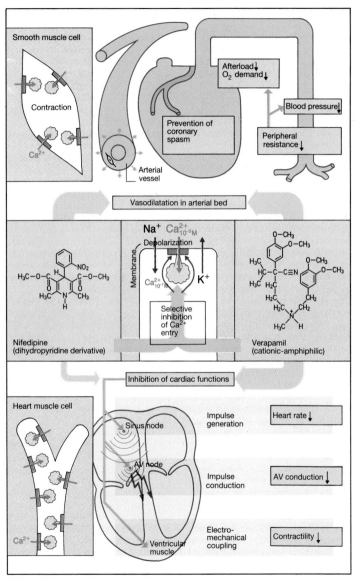

A. Vasodilators: calcium antagonists

ACE Inhibitors

Angiotensin-converting enzyme (ACE) is a component of the antihypotensive renin–angiotensin–aldosterone (RAA) system. Renin is produced by specialized cells in the wall of the afferent arterioles of the renal glomeruli. These belong to the juxtaglomerular apparatus of the nephron, the site of contact between afferent arteriole and distal tubule, which plays an important part in controlling nephron function. Stimuli eliciting *release of renin* are: a drop in renal perfusion pressure, decreased rate of delivery of Na^+ to the distal tubules, as well as β-adrenoceptor mediated sympatho-activation. The glycoprotein renin enzymatically cleaves the decapeptide angiotensin I from its circulating precursor substrate angiotensinogen. ACE, in turn, produces biologically active angiotensin II (Agt II) from angiotensin I (Agt I).

ACE is a rather nonspecific peptidase that can cleave C-terminal dipeptides from various peptides ("dipeptidyl carboxypeptidase"). As "kinase II," it contributes to the inactivation of kinins, such as bradykinin. ACE is also present in blood plasma; however, enzyme localized in the luminal side of vascular endothelium is primarily responsible for the formation of angiotensin II. The lung is rich in ACE, but kidneys, heart, and other organs also contain the enzyme.

Angiotensin II can raise blood pressure in different ways, including (1) vasoconstriction in both the arterial and venous limbs of the circulation; (2) stimulation of aldosterone secretion, leading to increased renal reabsorption of NaCl and water, hence an increased blood volume; (3) a central increase in sympathotonus and, peripherally, enhanced release and effects of norepinephrine.

ACE inhibitors, such as *captopril* and *enalaprilat,* the active metabolite of enalapril, occupy the enzyme as false substrates. Affinity significantly influences efficacy and rate of elimination. Enalaprilat has a stronger and longer-lasting effect than does captopril. **Indications** are *hypertension* and *cardiac failure.*

Lowering of an elevated blood pressure is predominantly brought about by diminished production of angiotensin II. Impaired degradation of kinins that exert vasodilating actions may contribute to the effect.

In heart failure, cardiac output rises again because ventricular afterload diminishes due to a fall in peripheral resistance. Venous congestion abates as a result of (1) increased cardiac output and (2) reduction in venous return (decreased aldosterone secretion, decreased tonus of venous capacitance vessels).

Undesired effects. The magnitude of the antihypertensive effect of ACE inhibitors depends on the functional state of the RAA system. When the latter has been activated by loss of electrolytes and water (e. g., resulting from treatment with diuretic drugs), cardiac failure, or renal arterial stenosis, administration of ACE inhibitors may initially cause an excessive fall in blood pressure. In renal arterial stenosis, the RAA system may be needed for maintaining renal function and ACE inhibitors may precipitate renal failure. Dry cough is a fairly frequent side effect, possibly caused by reduced inactivation of kinins in the bronchial mucosa. Rarely, disturbances of taste sensation, exanthema, neutropenia, proteinuria, and angioneurotic edema may occur.

In most cases, ACE inhibitors are well tolerated and effective.

Newer analogues include *lisinopril, perindopril,* and *ramipril.*

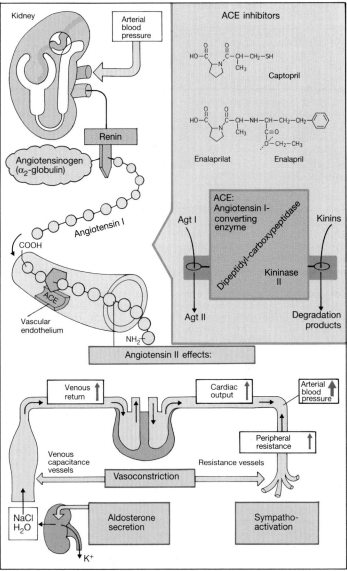

A. Renin-angiotensin-aldosterone system and ACE-inhibitors

Drugs Used to Influence Smooth Muscle Organs

Bronchodilators. Narrowing of bronchioles raises airway resistance, e.g., in bronchial or bronchitic asthma. Several substances that are employed as *bronchodilators* are described elsewhere in more detail: the methylxanthine, *theophylline* (p. 298, given parenterally or orally); β_2-sympathomimetics (p. 84, given by pulmonary, parenteral, or oral route); the parasympatholytic *ipratropium* (pp. 104, 107, given by inhalation).

Spasmolytics. *N-butylscopolamine* (p. 104, 107) is used for the relief of painful spasms of the biliary or ureteral ducts. Its poor absorption (NB: quaternary N; absorption rate < 10%) necessitates parenteral administration. Because the therapeutic effect is usually weak, a potent analgesic is given concurrently, e.g., the opioid meperidine. Note that some spasms of intestinal musculature can be effectively relieved by organic nitrates (in biliary colic) or by nifedipine (esophageal hypertension and achalasia).

Myometrial relaxants (Tocolytics). β_2-Sympatholytics, such as fenoterol and ritodrine, are suitable for preventing premature labor or for interrupting labor in progress when dangerous complications necessitate cesarean section (administration is parenteral or oral).

Myometrial stimulants. The neurohypophyseal hormone, *oxytocin* (p. 228) is given parenterally (or by the nasal or buccal route) before, during, or after labor in order to prompt uterine contractions or to enhance them. Certain *prostaglandins* or analogues of them (p. 188; $F_{2\alpha}$ = dinoprost; E_2 = dinoprostone, sulprostone) are capable of inducing rhythmic uterine contractions and cervical relaxation at any time. They are mostly employed as abortifacients (local or parenteral application).

Ergot alkaloids are obtained from *Secale cornutum* (ergot), the sclerotium of a fungus (*Claviceps purpurea*) parasitizing rye. Consumption of flour from contaminated grain was once the cause of epidemic poisonings (*ergotism*) characterized by gangrene of the extremities (St. Anthony's fire) and CNS disturbances (hallucinations).

Ergot alkaloids contain lysergic acid (formula in **A** shows an amide). They act on uterine and vascular muscle. *Ergometrine* particularly stimulates the uterus. It readily induces a tonic contraction of the myometrium (tetanus uteri). This jeopardizes placental blood flow and fetal O_2 supply. The semisynthetic derivative *methylergometrine* is, therefore, used only *after* delivery for uterine contractions that are too weak.

Ergotamine, as well as the ergotoxine alkaloids (ergocristine, ergocryptine, ergocornine), have a predominantly vascular action. Depending on the initial caliber, constriction or dilatation may be elicited. The mechanism of action is unclear; a partial agonism at α-adrenoceptors may be important. Ergotamine is used in the treatment of migraine (p. 294). Its congener, *dihydroergotamine*, is furthermore employed in orthostatic complaints (p. 288) and in combination with heparin for prevention of thrombosis (p. 146).

Other lysergic acid derivatives are the 5-HT antagonist, *methysergide*, the dopamine-agonist *bromocriptine* (pp. 114, 183), and the hallucinogen lysergic acid diethylamide (LSD, p. 227).

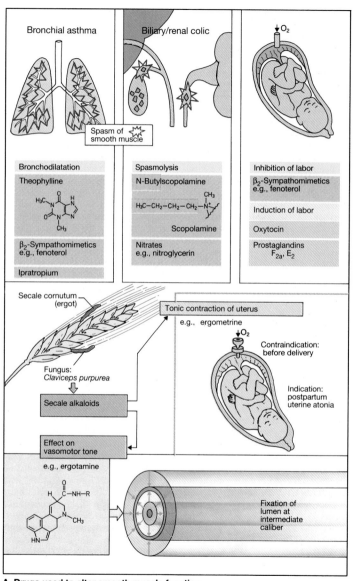

A. Drugs used to alter smooth muscle function

Overview of Modes of Action (A)

1. The pumping capacity of the heart is regulated by sympathetic and parasympathetic nerves (pp. 84, 104). Drugs capable of interfering with autonomic nervous function therefore provide a means of influencing cardiac performance. Thus, **anxiolytics** of the benzodiazepine type (p. 216), such as diazepam, can be employed in myocardial infarction in order to suppress sympathoactivation due to life-threatening distress. Under the influence of **antiadrenergic agents** (p. 96), used to lower an elevated blood pressure, cardiac work is decreased. **Ganglionic blockers** (p. 108) are used in managing hypertensive emergencies. **Parasympatholytics** (p. 104) and **β-blockers** (p. 92) prevent the transmission of autonomic nerve impulses to heart muscle cells by blocking the respective receptors.

2. An isolated mammalian heart whose extrinsic nervous connections have been severed will beat spontaneously for hours if it is supplied with a nutrient medium via the aortic trunk and coronary arteries (Langendorff preparation). In such a preparation, only those drugs that act directly on cardiomyocytes will alter contractile force and beating rate. **Parasympathomimetics** and **sympathomimetics** act at membrane receptors for visceromotor neurotransmitters. The plasmalemma also harbors the sites of action of **cardiac glycosides** (the Na^+/K^+-ATPases, p. 130), of calcium antagonists (Ca^{2+}-channels, p. 122), and of **agents that block Na-channels** (pp. 134, 194). An intracellular site is the target for **phosphodiesterase inhibitors** (e.g. amrinone, p. 132).

3. Mention should also be made of the possibility of affecting cardiac function in angina pectoris (p. 284) or congestive heart failure (p. 132) by reducing venous return, peripheral resistance, or both, with the aid of vasodilators.

Events Underlying Contraction and Relaxation (B)

The signal triggering **contraction** is a propagated action potential (AP) generated in the sinoatrial node. *Depolarization* of the plasmalemma leads to a rapid *rise in cytosolic Ca^{2+} levels,* which causes the contractile filaments to shorten (**electromechanical coupling**). The level of Ca^{2+} concentration attained determines the degree of shortening, i.e., the force of contraction. Sources of Ca^{2+} are: a) extracellular Ca^{2+} entering the cell through voltage-gated *Ca^{2+}-channels*; b) Ca^{2+} stored in membranous sacs of the *sarcoplasmic reticulum* (SR); c) Ca^{2+} bound to the inside of the plasmalemma. The plasmalemma of cardiomyocytes extends into the cell interior in the form of tubular invaginations (transverse tubuli).

The trigger signal for **relaxation** is the return of the membrane potential to its resting level. During repolarization Ca^{2+} levels fall below the threshold for activation of the myofilaments ($3 \times 10^{-7}M$), as the *plasmalemmal binding sites* regain their binding capacity; the SR pumps Ca^{2+} into its interior; and Ca^{2+} that entered the cell during systole is extruded by plasmalemmal Ca^{2+}-ATPases with expenditure of energy. In addition, a carrier, utilizing the transmembrane Na^+-gradient as energy source, transports Ca^{2+} out of the cell in exchange for Na^+ moving down its transmembrane gradient (*Na^+/Ca^{2+} exchange*).

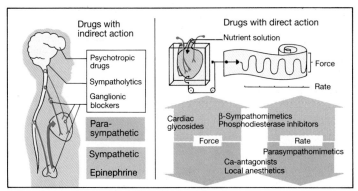

A. Possible mechanisms for influencing heart function

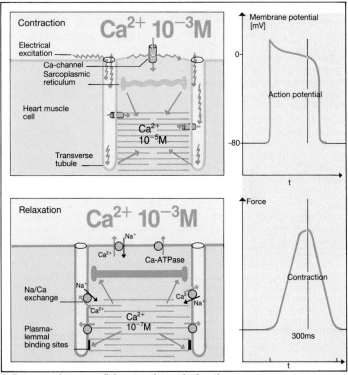

B. Processes in myocardial contraction and relaxation

Cardiac Glycosides

Diverse plants (**A**) are sources of sugar-containing compounds (glycosides) that also contain a steroid ring (structural formulas, p. 133) and augment the contractile force of heart muscle (**B**): *cardiotonic glycosides, cardiosteroids,* or *"digitalis."*

If the inotropic, "therapeutic" dose is exceeded by a small increment, signs of poisoning appear: arrhythmia and contracture (**B**). *The narrow therapeutic margin* can be explained by the **mechanism of action.**

Cardiac glycosides (CG) bind to the extracellular side of Na$^+$/K$^+$-ATPases of cardiomyocytes and inhibit enzyme activity. The Na$^+$/K$^+$-ATPases operate to pump out Na$^+$ leaked into the cell and to retrieve K$^+$ leaked from the cell. In this manner, they maintain the transmembrane gradients for K$^+$ and Na$^+$, the negative resting membrane potential, and the normal electrical excitability of the cell membrane. When part of the enzyme is occupied and inhibited by CG, the unoccupied remainder can increase its level of activity and maintain Na$^+$ and K$^+$ transport. The effective stimulus is a small elevation of intracellular Na$^+$ concentration (normally approx. 7 mM). Concomitantly, the amount of Ca^{2+} mobilized during systole and, thus, *contractile force increases.* It is generally thought that the underlying cause is the decrease in the Na$^+$ transmembrane gradient, i.e., the driving force for the Na$^+$/Ca^{2+} exchange (p. 128), allowing the intracellular Ca^{2+} level to rise. When too many ATPases are blocked, K$^+$- and Na$^+$-homeostasis is deranged; the membrane potential falls, *arrhythmias* occur. Flooding with Ca^{2+} prevents relaxation during diastole, resulting in *contracture.*

The **CNS effects** of CGs (**C**) are also due to binding to Na$^+$/K$^+$-ATPases. Enhanced vagal nerve activity causes a decrease in sinoatrial beating rate and velocity of atrioventricular conduction. In patients with heart failure, improved circulation also contributes to the reduction in heart rate. Stimulation of the area postrema leads to nausea and vomiting. Disturbances in color vision are evident.

Indications for CGs are: (1) *chronic congestive heart failure,* (2) *atrial fibrillation* or *flutter,* where inhibition of AV conduction protects the ventricles from excessive atrial impulse activity and thereby improves cardiac performance (**D**). Occasionally, sinus rhythm is restored.

Signs of intoxication are: (1) *Cardiac arrhythmias,* which under certain circumstances are life-threatening, e.g., sinus bradycardia, AV-block, ventricular extrasystoles, ventricular fibrillation; (2) *CNS disturbances:* altered color vision (e.g., xanthopsia); agitation, confusion, nightmares, hallucinations; (3) *gastrointestinal:* anorexia, nausea, vomiting, diarrhea; (4) *renal:* loss of electrolytes and water; this must be differentiated from the mobilization of accumulated edema fluid that occurs with therapeutic dosage.

Therapy of intoxication: *administration of K$^+$* which *inter alia* reduces binding of CG, but may impair AV-conduction; administration of antiarrhythmics, such as *phenytoin* or *lidocaine* (p. 136). Oral administration of *colestyramine* (p. 152) for binding and preventing absorption of digitoxin present in the intestines (enterohepatic cycle); injection of *antibody fragments* that bind and inactivate digitoxin and digoxin.

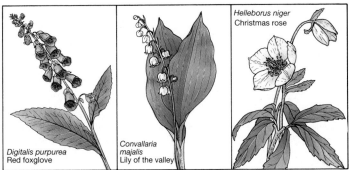

A. Plants containing cardiac glycosides

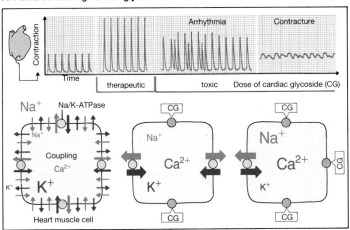

B. Therapeutic and toxic effects of cardiac glycosides (CG)

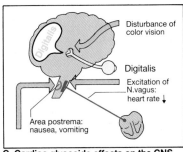

C. Cardiac glycoside effects on the CNS

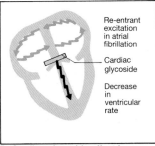

D. Cardiac glycoside effect in atrial fibrillation

Substance	Fraction absorbed %	Plasma Concentr. (ng/ml) free	total	Digitalizing dose (mg)	Elimination % per day	Maintenance dose (mg)
Digitoxin	100	~1	~20	~1	10	~0.1
Digoxin	50–90	~1	~ 1.5	~1	30	~0.3
Ouabain	< 1	~1	~ 1	0.5	no long-term use	

The **pharmacokinetics of cardiac glycosides (A)** are dictated by their polarity, i.e., the number of hydroxyl groups. Membrane penetrability is virtually nil in ouabain, high in digoxin, and very high in digitoxin. **Ouabain** (G-strophanthin) does not penetrate into cells, be they intestinal epithelial, renal tubular, or hepatic cells. At best, it is suitable for acute intravenous induction of glycoside therapy.

The absorption of **digoxin** depends on the kind of galenical preparation used and absorptive conditions in the intestine. Preparations are now of such quality that the derivatives *methyldigoxin* and *acetyldigoxin* no longer offer any advantage. Renal reabsorption is incomplete—approx. 30% of the total amount present in the body (s.c. full *"digitalizing"* dose) is eliminated per day. When renal function is impaired, there is a risk of accumulation. **Digitoxin** undergoes virtually complete reabsorption in the gut and kidneys. There is active hepatic biotransformation: cleavage of sugar moieties, hydroxylation at C12 (yielding digoxin), and conjugation to glucuronic acid. Conjugates secreted with bile are subject to enterohepatic cycling (p. 38); conjugates reaching the blood are renally eliminated. In renal insufficiency, there is no appreciable accumulation. When digitoxin is withdrawn following overdosage, its effect decays more slowly than that of digoxin.

Other positive inotropic drugs. The **phosphodiesterase inhibitors amrinone** (p. 64) can be administered only parenterally for a maximum of 14 days because it is poorly tolerated. A closely related compound is **milrinone**. They are only appropriate for the most severe conditions of heart failure. In terms of their positive inotropic effect, β-**sympathomimetics**, unlike dopamine (p. 114), are of little therapeutic use; they are also arrhythmogenic and the sensitivity of the β-receptor system declines during continuous stimulation.

Treatment Principles in Chronic Heart Failure
Myocardial insufficiency leads to a decrease in stroke volume and venous congestion with formation of edema. Administration of a **cardiac glycoside** for the purpose of augmenting cardiac force affords nearly causal therapy. Application of (**thiazide) diuretics** (p. 158) offers a second therapeutic approach. By lowering peripheral resistance, hence afterload, they also permit stroke volume to be increased. Beyond this effect, there occurs a decrease in circulating blood volume (decreased venous return) that contributes to a reduction in congestive signs. **ACE inhibitors** (p. 124) act similarly by preventing synthesis of angiotensin II (↓ vasoconstriction) and reducing secretion of aldosterone (↓ fluid retention).

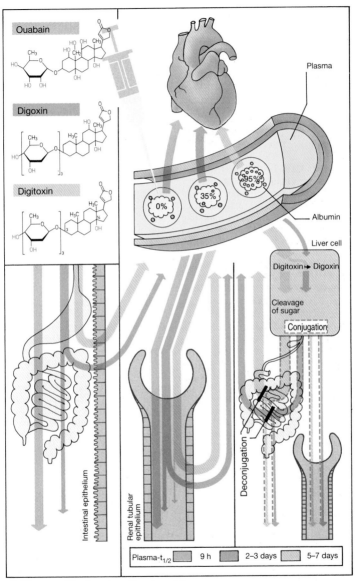

Ouabain

Digoxin

Digitoxin

Plasma

0%   35%   95%

Albumin

Liver cell

Digitoxin → Digoxin

Cleavage
of sugar

Conjugation

Intestinal epithelium

Renal tubular epithelium

Deconjugation

Plasma-$t_{1/2}$ 9 h   2–3 days   5–7 days

A. Pharmacokinetics of cardiac glycosides

Antiarrhythmic Drugs

The electrical impulse for contraction (propagated action potential; p. 136) originates in pacemaker cells of the sinoatrial node and spreads through the atria, atrioventricular (AV) node, and adjoining parts of the His–Purkinje fiber system to the ventricles (**A**). Irregularities of heart rhythm can interfere dangerously with cardiac pumping function.

I. Drugs for Selective Control of Sinoatrial and AV-Nodes

In some forms of arrhythmia, certain drugs can be used that are capable of selectively facilitating and inhibiting (green and red arrows, respectively) the pacemaker function of sinoatrial or atrioventricular cells.

Sinus bradycardia. An abnormally low sinoatrial impulse rate (< 60/min) can be raised by *parasympatholytics*. The quaternary *ipratropium* is preferable to atropine, because it lacks CNS-penetrability (p. 107). Sympathomimetics also exert a positive chronotropic action; they have the disadvantage of increasing myocardial excitability (and automaticity) and, thus, promoting ectopic impulse generation (tendency to extrasystolic beats). In **cardiac arrest,** *epinephrine* can be used to reinitiate heart beat.

Sinus tachycardia (resting rate > 100 beats/min). β-*Blockers* eliminate sympathetic nervous system excitation and lower cardiac rate.

Atrial flutter or fibrillation. An excessive ventricular rate can be decreased by *verapamil* (p. 122) or *cardiac glycosides* (p. 130). These drugs inhibit impulse propagation through the AV node, so that fewer impulses reach the ventricles.

II. Nonspecific Drug Actions on Impulse Generation and Propagation

Impulses originating at loci outside the sinus node are seen in *supraventricular* or *ventricular extrasystoles*, *tachycardia*; *atrial* or *ventricular flutter* and *fibrillation*. In these forms of rhythm disorders, **antiarrhythmics of the local anesthetic, Na^+ channel blocking type** (B) are used for both prophylaxis and therapy. Local anesthetics inhibit electrical excitation of nociceptive nerve fibers (p. 194); concomitant cardiac inhibition (*cardiodepression*) is an unwanted effect. However, in certain types of arrhythmias (see above), this effect is useful. Local anesthetics are readily cleaved (arrows) and unsuitable for oral administration (procaine, lidocaine). Given judiciously, intravenous lidocaine is an effective antiarrhythmic. *Procainamide* and *mexiletine*, congeners endowed with greater metabolic stability, are examples of orally effective antiarrhythmics. The desired and undesired effects are inseparable. Thus, these antiarrhythmics not only depress electrical excitability of cardiomyocytes (*negative bathmotropism, membrane stabilization*), but also lower sinoatrial rate (*negative chronotropism*), AV conduction (*negative dromotropism*), and force of contraction (*negative inotropism*). Interference with normal electrical activity can, not too paradoxically, also induce cardiac arrhythmias—*arrhythmogenic action*.

Inhibition of CNS neurons is the underlying cause of neurological effects such as vertigo, confusion, sensory disturbances, and motor disturbances (tremor, giddiness, ataxia, convulsions).

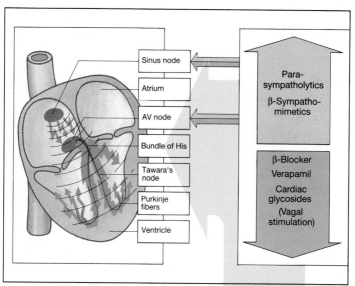

A. Cardiac impulse generation and conduction

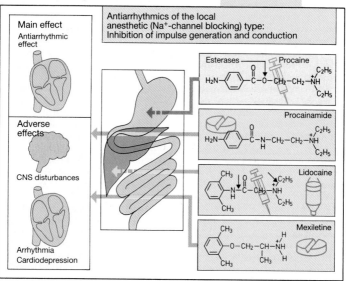

B. Antiarrhythmics of the Na⁺-channel blocking type

Electrophysiological Action of Antiarrhythmics of the Na⁺-Channel-Blocking Type (Class I)

Action potential and ionic currents. The transmembrane electrical potential of cardiomyocytes can be recorded through an intracellular microelectrode. Upon electrical excitation, a characteristic change occurs in membrane potential—the action potential (AP). Its underlying cause is a sequence of transient ionic currents. During *rapid depolarization* (Phase 0), there is a short-lived *influx of Na⁺* through the membrane. A subsequent transient *influx of Ca^{2+}* (as well as of Na⁺) maintains the depolarization (Phase 2, *plateau of AP*). A delayed *efflux of K⁺* returns the membrane potential (Phase 3, *repolarization*) to its resting value (Phase 4). The velocity of depolarization determines the speed at which the AP propagates through the myocardial syncytium.

The transmembrane ionic currents involve proteinaceous *membrane pores: Na⁺-, Ca^{2+}-, K⁺-channels*. In **A**, the phasic change in the functional state of Na⁺-channels during an action potential is illustrated.

Effects of antiarrhythmics. Class I antiarrhythmics block the opening of the Na⁺-channel and thus inhibit membrane depolarization, (**"membrane stabilization"**). The potential consequences are (**A**, bottom): a) A reduction in the *velocity of depolarization* and a decrease in the speed of impulse propagation; aberrant impulse propagation is impeded. b) *Depolarization is entirely absent;* pathological impulse generation, e.g., in the marginal zone of an infarction, is suppressed. c) The time required until a new depolarization can be elicited, i.e., the *refractory period, is increased*; prolongation of the AP (see below) contributes to the increase in refractory period and in consequence,

premature excitation with risk of fibrillation is prevented.

Mechanism of action. Class I antiarrhythmics resemble most local anesthetics in being cationic amphiphilic molecules (p. 198; exception: phenytoin, p. 184). Possible molecular mechanisms of their inhibitory effects are outlined on p. 194 in more detail. Their low structural specificity is reflected by a low selectivity towards different cation channels. Besides the Na⁺- channel, *Ca^{2+}- and K⁺-channels* are also likely to be blocked. Accordingly, cationic amphiphilic antiarrhythmics affect both the depolarization and repolarization phases. Depending on the substance, AP duration can be increased (Class IA), decreased (Class IB), or remain the same (Class IC).

Antiarrhythmics representative of these categories include: Class IA—quinidine, procainamide, ajmaline, disopyramide; Class IB—lidocaine, mexiletine, aprindine, tocainide, as well as phenytoin; Class IC—encainide, flecainide, propafenone.

Note: With respect to classification, β-blockers have been assigned to Class II and the Ca-channel blockers verapamil and diltiazem to Class IV.

Commonly listed under a separate rubric (Class III) are amiodarone and the non-β-blocking *d*-enantiomer of sotalol, which cause a marked prolongation of the AP with a lesser effect on Phase 0 rate of rise.

Therapeutic uses. Because of their *narrow therapeutic margin*, these antiarrhythmics are only employed when rhythm disturbances are of such severity as to impair the pumping action of the heart, or when there is a threat of other complications. The choice of drug is empirical. If the desired effect is not achieved, another drug is tried. Combinations of antiarrhythmics are not customary. Amiodarone is reserved for special cases.

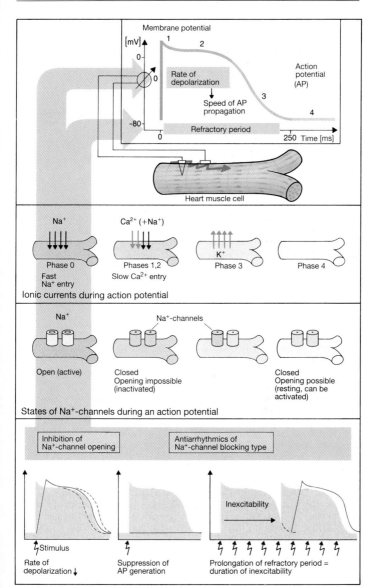

A. Effects of antiarrhythmics of the Na⁺-channel blocking type

Drugs for the Treatment of Anemias

Anemia denotes a reduction in red blood cell count, hemoglobin content, or both. Oxygen (O_2) transport capacity is decreased.

Erythropoiesis (A). Blood corpuscles develop from stem cells through several cell divisions. Hemoglobin is then synthesized and the cell nucleus is extruded. Erythropoiesis is stimulated by the hormone **erythropoietin** (a glycoprotein), which is released from the kidneys when renal O_2 tension declines, now also available as a drug produced by gene-manipulated bacteria.

Given an adequate production of erythropoietin, a **disturbance** of erythropoiesis is due to two principal causes. 1. **Cell multiplication** is **inhibited** because DNA synthesis is insufficient; this occurs in deficiencies of vitamin B_{12} or folic acid (macrocytic hyperchromic anemia). 2. **Hemoglobin synthesis** is **impaired**. This situation arises in iron deficiency, since Fe^{2+} is a constituent of hemoglobin (microcytic hypochromic anemia).

Vitamin B_{12} (cyanocobalamin) (B) is produced by bacteria; B_{12} generated in the colon, however, is unavailable for absorption (see below). Liver, meat, fish, and milk products are rich sources of the vitamin. The **minimal requirement** is about 1 μg/d. Enteral absorption of vitamin B_{12} requires the so-called **"intrinsic factor"** from parietal cells of the stomach. The complex formed with this glycoprotein undergoes endocytosis in the ileum. Bound to its transport protein, transcobalamin, vitamin B_{12} is destined for storage in the liver or uptake into tissues.

A frequent **cause of vitamin B_{12} deficiency** is atrophic gastritis, leading to a *lack of intrinsic factor*. Besides megaloblastic anemia, damage to mucosal linings and degeneration of myelin sheaths with neurological sequelae will occur (**pernicious anemia**).

The optimal **therapy** consists of **parenteral administration** of **cyanocobalamin** or **hydroxocobalamin** (Vitamin B_{12a}; exchange of –CN for –OH group). Adverse effects, in the form of hypersensitivity reactions, are very rare.

Folic Acid (B) Leafy vegetables and liver are rich in folic acid (FA). The **minimal requirement** is approx. 50 μg/day. Polyglutamine FA in food is hydrolyzed to monoglutamine-FA prior to being absorbed. FA is heat-labile. **Causes of deficiency** include: insufficient intake, malabsorption in gastrointestinal diseases, increased requirements during pregnancy. Antiepileptic drugs (phenytoin, primidone, phenobarbital) may decrease FA absorption, presumably by inhibiting the formation of monoglutamine-FA. Inhibition of dihydroFA reductase (e.g., by methotrexate, p. 280) depresses the formation of the active species, tetrahydro FA. *Symptoms* of deficiency are megaloblastic anemia and mucosal damage. **Therapy** consists of **oral administration** of FA.

Administration of FA can mask a vitamin B_{12} deficiency. Vitamin B_{12} is required for the conversion of methyltetrahydroFA to tetrahydroFA, which is important for DNA synthesis (**B**). Inhibition of this reaction due to B_{12} deficiency can be compensated by increased FA intake. The anemia is readily corrected; however, nerve degeneration progresses unchecked and its cause made more difficult to diagnose by the absence of hematological changes. Indiscriminate use of FA-containing multivitamin preparations can, therefore, be harmful.

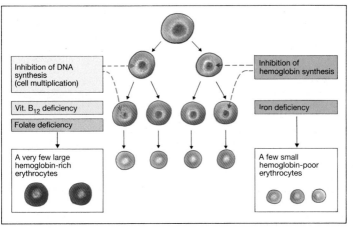

A. Erythropoiesis in bone marrow

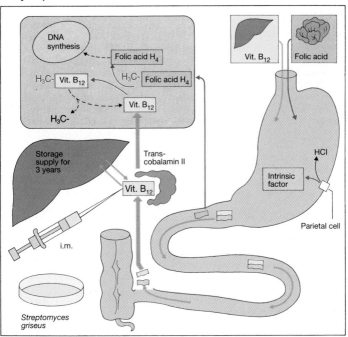

B. Vitamin B$_{12}$ and folate metabolism

Iron Compounds

Not all iron ingested in food is equally absorbable. Trivalent Fe^{3+} is virtually not taken up from the neutral milieu of the small bowel, where the divalent Fe^{2+} is **markedly better absorbed**. Uptake is particularly efficient in the form of heme (present in hemo- and myoglobin). Within the mucosal cells of the gut, iron is oxidized and either deposited as ferritin (see below) or passed on to the transport protein, transferrin, a β_1-glycoprotein. The amount absorbed does not exceed that needed to balance losses due to epithelial shedding from skin and mucosae or to hemorrhage ("**mucosal block**"). In men, this amount is approx. 1 mg/day, in women, it is approx. 2 mg/day (menstrual blood loss). It corresponds to about 10% of the dietary intake. The transferrin–iron complex undergoes endocytotic uptake mainly into erythroblasts to be utilized for hemoglobin synthesis.

About 70% of the **total body store of iron** (~5 g) is contained within the erythrocytes. When these are degraded by macrophages of the reticuloendothelial system (mononuclear phagocyte system), iron is liberated from hemoglobin. Fe^{3+} can be stored as ferritin (= protein apoferritin + Fe^{3+}) or be returned to erythropoiesis sites via transferrin.

A frequent **cause of iron deficiency** is chronic blood loss due to gastric/intestinal ulcers or tumors. One liter of blood contains 500 mg of iron. Despite a significant increase of the fraction absorbed (up to 50%), absorption is unable to keep up with losses and the body store of iron falls. Iron deficiency results in impaired synthesis of hemoglobin and **anemia** (p. 138).

The **treatment** of choice (after the cause of bleeding has been found and eliminated) consists of the **oral administration** of Fe^{2+} compounds, e.g., ferrous sulfate (daily dose 100 mg of iron, equivalent to 300 mg of $FeSO_4$, divided into multiple doses). Replenishing of iron stores may take several months. Oral administration, however, is advantageous in that it is impossible to overload the body with iron through an intact mucosa because of its demand-regulated absorption (mucosal block).

Adverse effects. The frequent gastrointestinal complaints (epigastric pain, diarrhea, and constipation) necessitate intake of iron with or after meals, although absorption is higher from the empty stomach.

Interactions. Antacids inhibit iron absorption. Combination with ascorbic acid (vitamin C), for protecting Fe^{2+} from oxidation to Fe^{3+}, is theoretically sound, but practically is not needed.

Parenteral administration of Fe^{3+} salts is indicated only when adequate oral replacement is not possible. There is a risk of overdosage with iron deposition in tissues (**hemosiderosis**). The binding capacity of transferrin is limited and free Fe^{3+} is toxic. Therefore, Fe^{3+} complexes are employed that can donate Fe^{3+} directly to transferrin or can be phagocytosed by macrophages, enabling iron to be incorporated into the ferritin store. Possible *adverse effects* are, with i.m. injection, persistent pain at the injection site and skin discoloration; with i.v. injection, flushing, hypotension, and anaphylactic shock.

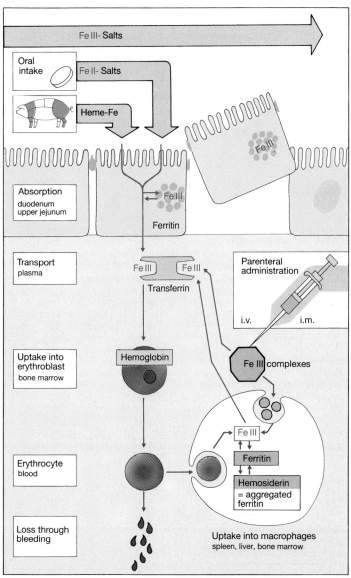

A. Iron: possible routes of administration and fate in the organism

Prophylaxis and Therapy of Thromboses

Upon vascular injury, the coagulation system is activated: thrombocytes and fibrin molecules coalesce into a "plug" that seals the defect and halts bleeding (**hemostasis**). Unnecessary formation of an intravascular clot—a **thrombosis**—can be life-threatening. If the clot forms on an atheromatous plaque in a coronary artery, myocardial infarction is imminent; a thrombus in a deep leg vein can be dislodged, carried into a lung artery, and cause pulmonary embolism.

Drugs that *decrease the coagulability of blood*, such as **coumarins** and **heparin** (A), are employed for the **prophylaxis** of thromboses. In addition, attempts are directed at inhibiting, by means of **acetylsalicylic acid**, the aggregation of blood platelets, which are prominently involved in intra-arterial thrombogenesis (p. 148). For the **therapy** of thrombosis, drugs are used that dissolve the fibrin meshwork—**fibrinolytics** (p. 146).

An overview of the **coagulation cascade** and the sites of action for coumarins and heparin is shown in A. There are two ways to initiate the cascade (**B**): 1) conversion of factor XII into its active form (XIIa, intrinsic system) at intravascular sites denuded of endothelium; 2) conversion of factor VII into VIIa (extrinsic system) under the influence of a tissue-derived lipoprotein (tissue thromboplastin). Both mechanisms converge via factor X into a common final pathway.

The **clotting factors** are protein molecules. "Activation" mostly means proteolysis (cleavage of protein fragments) and, with the exception of fibrin, conversion into protein-hydrolyzing enzymes (*proteases*). Some activated factors require the presence of phospholipids (Pl) and Ca^{2+} for their proteolytic activity. Conceivably, Ca^{2+} ions cause the adhesion of a factor to a phospholipid surface, as depicted in **C**. Phospholipids are contained in platelet factor 3 (PF3), which is released from aggregated platelets, and in tissue thromboplastin (**B**). The sequential activation of several enzymes allows the aforementioned reactions to "snowball," culminating in massive production of fibrin.

The progression of the coagulation cascade can be inhibited as follows: 1) **coumarin derivatives** decrease the blood concentrations of inactive factors II, VII, IX, and X, by inhibiting their synthesis; 2) the complex consisting of **heparin** and antithrombin III neutralizes the protease activity of activated factors; 3) **Calcium chelators** prevent the enzymatic activity of Ca^{2+}-dependent factors; they contain $-COO^-$ groups that bind Ca^{2+} ions (**C**): **citrate** and **EDTA** (ethylenediaminetetraacetic acid) form soluble complexes with calcium, **oxalate** precipitates Ca^{2+} as insoluble calcium oxalate. Chelation of Ca^{2+} cannot be used for therapeutic purposes because Ca^{2+} concentrations would have to be lowered to a level incompatible with life (hypocalcemic tetany). These compounds (sodium salts) are, therefore, used only for rendering blood incoagulable outside the body.

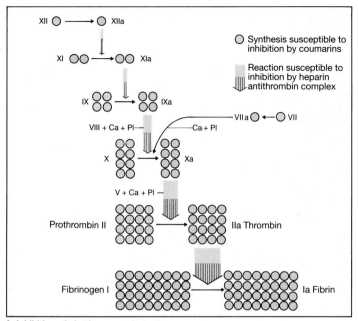

A. Inhibition of clotting cascade in vivo

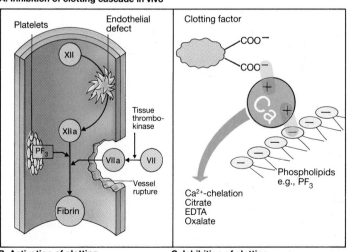

B. Activation of clotting

C. Inhibition of clotting by removal of Ca^{2+}

Coumarin Derivatives (A)

Vitamin K promotes the hepatic γ-carboxylation of glutamate residues on the precursors of factors II, VII, IX, X. Carboxyl groups are required for Ca^{2+}-mediated binding to phospholipid surfaces (p. 142). There are several vitamin K derivatives of different origins: K_1 (phytomenadione) from chlorophyllous plants; K_2 from gut bacteria; and K_3 (menadione) synthesized chemically. All are hydrophobic and require bile acids for absorption.

Oral anticoagulants. Structurally related to vitamin K, **4-hydroxycoumarins** prevent regeneration of reduced (active) vitamin K and inhibit the synthesis of vitamin K-dependent clotting factors.

Coumarins are well absorbed after oral administration. Their duration of action varies considerably. Synthesis of clotting factors depends on the intrahepatocytic concentration ratio between coumarins and vitamin K. The dose required for an adequate anticoagulant effect must be determined individually for each patient (*one-stage prothrombin time*). Subsequently, the patient must avoid changing dietary consumption of green vegetables (alteration in vitamin K levels), refrain from taking additional drugs likely to affect absorption or elimination of coumarins (alteration in coumarin levels), and not risk inhibiting platelet function by ingesting acetylsalicylic acid.

The most **important adverse effect is bleeding**. With coumarins, this can be counteracted by giving vitamin K_1. Coagulability of blood returns to normal only after hours or days, when the liver has resumed synthesis and restored sufficient blood levels of clotting factors. In urgent cases, deficient factors must be replenished directly (e.g., by transfusion of whole blood or of prothrombin concentrate).

Because of their very narrow therapeutic margin and liability to interact with other drugs, oral anticoagulants are being replaced by safer agents.

Heparin (B)

A clotting factor is activated when the factor that precedes it in the clotting cascade splits off a protein fragment and thereby exposes an enzymatic center. The latter can again be inactivated physiologically by complexing with **antithrombin III (AT III)**, a circulating glycoprotein. Heparin acts to inhibit clotting by accelerating formation of this complex more than 1000-fold. Heparin is present (together with histamine) in the vesicles of mast cells. Its physiological role is unclear. Therapeutically used heparin is obtained from porcine gut or bovine lung. Heparin molecules are chains of amino sugars bearing $-COO^-$ and $-SO_3^-$ groups; they contain approx. 10 to 20 of the units depicted in **(B)**; mean molecular weight 20,000. Anticoagulant efficacy varies with chain length. The potency of a preparation is standardized in international units of activity (IU) by bioassay and comparison with a reference preparation.

The numerous negative charges are significant in several respects: (1) they contribute to the poor membrane penetrability—heparin is ineffective by the oral or cutaneous routes and must be injected; (2) attraction to positively charged lysine residues is involved in complex formation with ATIII; (3) they permit binding of heparin to its antidote, **protamine** (polycationic protein from salmon sperm).

If protamine is given in heparin-induced bleeding, the effect of heparin is immediately reversed.

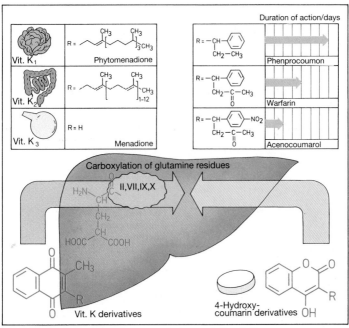

A. Vitamin K-antagonists of the coumarin type and vitamin K

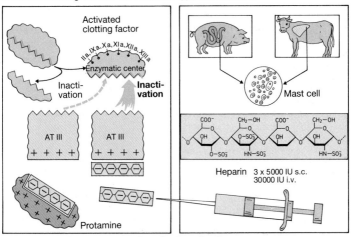

B. Heparin: origin, structure, and mechanism of action

For effective thromboprophylaxis, a low dose of 5000 IU is injected subcutaneously two to three times daily. *Low-molecular-weight heparin* (average MW ~5000) has a longer duration of action and needs to be given only once daily. With a low dosage of heparin, the risk of bleeding is sufficiently small to allow the first injection to be given as early as 2 h prior to surgery. Higher daily i.v. doses are required in order to prevent growth of clots. Besides bleeding, other potential adverse effects are: allergic reactions (e.g., thrombocytopenia); and with chronic administration, reversible hair loss and osteoporosis.

Fibrinolytic Therapy (A)

Fibrin is formed from fibrinogen through thrombin (factor IIa)-catalyzed proteolytic removal of two oligopeptide fragments. Individual fibrin molecules polymerize into a fibrin mesh that can be split into fragments and dissolved by **plasmin**. Plasmin derives by proteolysis from an inactive precursor, plasminogen. **Plasminogen activators** can be infused for the purpose of dissolving clots (e.g., in myocardial infarction). Thrombolysis is not likely to be successful unless the activators can be given very soon after thrombus formation. **Urokinase** is an endogenous plasminogen activator obtained from cultured human kidney cells. Urokinase is better tolerated than is **streptokinase**. By itself, the latter is enzymatically inactive; only after binding to a plasminogen molecule does the complex become effective in converting plasminogen to plasmin. Streptokinase is produced by streptococcal bacteria, which probably accounts for the frequently adverse reactions. Streptokinase antibodies may be present as a result of prior streptococcal infections. Binding to such antibodies would neutralize streptokinase molecules.

Another thrombolytic factor is tissue plasminogen activator (t-PA), which preferentially acts on plasminogen bound to fibrin. Albeit undesired, an expected effect of fibrinolytics is to promote a tendency to bleed.

Inactivation of the fibrinolytic system can be achieved by "**plasmin inhibitors**," such as ε-*aminocaproic acid, p-aminomethylbenzoic acid (PAMBA), tranexamic acid,* and *aprotinin*, which also inhibits other proteases.

Lowering of Blood Fibrinogen Concentration

Ancrod is a constituent of the venom from a Malaysian pit viper. It enzymatically cleaves a fragment from fibrinogen, resulting in the formation of a degradation product that cannot undergo polymerization. Reduction in blood fibrinogen level decreases the coagulability of the blood. Since fibrinogen (MW ~340,000) contributes to the viscosity of blood, an improved "fluidity" of the blood would be expected. Both effects are felt to be of benefit in the treatment of certain disorders of blood flow.

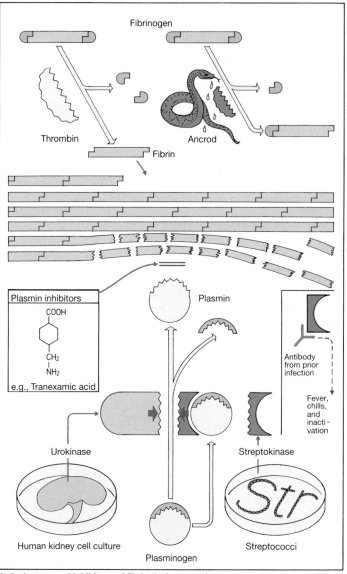

A. Activators and inhibitors of fibrinolysis; ancrod

Inhibition of Platelet Aggregation (A)

In arterial beds, white thrombi consist mainly of platelet aggregates. Because platelets tend to adhere to atherosclerotic intimal plaques in coronary or cerebral arteries, there is risk of myocardial and cerebral infarction, respectively. **Acetylsalicylic acid** (ASA; p. 190) inhibits platelet aggregation. The labile *acetyl residue* binds *covalently* to cyclooxygenase in platelets, resulting in an *irreversible* inhibition and prevention of thromboxane A_2 synthesis (p. 188). Released **thromboxane A_2** promotes two processes that are necessary for hemostasis after vascular damage, but are inopportune in the presence of atherosclerosis: *aggregation of platelets* and *vasoconstriction*.

Indications for administration of ASA to inhibit platelet aggregation are: prophylaxis of myocardial infarction, e.g., in unstable angina pectoris (preinfarction angina), or treatment of myocardial infarction; prophylaxis of stroke in transient cerebral ischemic attacks. **Unwanted effects** result from the principal action: risk of bleeding (cerebrovascular accident, severe hemorrhagic stroke); likewise, from inhibition of prostaglandin synthesis (p. 190), erosions of gastric or intestinal mucosa, among other effects.

The therapeutic success of ASA in the above indications is not too impressive, conceivably because of the concomitant inhibition of the synthesis of **prostacyclin,** the *endogenous functional antagonist of thromboxane*. Prostacyclin is formed in *endothelial cells* through the action of cyclooxygenase (p. 188). However, endothelial cells can replace inactivated enzyme by *de novo* synthesis, which is not possible in the anuclear

platelets. Thus, the effect of acetylation persists for the lifetime of the platelet (approx. 1 week). Preferential inhibition of thromboxane formation occurs with low dosage of ASA, e.g., 300 mg/day or even twice weekly.

Inhibition of Erythrocyte Aggregation (B)

Because speed of blood flow is lowest in postcapillary venules, red blood cells have a marked tendency to aggregate in this region. There is a danger of microcirculatory disturbance with stagnation of blood flow (venostasis) and concomitant insufficient O_2 supply. Low velocity of flow also favors thrombogenesis.

Velocity of blood flow can be raised by **lowering red blood cell concentration**. Controlled **hemodilution** can be achieved by means of withdrawal of blood and replacement with a plasma substitute (p. 150). In order to maintain O_2 supply of tissues despite the hemodilution, flow volume per unit of time must be increased. Therefore, resistance vessels dilate, peripheral resistance falls, and cardiac output rises. In addition to increased flow velocity, the reduction in erythrocyte concentration contributes to decreasing the tendency to aggregate. **Indications** for hemodilution are: severe impairment of blood flow in the legs; status after cerebrovascular accident; thromboprophylaxis. A competent heart capable of carrying the extra volume load is a precondition (see above).

It should be noted that erythrocyte flexibility and, therefore, rheological properties of blood are said to be improved by **pentoxifylline.**

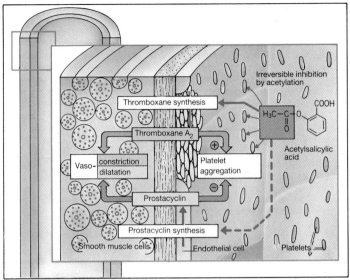

A. Inhibition by ASA of platelet aggregation

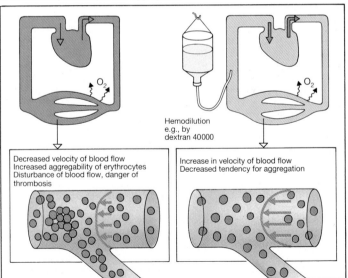

B. Inhibition of erythrocyte aggregation by hemodilution with plasma substitutes

Plasma Volume Expanders

Major blood loss entails the danger of life-threatening circulatory failure, i.e., hypovolemic shock. The immediate threat results not so much from the loss of erythrocytes, i.e., oxygen carriers, as from the reduction in volume of circulating blood.

To eliminate the threat of shock, replenishment of the circulation is essential. With moderate loss of blood, administration of a plasma volume expander may be sufficient. Blood plasma consists basically of water, electrolytes, and plasma proteins. However, a plasma substitute need not contain **plasma proteins**. These can be suitably **replaced** with **macromolecules** ("colloids") that, like plasma proteins, (1) *do not readily leave the circulation* and are *poorly filtrable in the renal glomerulus*, and (2) bind water along with its solutes due to their *colloid osmotic properties*. In this manner, they will maintain circulatory filling pressure for many hours. On the other hand, complete elimination of these colloids from the body is clearly desirable.

Compared with whole blood or plasma, plasma substitutes offer several *advantages*: they can be produced more easily and at lower cost, have a longer shelf-life, and are free of pathogens such as the hepatitis B or AIDS viruses.

Three colloids are currently employed as plasma volume expanders—the two polysaccharides, dextran and hydroxyethyl starch, as well as the polypeptide, gelatin.

Dextran is a glucose polymer formed by bacteria and linked by a $1 \rightarrow 6$ instead of the typical $1 \rightarrow 4$ bond. Commercial solutions contain dextran of a mean molecular weight of 70 kDa (**dextran 70**) or 40 kDa (**lower-molecular-weight dextran, dextran 40**).

The chain length of single molecules, however, varies widely. Smaller dextran molecules can be filtered at the glomerulus and slowly excreted in urine; the larger ones are eventually taken up and degraded by cells of the reticuloendothelial (mononuclear phagocyte) system. Apart from restoring blood volume, dextran solutions are used for hemodilution in the management of blood flow disorders (p. 148).

As for microcirculatory improvement, it is occasionally emphasized that low-molecular dextran, unlike dextran 70, may directly reduce the aggregability of erythrocytes by altering their surface properties. With prolonged use, however, larger molecules will accumulate because of the more rapid renal excretion of the smaller ones. Consequently, the molecular weight of dextran circulating in blood will tend towards a higher mean molecular weight with the passage of time.

The most important adverse effect results from the antigenicity of dextrans and consists of an **anaphylactic reaction**. This can be preempted by injection of very small dextran molecules (MW 1000; **dextran 1**), because these bind and inactivate any antibodies present without provoking an immune reaction.

Hydroxyethyl starch (hetastarch) is produced from starch. By virtue of its hydroxyethyl groups, it is metabolized more slowly and retained significantly longer in blood than would be the case with infused starch. Hydroxyethyl starch resembles dextrans in terms of its pharmacological properties and therapeutic applications.

Gelatin colloids consist of crosslinked peptide chains obtained from collagen. They are employed for blood replacement, but not for hemodilution in circulatory disturbances.

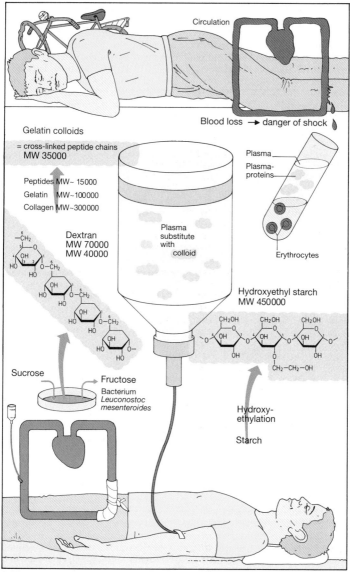

A. Plasma substitutes

Drugs Used
in Hyperlipoproteinemias

Lipoproteins serve to transport water-insoluble lipids in blood. According to density, one distinguishes: (1) chylomicrons; (2) very low-density lipoproteins (VLDL); (3) low-density lipoproteins (LDL) and (4) high-density lipoproteins (HDL). The structure of lipoproteins is shown diagrammatically in (A).

Lipoprotein metabolism. Enterocytes release absorbed lipids in the form of triglyceride-rich chylomicrons into the lymph. Bypassing the liver, these enter the circulation where they are hydrolyzed by extrahepatic endothelial lipoprotein lipases to liberate fatty acids. The remnant particles move on into liver cells and supply these with cholesterol of dietary origin. As additional *sources of cholesterol*, the liver uses HDL and LDL particles. Moreover, it synthesizes cholesterol. The key enzyme is hydroxymethylglutaryl coenzyme A reductase (HMG CoA reductase). End-product feedback inhibition enables activity of the enzyme to rise when the cellular cholesterol level falls. Cholesterol is used also in bile acid synthesis. The liver releases VLDL and HDL into the blood. Upon giving up fatty acids, the triglyceride-rich VLDL shrinks into the cholesterol-rich LDL, which undergoes receptor-mediated endocytosis into tissue cells, including hepatocytes. Cholesterol from tissue cells can be transferred to HDL and then to VLDL and LDL.

Hyperlipoproteinemias can be caused genetically (primary h.) or can occur in obesity and metabolic disorders (secondary h.). Elevated LDL–cholesterol serum concentrations are associated with an increased risk of atherosclerosis, especially when there is a concomitant decline in HDL con-centration (increase in LDL:HDL ratio).

Treatment. Various drugs are available that have different mechanisms of action and effects on LDL and VLDL (**A**). Their use is indicated in the therapy of *primary hyperlipoproteinemias*. In secondary hyperlipoproteinemias, it is imperative to lower lipoprotein levels by dietary restriction, treatment of the primary disease, or both. Trials with colestyramine, clofibrate, or nicotinic acid have failed to establish a positive effect on overall mortality, beyond a reduction in lipid concentration and slowing of the progression of atheromatosis.

Drugs. *Colestyramine* and *colestipol* are nonabsorbable anion-exchange resins. By virtue of inactivating bile acids, they promote consumption of cholesterol for the synthesis of bile acids; in addition, they can interfere with the absorption not only of cholesterol, but also of fats and fat-soluble vitamins (A, D, E, K). They also adsorb drugs such as digitoxin, and decrease their absorption. At the required dosage (approx. 3 x 5 to 10 g/day) they cause diverse gastrointestinal disturbances.

Lovastatin is of fungal origin. Its active metabolite resembles HMG and inhibits HMG CoA reductase, resulting in a particularly large decline in LDL-cholesterol concentration. Simvastatin and pravastatin are related substances.

β-*Sitosterol*, a plant cholesterol derivative that is absorbed poorly inhibits enteral cholesterol uptake.

Clofibrate and derivatives (such as bezafibrate, etofibrate, gemfibrozil) lower plasma lipids by an unknown mechanism. They may damage the liver and skeletal musculature. *Nicotinic acid* and derivatives are not well tolerated because of cutaneous vasodilation ("flushing") and hypotension that may be associated with it.

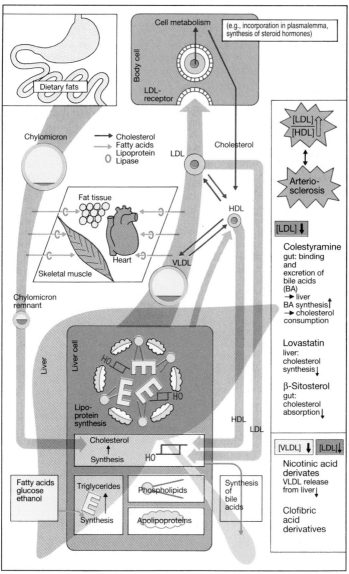

A. Drug treatment of hyperlipoproteinemias

Diuretics—an Overview

Diuretics (saluretics) elicit increased production of urine (diuresis). In the strict sense, the term is applied to drugs with a direct renal action. The predominant action of such agents is to augment urine excretion by inhibiting the reabsorption of NaCl and water.

The most important **indications** for the use of diuretics are:

Mobilization of edemas (A). In edema there is swelling of tissues due to accumulation of fluid, chiefly in the extracellular (interstitial) space. When a diuretic is given, increased renal excretion of Na^+ and H_2O causes a reduction in plasma volume with hemoconcentration. As a result, plasma protein concentration rises along with oncotic pressure. As the latter operates to attract water, fluid will shift from interstitium into the capillary bed. The fluid content of tissues thus falls and the edemas recede. The decrease in plasma volume and interstitial volume means a diminution of the extracellular fluid volume (EFV). Depending on the condition, use is made of: thiazides, loop diuretics, aldosterone antagonists, and osmotic diuretics.

Antihypertensive therapy. Diuretics have been used as drugs of first choice for lowering elevated blood pressure (p. 286). Even at low dosage, they decrease peripheral resistance (without significantly reducing EFV) and thereby normalize blood pressure.

Therapy of congestive heart failure. By lowering peripheral resistance, diuretics aid the heart in ejecting blood (reduction in afterload, p. 282); cardiac output and exercise tolerance are increased. Due to the increased excretion of fluid, EFV and venous return decrease (reduction in preload, p. 282). Symptoms of venous congestion, such as ankle edema and hepatic enlargement, subside. The drugs principally used are thiazides (possibly combined with K^+-sparing diuretics) and loop diuretics.

Prophylaxis of renal failure. In circulatory failure (shock), e.g., secondary to massive hemorrhage, renal production of urine may cease (anuria). By means of diuretics, an attempt is made to maintain urinary flow. Use of either osmotic or loop diuretics is indicated.

Massive use of diuretics entails a hazard of **adverse effects**: (1) the decrease in blood volume can lead to hypotension and *collapse*; (2) blood viscosity rises due to the increase in erythro- and thrombocyte concentration, bringing an increased risk of intravascular coagulation or *thrombosis.*

When depletion of NaCl and water (EFV reduction) occurs as a result of diuretic therapy, the body can initiate **counter-regulatory responses (B)**, viz., activation of the renin–angiotensin–aldosterone system (p. 124). Because of the diminished blood volume, renal blood flow is jeopardized. This leads to release from the kidneys of the hormone, renin, which enzymatically catalyzes the formation of angiotensin I. Angiotensin I is converted to angiotensin II by the action of angiotensin-converting enzyme (ACE). Angiotensin II stimulates release of aldosterone. The mineralocorticoid promotes renal reabsorption of NaCl and water and thus counteracts the effect of diuretics. ACE inhibitors augment the effectiveness of diuretics by preventing this counter-regulatory response.

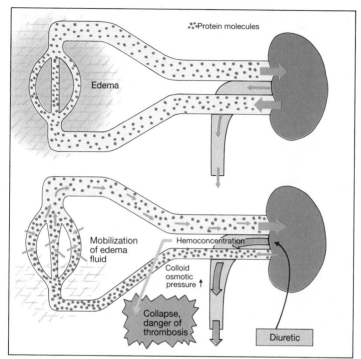

A. Mechanism of edema fluid mobilization by diuretics

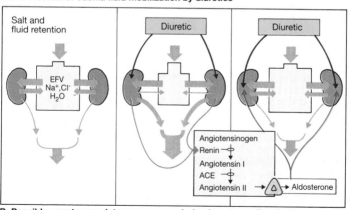

B. Possible counter-regulatory responses during long-term diuretic therapy

NaCl Reabsorption
in the Kidney (A)

The smallest functional unit of the kidney is the **nephron**. In the glomerular capillary loops, ultrafiltration of plasma fluid into Bowman's capsule (BC) yields primary urine. In the proximal tubules (pT), approx. 70% of the ultrafiltrate is retrieved by iso-osmotic reabsorption of NaCl and water. In the thick portion of the ascending limb of Henle's loop (HL), NaCl is absorbed unaccompanied by water. This is the prerequisite for the hairpin countercurrent mechanism that allows build-up of a very high NaCl concentration in the renal medulla. In the distal tubules (dT), NaCl and water are again jointly reabsorbed. At the end of the nephron, this process involves an aldosterone-controlled exchange of Na^+ against K^+ or H^+. In the collecting tubule (C), vasopressin (antidiuretic hormone, ADH) increases the epithelial permeability for water, which is drawn into the hyperosmolar milieu of the renal medulla and thus retained in the body. As a result, a concentrated urine enters the renal pelvis.

Na^+ transport through the tubular cells basically occurs in similar fashion in all segments of the nephron. The intracellular concentration of Na^+ is significantly below that in primary urine. This concentration gradient is the driving force for entry of Na^+ into the cytosol of tubular cells. A carrier mechanism moves Na^+ across the membrane. Energy liberated during this influx can be utilized for the coupled outward transport of another particle against a gradient. From the cell interior, Na^+ is moved under expenditure of energy (ATP hydrolysis) by Na^+/K^+-ATPase into the extracellular space. The enzyme molecules are confined to the basolateral parts of the cell membrane, facing the interstitium; Na^+ can, therefore, not escape back into tubular fluid.

All diuretics inhibit Na^+ reabsorption. Basically, either the inward or the outward transport of Na^+ can be affected.

Osmotic Diuretics (B)

Agents: mannitol, sorbitol. *Site of action*: mainly the proximal tubules. *Mode of action*: since NaCl and H_2O are reabsorbed together in the proximal tubules, Na^+ concentration in the tubular fluid does not change despite the extensive reabsorption of Na^+ and H_2O. Body cells lack transport mechanisms for polyhydric alcohols such as mannitol (structure on p. 167) and sorbitol, which are thus prevented from penetrating cell membranes. Therefore, they need to be given by intravenous infusion. They also cannot be reabsorbed from the tubular fluid after glomerular filtration. These agents bind water osmotically and retain it in the tubular lumen. When Na ions are taken up into the tubule cell, water cannot follow in the usual amount. The fall in urine Na^+ concentration reduces Na^+ reabsorption, in part because the reduced concentration gradient towards the interior of tubule cells means a reduced driving force for Na^+ influx. The result of osmotic diuresis is a large volume of dilute urine.

Indications: prophylaxis of renal hypovolemic failure, mobilization of brain edema, and acute glaucoma.

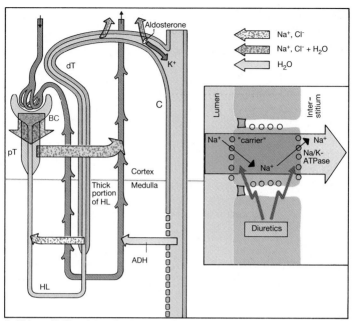

A. Kidney: NaCl reabsorption in nephron and tubular cell

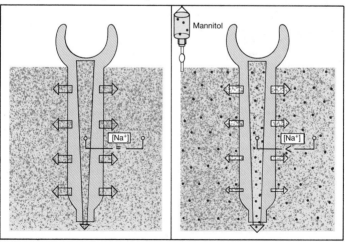

B. NaCl reabsorption in proximal tubule and effect of mannitol

Diuretics of the Sulfonamide Type

These drugs contain the sulfonamide group $-SO_2NH_2$. They are suitable for oral administration. In addition to being filtered at the glomerulus, they are subject to tubular secretion. Their concentration in urine is higher than in blood. They act on the luminal membrane of the tubule cells. Loop diuretics have the highest efficacy. Thiazides are most frequently used. Their forerunners, the carbonic anhydrase inhibitors, are now restricted to special indications.

Carbonic anhydrase (CAH) inhibitors, such as acetazolamide and sulthiame, act predominantly in the proximal tubule. CAH catalyzes CO_2 hydration/dehydration reactions:

$$H^+ + HCO_3^- \rightleftharpoons H_2CO_3 \rightleftharpoons H_2O + CO_2.$$

The enzyme is used in tubule cells to generate H^+, which is secreted into the tubular fluid in exchange for Na^+. There, H^+ captures HCO_3^-, leading to formation of CO_2 via the unstable carbonic acid. Membrane-permeable CO_2 is taken up into the tubule cell and is used to regenerate H^+ and HCO_3^-. When the enzyme is inhibited, these reactions are retarded so that less Na^+, HCO_3^-, and water are reabsorbed from the fast-flowing tubular fluid. Loss of HCO_3^- leads to acidosis. The diuretic effectiveness of CAH inhibitors decreases with prolonged use. CAH is also involved in the production of ocular aqueous humor. Present *indications* for drugs in this class include: acute glaucoma, acute mountain sickness, and epilepsy.

Loop diuretics include furosemide (frusemide), piretanide, and bumetanide. With oral administration, a strong diuresis occurs within 1 h but persists for only about 4 h. The effect is rapid, intense, and brief (high-ceiling diuresis). The site of action of these agents is the thick portion of the ascending limb of Henle's loop, where they inhibit $Na^+/K^+/2Cl^-$-cotransport. As a result, these electrolytes, together with water, are excreted in larger amounts. Excretion of Ca^{2+} and Mg^{2+} also increases. Special *toxic effects* include: (reversible) hearing loss, enhanced sensitivity to renotoxic agents. *Indications*: pulmonary edema (added advantage of i.v. injection in left ventricular failure: immediate dilatation of venous capacitance vessels → preload reduction); refractoriness to thiazide diuretics, e.g., in renal hypovolemic failure with creatinine clearance reduction (<30 mL/min); prophylaxis of acute renal hypovolemic failure; hypercalcemia.

Thiazide diuretics (benzothiadiazines) include hydrochlorothiazide, benzthiazide, trichlormethiazide, and cyclothiazide. A long-acting analogue is chlorthalidone. These drugs affect the intermediate segment of the distal tubules, where they inhibit a Na^+/Cl^-cotransport. Thus, reabsorption of NaCl and water is inhibited. Renal excretion of Ca^{2+} decreases, that of Mg^{2+} increases. *Indications* are hypertension, cardiac failure, and mobilization of edema.

Unwanted effects of sulfonamide-type diuretics: (a) *hypokalemia* is a consequence of excessive K^+ loss in the terminal segments of the distal tubule, where increased amounts of Na^+ are available for exchange with K^+; (b) hyperglycemia and glycosuria; (c) hyperuricemia—increase in serum urate levels may precipitate gout in predisposed patients. Sulfonamide diuretics compete with urate for the tubular organic anion secretory system.

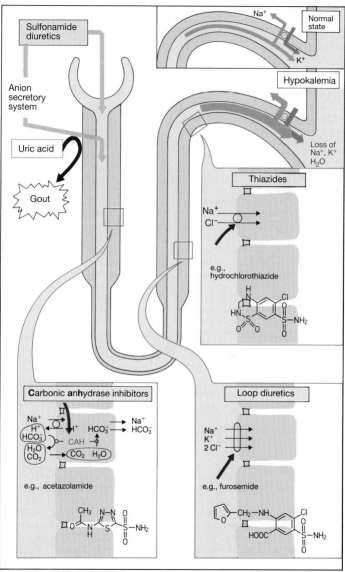

A. Diuretics of the sulfonamide type

Potassium-Sparing Diuretics (A)

These agents act in the distal portion of the distal tubule and the proximal part of the collecting ducts where Na$^+$ is reabsorbed in exchange for K$^+$ or H$^+$. Their diuretic effectiveness is relatively minor. In contrast to sulfonamide diuretics (p. 158), there is no increase in K$^+$ secretion; rather, there is a risk of hyperkalemia. These drugs are suitable for oral administration.

a) *Triamterene* and *amiloride*, in addition to glomerular filtration, undergo secretion in the proximal tubule. They act on the luminal membrane of tubule cells. Both inhibit the entry of Na$^+$, hence its exchange for K$^+$ and H$^+$. They are mostly used in combination with thiazide diuretics, e.g., hydrochlorothiazide, because the opposing effects on K$^+$ excretion cancel each other, while the effects on secretion of NaCl and water are complementary.

b) *Aldosterone antagonists.* The mineralocorticoid aldosterone promotes the reabsorption of Na$^+$ (Cl$^-$ and H$_2$O follow) in exchange for K$^+$. Its hormonal effect on protein synthesis leads to augmentation of the reabsorptive capacity of tubule cells. *Spironolactone*, as well as its *metabolite canrenone*, are antagonists at the aldosterone receptor and attenuate the effect of the hormone. The diuretic effect of spironolactone develops fully only with continuous administration for several days. Two possible explanations are: (i) the conversion of spironolactone into and accumulation of the more slowly eliminated metabolite canrenone; (ii) an inhibition of aldosterone-stimulated protein synthesis would become noticeable only if existing proteins had become nonfunctional and needed to be replaced by *de novo* synthesis. A particular *adverse effect* results from interference with gonadal hormones, as evidenced by the development of gynecomastia (enlargement of male breast). *Clinical uses* include conditions of increased aldosterone secretion, e.g., liver cirrhosis with ascites.

Ethacrynic Acid

This substance affects tubular cell function along the entire nephron, presumably by inhibiting Na$^+$/K$^+$-ATPases. Ethacrynic acid resembles loop diuretics in terms of pharmacokinetics, time course, and intensity of effect, as well as toxicity (e.g., ototoxicity).

Antidiuretic Hormone (ADH) and Derivatives (B)

ADH, a nonapeptide, is released from the posterior pituitary gland and promotes reabsorption of water in the kidney. It enhances the permeability of collecting duct epithelium for water (but not for electrolytes). As a result, water is drawn from urine into the hyperosmolar interstitium of the medulla. Nicotine augments (p. 110) and ethanol decreases ADH release. At concentrations above those required for antidiuresis, ADH stimulates smooth musculature, including that of blood vessels ("**vasopressin**"). Blood pressure rises; coronary vasoconstriction can precipitate angina pectoris. *Lypressin* (8-L-lysine-vasopressin) acts like ADH. Other derivatives may display only one of the two actions. *Desmopressin* is used for the therapy of diabetes insipidus (ADH deficiency) and nocturnal enuresis; it is given by injection or via the nasal mucosa (as "snuff"). *Felypressin* and *ornipressin* serve as adjunctive vasoconstrictors in infiltration local anesthesia (p. 198).

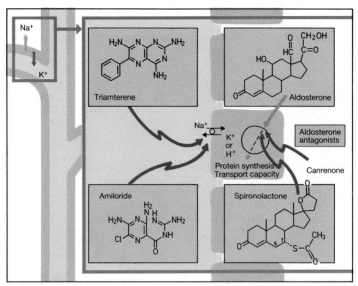

A. Potassium-sparing diuretics

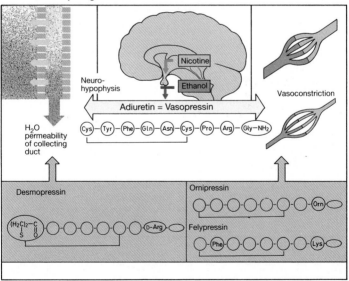

B. Antidiuretic hormone (ADH) and derivatives

Drugs for Gastric
and Duodenal Ulcers

In the area of a gastric or duodenal peptic ulcer, the mucosa has been attacked by digestive juices to such an extent as to expose the subjacent connective tissue layer (submucosa). This self-digestion occurs when the equilibrium between the corrosive hydrochloric acid and the acid-neutralizing mucus, which forms a protective cover on the mucosal surface, is shifted in favor of hydrochloric acid. The acid (H^+) concentration may be too high or mucus production may be too low. Although an ulcer will heal without treatment, usually within about 6 weeks, drugs are employed with the following **therapeutic aims**: (1) relief of pain; and (2) acceleration of healing to lessen the risk of dangerous complications. Two therapeutic approaches are available: (1) reduction of H^+ concentration (**A**); (2) mucosal protection (p. 164).

I. Drugs for Lowering
Acid Concentration

Ia. Acid neutralization. H^+-binding groups, such as CO_3^{2-}, HCO_3^-, or OH^-, together with their counter ions, are contained in the **antacid drugs** calcium carbonate ($CaCO_3$), sodium bicarbonate ($NaHCO_3$), magnesium hydroxide ($Mg(OH)_2$), and aluminum hydroxide ($Al(OH)_3$). Neutralization reactions occurring after intake of $CaCO_3$ and $NaHCO_3$, respectively, are shown in (**A**) at left. With nonabsorbable antacids, the counter ion is dissolved in the acidic gastric juice in the process of neutralization. Upon mixture with the alkaline pancreatic secretion in the duodenum, it is largely precipitated again by basic groups, e.g., as $CaCO_3$ or $AlPO_4$, and excreted in the feces. Therefore, systemic absorption of counter ions or basic residues is minor. In the presence of renal insufficiency, however, absorption of even small amounts may cause an increase in plasma levels of counter ions (e.g., magnesium intoxication with paralysis and cardiac disturbances).

Intake of large amounts of $Al(OH)_3$ can deplete the body store of phosphate by precipitation of $AlPO_4$. Adsorption of a concomitantly present drug to this precipitate can withdraw it from absorption.

Na^+ ions remain in solution even in the presence of HCO_3^--rich pancreatic secretions and are subject to absorption, like HCO_3^-. Because of the uptake of Na^+, use of $NaHCO_3$ must be avoided in conditions requiring restriction of NaCl intake, such as hypertension, cardiac failure, or edema.

Since food has a buffering effect, antacids are taken between meals (e.g., 1 and 3 h after meals and at bedtime). Nonabsorbable antacids are preferred. Because $Mg(OH)_2$ produces a laxative effect (cause: osmotic action, p. 166, and/or release of cholecystokinin by Mg^{2+}) and $Al(OH)_3$ produces constipation (cause: astringent action of Al^{3+}, p. 174), these two antacids are frequently used in combination.

Ib. Inhibitors of acid production. Acting on their respective receptors, the transmitter acetylcholine, the hormone gastrin, and histamine released intramucosally stimulate the parietal cells of the gastric mucosa to increase output of HCl. The effects of acetylcholine and histamine can be abolished by oral administration of antagonists that reach the parietal cells via the blood.

The cholinoceptor antagonist **pirenzepine**, unlike atropine, prefers cholinoceptors of the M_1 type, does not act in the CNS, and produces fe-

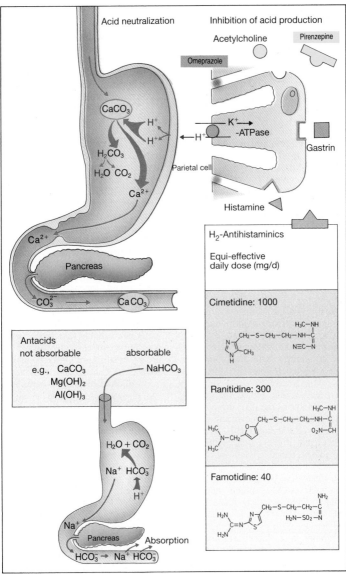

A. Drugs used to lower gastric acid concentration or production

wer anticholinergic side effects (p. 104). The cholinoceptors on the parietal cell probably belong to the M_3-subtype, and the site of action of pirenzepine in the gastric mucosa is not precisely known.

Histamine receptors on the parietal cells belong to the H_2-type (p. 114) and are blocked by **H_2-antihistaminics** (p. 163). Remarkably, antihistaminics also diminish responsivity to other stimulants, e.g., gastrin (in gastrin-producing pancreatic tumors, Zollinger–Ellison syndrome). The explanation may be that gastrin and acetylcholine also stimulate the parietal cells indirectly by promoting the release of histamine in the gastric mucosa. *Cimetidine*, the first H_2-antihistaminic used therapeutically, only rarely produces side effects (CNS disturbances such as confusion; endocrine effects in the male such as gynecomastia, decreased libido, impotence). Cimetidine may inhibit hepatic biotransformation of other drugs. More recently introduced congeners, *ranitidine, famotidine* and *nizatidine*, exhibit higher potency and do not interfere with the biotransformation of other drugs.

Omeprazole (p. 163), via an active metabolite, acts at the decisive site: it inhibits the ATP-driven pump that transports H^+ in exchange for K^+ into the gastric juice (H^+/K^+-ATPase). This agent affords maximal inhibition of acid secretion.

II. Protective Drugs

Sucralfate (A) contains numerous aluminum hydroxide residues that can buffer H^+. However, it is not an antacid because it fails to lower the acidity of gastric juice. After oral administration, sucralfate molecules undergo cross-linking in gastric juice, forming a paste that adheres to mucosal defects and exposed deeper layers. Here sucralfate intercepts H^+. Protected from acid, and also from pepsin, trypsin, and bile acids, the mucosal defect can heal more rapidly. Sucralfate is taken on an empty stomach (1 h before meals and at bedtime). It is well tolerated; however, released Al^{3+} ions can cause constipation.

Misoprostol (B) is a semisynthetic prostaglandin derivative with greater stability than natural prostaglandin, permitting absorption after oral administration. Like locally released prostaglandins, it promotes mucus production and inhibits acid secretion. Additional systemic effects (frequent diarrhea; risk of precipitating contractions of the gravid uterus) significantly restrict its therapeutic utility.

Carbenoxolone (B) is a derivative of glycyrrhetinic acid, which occurs in the sap of licorice root (succus liquiritiae). Carbenoxolone stimulates mucus production. At the same time, it has an aldosterone-like action that promotes renal reabsorption of NaCl and water and may, therefore, exacerbate hypertension, congestive heart failure, or edemas. It is practically obsolete.

Colloidal bismuth compounds, e.g., bismuth subsalicylate and subcitrate kill *Helicobacter pylori* bacteria that may colonize the gastric mucosa and that promote mucosal injury (e.g., gastritis) as an aggressive factor. It is still unclear whether bismuth compounds have any special value in antiulcer therapy.

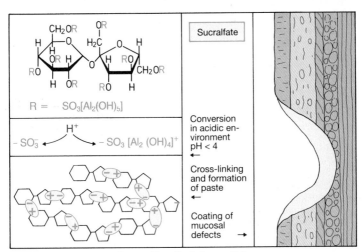

A. Chemical structure and protective effect of sucralfate

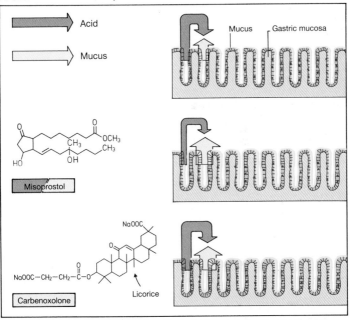

B. Chemical structure and protective effect of misoprostol and carbenoxolone

Laxatives

Laxatives promote and facilitate bowel evacuation by acting locally to stimulate intestinal peristalsis, to soften bowel contents, or both.

1. Bulk laxatives. Distention of the intestinal wall by bowel contents stimulates propulsive movements of the gut musculature (peristalsis). Activation of intramural mechanoreceptors induces a neurally mediated ascending reflex contraction (red in **A**) and descending relaxation (blue) whereby the intraluminal bolus is moved in the anal direction.

Hydrophilic colloids or bulk gels (B) comprise insoluble and nonabsorbable carbohydrate substances that expand on taking up water in the bowel. *Vegetable fibers* in the diet act in this manner. They consist of the indigestible plant cell walls containing homoglycans that are resistant to digestive enzymes, e.g., *cellulose* (1 → 4β-linked glucose molecules vs. 1 → 4α glucoside bond in starch, p. 151).

Bran, a grain milling waste product, and *linseed* (flaxseed) are both rich in cellulose. Other hydrophilic colloids derive from the seeds of *Plantago* species or *karaya gum*. Ingestion of hydrophilic gels for the prophylaxis of constipation usually entails a low risk of side effects. However, with low fluid intake in combination with a pathological bowel stenosis, mucilaginous viscous material could cause bowel occlusion (ileus).

Osmotically active laxatives (C) are soluble but nonabsorbable particles that retain water in the bowel by virtue of their osmotic action. The osmotic pressure (particle concentration) of bowel contents always corresponds to that of the extracellular space. The intestinal mucosa is unable to maintain a higher or lower osmotic pressure of the luminal contents. Therefore, absorption of molecules (e.g., glucose, NaCl) occurs iso-osmotically, i.e., solute molecules are followed by a corresponding amount of water. Conversely, water remains in the bowel when molecules cannot be absorbed.

With *Epsom and Glauber's salts* ($MgSO_4$ and Na_2SO_4, respectively), the SO_4^{2-} anion is nonabsorbable and retains cations to maintain electroneutrality. Mg^{2+} ions are also believed to promote release from the duodenal mucosa of cholecystokinin/pancreozymin, a polypeptide that also stimulates peristalsis. These so-called saline cathartics elicit a watery bowel discharge 1—3 h after administration (preferably in isotonic solution). They are used to purge the bowel (e.g., before bowel surgery) or to hasten the elimination of ingested poisons. Glauber's salt (high Na^+ content) is contraindicated in hypertension, congestive heart failure, or edema; Epsom salt is contraindicated in renal failure (risk of magnesium intoxication).

Osmotic laxative effects are also produced by the *polyhydric alcohols*, *mannitol* and *sorbitol*, which unlike glucose cannot be transported through the intestinal mucosa, as well as by the nonhydrolyzable disaccharide, *lactulose*. Fermentation of lactulose by colon bacteria results in acidification of bowel contents and microfloral damage. Lactulose is used in hepatic failure in order to prevent bacterial production of ammonia and its subsequent absorption (absorbable NH_3 → nonabsorbable NH_4^+), so as to forestall hepatic coma.

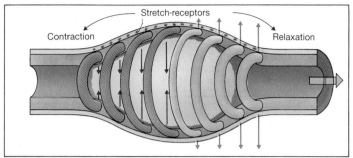

A. Stimulation of peristalsis by an intraluminal bolus

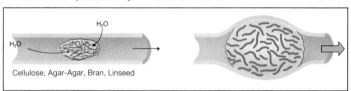

B. Bulk laxatives

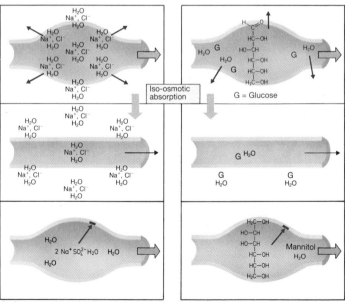

C. Osmotically active laxatives

2. Irritant laxatives—purgatives/ cathartics.

Laxatives in this group exert an irritant action on the enteric mucosa (**A**). Consequently, less fluid is absorbed than is secreted. The increased filling of the bowel promotes peristalsis; excitation of sensory nerve endings elicits enteral hypermotility. According to the site of irritation, one distinguishes the small bowel irritant castor oil from the large bowel irritants anthraquinone and diphenolmethane derivatives (for details see p. 170).

Misuse of laxatives. It is a widely held belief that at least one bowel movement per day is essential for health, yet three bowel evacuations per week are quite normal. The desire for frequent bowel emptying probably stems from the time-honored, albeit mistaken, notion that absorption of colon contents is harmful. Thus, purging has long been part of standard therapeutic practice. Nowadays it is known that intoxication from intestinal substances is impossible as long as the liver functions normally. Nonetheless, purgatives continue to be sold as remedies to "cleanse the blood" or to rid the body of "corrupt humors."

There can be no objection to ingestion of bulk substances for the purpose of supplementing low-residue "modern diets." However, use of irritant purgatives or cathartics is not without hazards. Specifically, there is a risk of laxative dependence, i.e., the inability to do without them. Chronic intake of irritant purgatives disrupts the water and electrolyte balance of the body and can thus cause symptoms of illness (e.g., cardiac arrhythmias secondary to hypokalemia).

Causes of purgative dependence (B). The defecation reflex is triggered when the sigmoid colon and rectum are filled. A natural defecation empties the large bowel up to and including the descending colon. The interval between natural stool evacuations depends on the speed with which these colon segments are refilled. A large bowel irritant purgative clears out the entire colon. Accordingly, a longer period is needed until the next natural defecation can occur. Fearing constipation, the user becomes impatient and again resorts to the laxative, which then produces the desired effect as a result of emptying out the upper colonic segments. Therefore, a "compensatory pause" following cessation of laxative use must not give cause for concern (1).

In the colon, semifluid material entering from the small bowel is thickened by absorption of water and salts (from about 1 000 mL to 150 mL per day). If, due to the action of an irritant purgative, the colon empties prematurely, an enteral loss of NaCl, KCl, and water will be incurred. In order to forestall depletion of NaCl and water, the body responds with an increased release of aldosterone (p. 160), which stimulates their resorption in the kidney. The action of aldosterone is, however, associated with an increased renal excretion of KCl. The enteral and renal K^+ loss add up to a K^+ depletion of the body, evidenced by a fall in serum K^+ concentration (hypokalemia). This condition is accompanied by a reduction in intestinal peristalsis (bowel atonia). The affected individual infers "constipation," again partakes of the purgative and the vicious circle is closed (2).

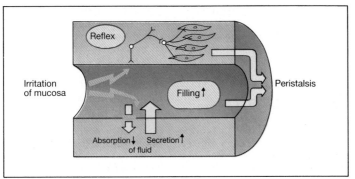

A. Stimulation of peristalsis by mucosal irritation

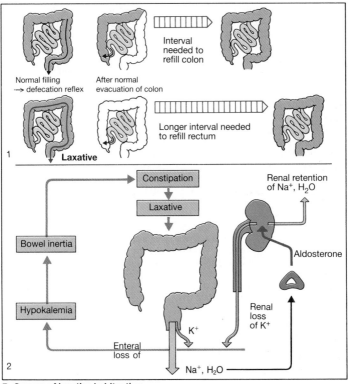

B. Causes of laxative habituation

Small Bowel Irritant Purgative, Ricinoleic Acid

Castor oil comes from *Ricinus communis* (castor plants; Fig: sprig, panicle, seed); it is obtained from the first cold-pressing of the seed (shown in natural size). Oral administration of 10–30 mL of castor oil is followed within 0.5 to 3 h by discharge of a watery stool. Ricinoleic acid, but not the oil itself, is active. The former arises as a result of the regular processes involved in fat digestion: the duodenal mucosa releases the enterohormone cholecystokinin/pancreozymin into the blood. The hormone elicits contraction of the gallbladder and discharge of bile acids via the bile duct, as well as release of lipase from the pancreas (intestinal peristalsis is also stimulated). Because of its massive effect, castor oil is hardly suitable for the treatment of ordinary constipation. It can be employed after oral ingestion of a toxin in order to hasten elimination and to reduce absorption of the toxin from the gut. Castor oil is not indicated after the ingestion of lipophilic toxins likely to depend on bile acids for their absorption.

Large Bowel Irritant Purgatives
(pp. 172ff)

Anthraquinone derivatives (p. 173 A) are of plant origin. They occur in the leaves (*Folia sennae*) or fruits (*Fructus sennae*) of the *Senna* plant, the bark of *Rhamnus frangulae* and *Rh. purshiana* (*Cortex frangulae, Cascara sagrada*), the roots of rhubarb (*Rhizoma rhei*), or the leaf extract from *Aloe* species (p. 172). The structural features of anthraquinone derivatives are illustrated by the prototype structure depicted on p. 173 A. Among other substituents, the anthraquinone nucleus contains hydroxyl groups, one of which is bound to a sugar (glucose, rhamnose). Following ingestion of galenical preparations or of the anthraquinone glycosides, discharge of soft stool occurs after a latency of 6–8 h. The anthraquinone glycosides themselves are inactive, but are converted by colon bacteria to the active free aglycones.

Diphenolmethane derivatives (p. 173 B) were developed from *phenolphthalein*, an accidentally discovered laxative, use of which had been noted to result in rare but severe allergic reactions. *Bisacodyl* and *sodium picosulfate* are converted by gut bacteria into the active colon-irritant principle. Given by the enteral route, bisacodyl is subject to hydrolysis of acetyl residues, absorption, conjugation in the liver, and biliary secretion into the duodenum. Oral use is followed after approx. 6–8 h by discharge of soft formed stool. When given by suppository, bisacodyl produces its effect within 1 h.

Indications for colon-irritant purgatives are the prevention of straining at stool following surgery, myocardial infarction, or stroke; provision of relief in painful diseases of the anus, e.g., fissure, hemorrhoids.

Purgatives must not be given in abdominal complaints of unclear origin.

3. Lubricant laxatives. Liquid paraffin (paraffinum subliquidum) is almost nonabsorbable and makes feces softer and more easily passed. It interferes with the absorption of fat-soluble vitamins by trapping them. The few absorbed paraffin particles may induce formation of foreign-body granulomas in enteric lymph nodes (paraffinomas). Aspiration into the bronchial tract can result in lipoid pneumonia. Because of these adverse effects, its use is not advisable.

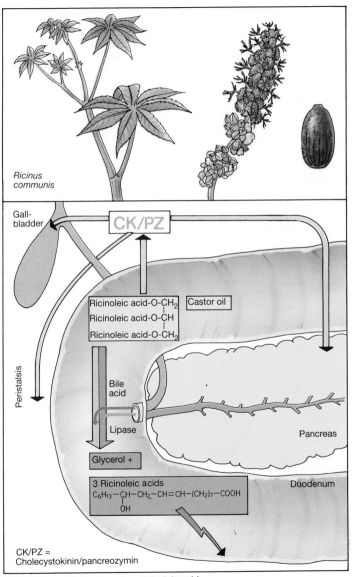

Ricinus
communis

Gall-
bladder

CK/PZ

Peristalsis

Ricinoleic acid-O-CH₂
Ricinoleic acid-O-CH   Castor oil
Ricinoleic acid-O-CH₂

Bile
acid

Lipase

Glycerol +

3 Ricinoleic acids
$C_6H_{13}-CH-CH_2-CH=CH-(CH_2)_7-COOH$
         OH

Pancreas

Duodenum

CK/PZ =
Cholecystokinin/pancreozymin

A. Small-bowel irritant laxative: ricinoleic acid

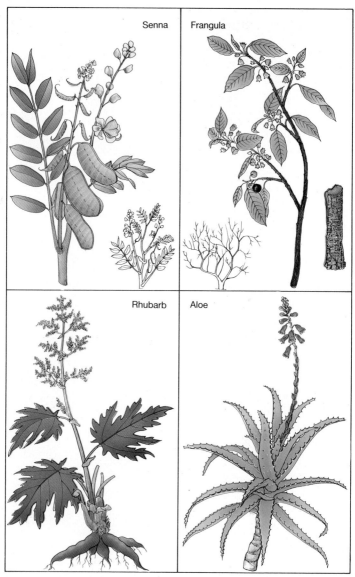

Senna

Frangula

Rhubarb

Aloe

A. Plants containing anthraquinone glycosides

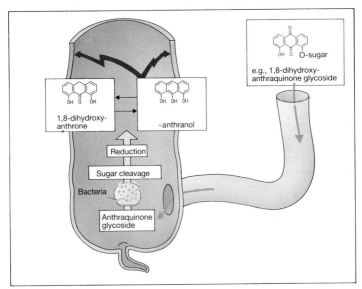

A. Large bowel irritant laxatives: anthraquinone derivatives

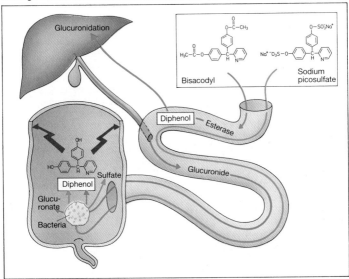

B. Large bowel irritant laxatives: diphenylmethane derivatives

Antidiarrheal Agents

Causes of diarrhea (in red): Many bacteria (e.g., *Vibrio cholerae*) secrete **toxins** that inhibit the ability of mucosal enterocytes to absorb NaCl and water and, at the same time, stimulate mucosal secretory activity. **Bacteria** or **viruses** that invade the gut wall cause inflammation characterized by increased fluid secretion into the lumen. The enteric musculature reacts with increased peristalsis.

The **aims** of antidiarrheal **therapy** are to prevent (1) dehydration and electrolyte depletion, and (2) excessively high stool frequency. The different **therapeutic approaches** (in green) listed are variously suited for these purposes.

Adsorbent powders are nonabsorbable materials with a large surface area. These bind diverse substances including toxins, permitting them to be inactivated and eliminated. *Medicinal charcoal* possesses a particularly large surface because of the preserved cell structures. The recommended effective antidiarrheal dose is in the range of 4–8 g. Other adsorbents are kaolin (hydrated aluminum silicate) and chalk.

Oral rehydration solution (g/L of boiled water: NaCl 3.5, glucose 20, NaHCO$_3$ 2.5, KCl 1.5). Oral administration of glucose-containing salt solutions enables fluids to be absorbed because toxins do not impair the cotransport of Na$^+$ and glucose (as well as of H$_2$O) through the mucosal epithelium. In this manner, although frequent discharge of stool is not prevented, dehydration is successfully corrected.

Opioids. Activation of opioid receptors in the enteric nerve plexus results in inhibition of propulsive motor activity and enhancement of segmentation activity. This antidiarrheal effect was formerly induced by application of *opium tincture* (*paregoric*) containing *morphine*. Because of the CNS effects (sedation, respiratory depression, physical dependence), derivatives with peripheral actions have been developed. Whereas *diphenoxylate* can still produce clear CNS effects, *loperamide* does not affect brain functions at normal dosage. Loperamide is, therefore, the opioid antidiarrheal of first choice. The prolonged contact time of intestinal contents and mucosa may also improve absorption of fluid. With overdosage, there is a hazard of ileus.

Antibacterial drugs. Use of these agents (e.g., co-trimoxazole, p. 258) is only rational when bacteria are the cause of diarrhea. This is rarely the case. It should be kept in mind that antibiotics also damage the intestinal flora, which in turn can give rise to diarrhea.

Astringents such as tannic acid (home remedy: black tea) or metal salts precipitate surface proteins and are thought to help seal the mucosal epithelium. Protein denaturation must not include cellular proteins, for this would mean cell death. Although astringents induce constipation (cf. Al^{3+} salts, p. 162), a therapeutic effect in diarrhea is doubtful.

Demulcents, e.g., pectin (home remedy: grated apples) are carbohydrates that expand on absorbing water. They improve the consistency of bowel contents; beyond that they are devoid of any favorable effect.

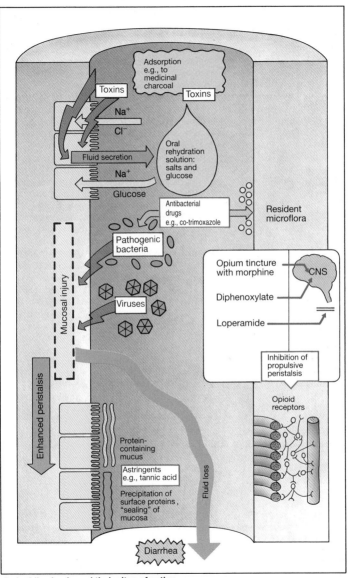

A. Antidiarrheals and their sites of action

Drugs Affecting Motor Function

The smallest structural unit of skeletal musculature is the striated muscle fiber. It contracts in response to an impulse of its motor nerve. In executing motor programs, the brain sends impulses to the spinal cord. These converge on α-motoneurons in the anterior horn of the spinal medulla. Efferent axons course, bundled in motor nerves, to skeletal muscles. Simple reflex contractions to sensory stimuli, conveyed via the dorsal roots to the motoneurons, occur without participation of the brain. Neural circuits that propagate afferent impulses into the spinal cord contain inhibitory interneurons. These serve to prevent a possible overexcitation of motoneurons (or excessive muscle contractions) due to the constant barrage of sensory stimuli.

Neuromuscular transmission (B) of motor nerve impulses to the striated muscle fiber takes place at the motor end plate. The nerve impulse liberates acetylcholine (ACh) from the axon terminal, and it binds to *nicotinic cholinoceptors* (p. 64) at the motor end plate. Activation of the receptors leads to depolarization of the end plate, which elicits a propagated action potential (AP) in the surrounding sarcolemma. The AP triggers a release of Ca^{2+} from its storage organelles, the sarcoplasmic reticulum (SR), within the muscle fiber; the rise in Ca^{2+} concentration induces a contraction of the myofilaments (electromechanical coupling). Meanwhile, ACh is hydrolyzed by acetylcholinesterase (p. 100); excitation of the end plate subsides. If no AP follows, Ca^{2+} is taken up again by the SR and the myofilaments relax.

Clinically important drugs (with the exception of dantrolene) all interfere with neural control of the muscle cell (A, B, p. 178).

Centrally acting muscle relaxants (A) lower muscle tone by augmenting the activity of intraspinal inhibitory interneurons. They are used in the treatment of painful muscle spasm, e.g., in spinal disorders. *Benzodiazepines* enhance the effectiveness of the inhibitory transmitter GABA (p. 216). *Baclofen* stimulates $GABA_B$ receptors.

The **convulsant toxins**, *tetanus toxin* (cause of wound tetanus) and *strychnine* diminish the efficacy of interneuronal synaptic inhibition mediated by the amino acid glycine (A). As a consequence of an unrestrained spread of nerve impulses in the spinal cord, motor convulsions develop. The involvement of respiratory muscle groups endangers life.

Botulinus toxin from Clostridium botulinum is the most potent poison known. The lethal dose in an adult is approx. 3×10^{-6} mg. The toxin inhibits the release of ACh from motor (and also parasympathetic) nerve endings. Death is caused by paralysis of respiratory muscles.

A pathological *rise in serum Mg^{2+}* levels also causes inhibition of neuromuscular transmission.

Dantrolene interferes with electromechanical coupling in the muscle cell by inhibiting Ca^{2+} release from the SR. It is employed in spinal diseases giving rise to painful muscle spasms and in skeletal muscle disorders involving excessive release of Ca^{2+} (malignant hyperthermia).

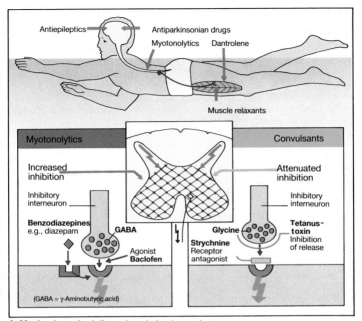

A. Mechanisms for influencing skeletal muscle tone

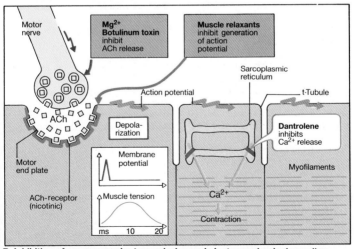

B. Inhibition of neuromuscular transmission and electromechanical coupling

Muscle Relaxants

Muscle relaxants cause a *flaccid paralysis of skeletal musculature* by binding to motor end plate cholinoceptors, thus blocking *neuromuscular transmission* (p. 176). According to whether receptor occupancy leads to a blockade or an excitation of the end plate, one distinguishes *nondepolarizing* from *depolarizing* muscle relaxants (p. 180). As adjuncts to general anesthetics, muscle relaxants help to ensure that surgical procedures are not disturbed by muscle contractions of the patient (p. 208).

Nondepolarizing Muscle Relaxants

Curare is the term for plant-derived arrow poisons of South American natives. When struck by a curare-tipped arrow, an animal suffers paralysis of skeletal musculature within a short time after the poison spreads through the body; death follows because respiratory muscles fail (respiratory paralysis). Killed game can be eaten without risk because absorption of the poison from the gastrointestinal tract is virtually nil.

The curare ingredient of greatest medicinal importance is **d-tubocurarine**. This compound contains a quaternary nitrogen atom (N) and, at the opposite end of the molecule, a tertiary N that is protonated at physiological pH. These two positively charged N atoms are common to all other muscle relaxants. The fixed positive charge of the quaternary N accounts for the poor enteral absorbability.

d-Tubocurarine is given by i.v. injection (average dose approx. 10 mg). It binds to the end plate nicotinic cholinoceptors without exciting them, acting as a *competitive antagonist* towards ACh. By preventing the binding of released ACh, it blocks neuromuscular transmission. Muscular paralysis develops within about 4 min. d-Tubocurarine does not penetrate into the CNS. The patient would thus experience motor paralysis and inability to breathe, while remaining fully conscious but incapable of expressing anything. For this reason, care must be taken to eliminate consciousness by administration of an appropriate drug before using a muscle relaxant. The effect of a single dose lasts about 30 min.

The duration of the effect of d-tubocurarine can be shortened by administering an *acetylcholinesterase inhibitor*, such as *neostigmine* (p. 102). Inhibition of ACh breakdown causes the concentration of ACh released at the end plate to rise. Competitive "displacement" by ACh of d-tubocurarine from the receptor allows transmission to be restored.

Unwanted effects produced by d-tubocurarine result from a non-immune-mediated release of histamine from mast cells leading to bronchospasm, urticaria, and hypotension. More commonly, a fall in blood pressure can be attributed to ganglionic blockade by d-tubocurarine.

Pancuronium is a synthetic compound now frequently used and not likely to cause histamine release or ganglionic blockade. It is approx. 5-fold more potent than d-tubocurarine, with a somewhat longer duration of action. Increased heart rate and blood pressure are attributed to blockade of cardiac M_2-cholinoceptors, an effect not shared by newer pancuronium congeners such as *vecuronium* and *pipecuronium*.

Other nondepolarizing muscle relaxants include **alcuronium,** derived from the alkaloid toxiferin, **gallamine,** and **atracurium**. The latter undergoes spontaneous cleavage and does not depend on hepatic or renal elimination.

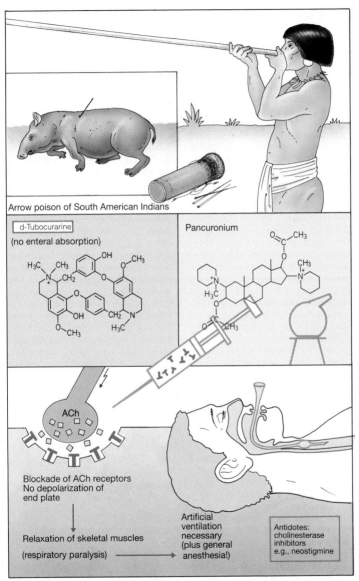

Arrow poison of South American Indians

d-Tubocurarine
(no enteral absorption)

Pancuronium

ACh

Blockade of ACh receptors
No depolarization of
end plate

↓

Relaxation of skeletal muscles

(respiratory paralysis) ⟶

Artificial
ventilation
necessary
(plus general
anesthesia!)

Antidotes:
cholinesterase
inhibitors
e.g., neostigmine

A. Non depolarizing muscle relaxants

Depolarizing Muscle Relaxants

In this drug class, only **succinylcholine** (succinyldicholine, suxamethonium, **A**) is of clinical importance. Structurally, it can be described as a double ACh molecule. Like ACh, succinylcholine acts as agonist at end plate nicotinic cholinoceptors, yet it produces muscle relaxation. Unlike ACh, it is not hydrolyzed by acetylcholinesterase. However, it is a substrate of nonspecific plasma cholinesterase (serum cholinesterase, p. 100). Succinylcholine is degraded more slowly than is ACh and therefore remains in the synaptic cleft for several minutes, causing an end plate depolarization of corresponding duration. This depolarization initially triggers a propagated action potential (AP) in the surrounding muscle cell membrane leading to contraction of the muscle fiber. After its i.v. injection, fine muscle twitches can be observed. A new AP can be elicited near the end plate only if the membrane has been allowed to repolarize.

The AP is due to opening of Na-channel proteins, allowing Na^+ ions to flow through the sarcolemma and to cause depolarization. After a few milliseconds, the Na channels close automatically ("inactivation"), the membrane potential returns to resting levels, and the AP is terminated. As long as the membrane potential remains incompletely repolarized, renewed opening of Na channels, hence a new AP, is impossible. In the case of released ACh, rapid breakdown by ACh esterase allows repolarization of the end plate and hence a return of Na channel excitability in the adjacent sarcolemma. With succinylcholine, however, there is a persistent depolarization of the end plate and adjoining membrane regions. Because the Na channels remain inactivated, an AP cannot be triggered in the adjacent membrane.

Because most skeletal muscle fibers are innervated only by a single end plate, activation of such fibers, with lengths up to 30 cm, entails propagation of the AP through the entire cell. If the AP fails, the muscle fiber remains in a relaxed state.

The effect of a standard dose of succinylcholine lasts only about 10 minutes. It is often given at the start of anesthesia to facilitate intubation of the patient. As expected, cholinesterase inhibitors are unable to counteract the effect of succinylcholine. In the few patients with a genetic deficiency in pseudocholinesterase (= nonspecific cholinesterase), the succinylcholine effect is significantly prolonged.

Since the persistent depolarization of end plates is associated with an efflux of K^+ ions, hyperkalemia can result (risk of cardiac arrhythmias). Only in a few muscle types (e.g., extraocular muscle) are muscle fibers supplied with multiple endplates. Here succinylcholine causes depolarization distributed over the entire fiber, which responds with a contracture. Intraocular pressure rises, which must be taken into account during eye surgery.

In skeletal muscle fibers whose motor nerve has been severed, ACh receptors spread in a few days over the entire cell membrane. In this case, succinylcholine would evoke a persistent depolarization with contracture and hyperkalemia.

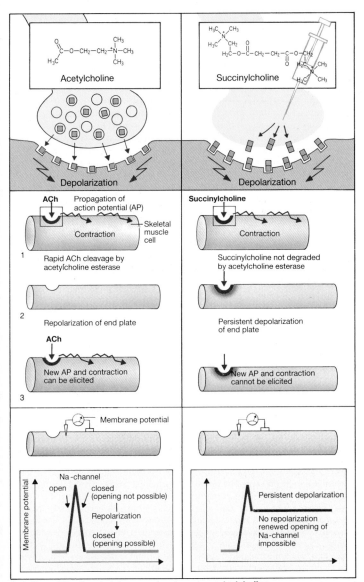

A. Action of the depolarizing muscle relaxant succinylcholine

Antiparkinsonian Drugs

Parkinson's disease (shaking palsy) and the eponymous syndrome are caused by a destruction of dopaminergic neurons that project from the *substantia nigra* to the *corpus striatum*, where they play a part in the telencephalic regulation of motor function by modulating the activity of cholinergic neurons. Dopamine deficiency and relative preponderance of cholinergic activity are considered critical pathogenetic factors. Cardinal signs of the disorder include poverty of movement (akinesia), muscle stiffness (rigidity), and tremor at rest.

Pharmacotherapeutic measures are aimed at restoring dopaminergic function or suppressing cholinergic hyperactivity.

L-dopa. Dopamine itself cannot penetrate the blood–brain barrier; however, its natural precursor, L-**d**ihydr**o**xy **p**henyl**a**lanine (L-dopa), can be used for the purpose of replenishing striatal dopamine levels, because it undergoes transport across the blood–brain barrier via an amino acid carrier and is subsequently decarboxylated by dopa-decarboxylase present in striatal tissue. Decarboxylation also takes place in peripheral organs where dopamine is not needed and is likely to cause undesirable effects (tachycardia, arrhythmias resulting from activation of β_1-adrenoceptors (p. 84), hypotension and vomiting). Extracerebral production of dopamine can be prevented by inhibitors of dopa decarboxylase (carbidopa, benserazide) that do not penetrate the blood–brain barrier, leaving intracerebral decarboxylation unaffected. Excessive elevation of brain dopamine levels may lead to undesirable reactions, such as choreoathetoid dyskinesias and mental disturbances.

Dopamine D_2-Receptor Agonists. Striatal dopamine deficiency can also be alleviated by ergot derivatives, such as *bromocriptine* (p. 114), *lisuride,* or *pergolide.* Due to their efficacy at D_2 receptors, these agents preferentially stimulate brain postsynaptic dopamine receptors. D_2 agonists may produce the same adverse effects as L-dopa.

Inhibitors of Monoamine Oxidase-B (MAO$_B$). Inactivation of monoamines by oxidation may be catalyzed by the isoenzymes MAO$_A$ and MAO$_B$. The corpus striatum is rich in MAO$_B$. This isoenzyme can be selectively inhibited by *selegiline*, which may slow the progression of Parkinson's disease. Inactivation of biogenic amines via MAO$_A$ is unaffected.

Anticholinergics. Centrally acting antagonists at muscarinic cholinoceptors, such as *benztropine* and *biperiden* (p. 106), suppress the disinhibited cholinergic activity, especially tremor. Other parkinsonian symptoms, especially akinesia, are not relieved or are even exacerbated. Atropine-like side effects limit the tolerable dosage.

Amantadine. In the early stages of the disease, symptoms can be relieved by amantadine; however, this treatment soon becomes ineffective. The mechanisms of action may involve facilitation of dopamine release, inhibition of re-uptake, or stimulation of postsynaptic receptors, as well as an anticholinergic action.

Administration of L-dopa plus carbidopa (or benserazide) is the most effective treatment during the first 5 years after disease onset. Monotherapy with amantadine or anticholinergics is restricted to the initial stages or when tremor is the prevalent symptom. As the disease progresses, the effectiveness of L-dopa gradually wanes, but it can be extended by the addition of dopamine D_2 agonists, anticholinergics, or selegiline.

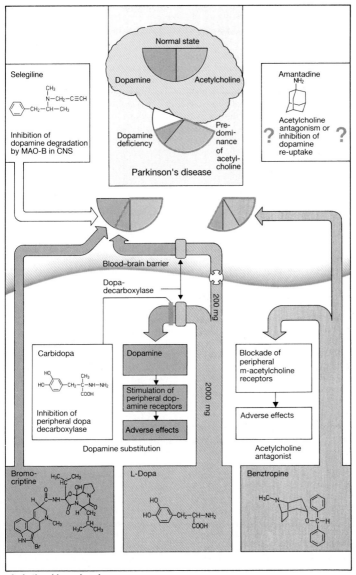

A. Antiparkinsonian drugs

Antiepileptics

An epileptic seizure is caused by a sudden burst and spread of paroxysmal electrical activity in the brain. With the aid of scalp electrodes, these events can be registered (electroencephalography; EEG). The pathological discharges may be locally restricted (focal seizures) or may involve the entire cerebral cortex (generalized seizures). Generalized seizures are classified into grand mal type fits causing generalized convulsions and petit mal type fits, the manifestations of which vary with age.

Because of its short duration, an individual seizure does not require acute pharmacotherapeutic intervention. Antiepileptics are employed for the **prophylaxis** of epileptic seizures and are administered chronically (oral route). However, in **status epilepticus** (a succession of grand mal seizures), anticonvulsants must be given acutely (preferably benzodiazepines given i.v. or rectally).

Anticonvulsant drugs are tabulated in (**A**) according to structure and clinical uses. Their mechanism of action is not fully understood, except for the benzodiazepines (p. 216). The therapeutic goal is complete seizure control, preferably with a single drug. Drug dosage is increased until there is freedom from seizures or until side effects can no longer be tolerated. Monitoring of plasma levels may be helpful in optimizing dosage adjustment. After a seizure-free period of 3 years, gradual lowering of the dosage can be attempted in order to determine if medication can be withdrawn.

Antiepileptic therapy entails more or less pronounced **adverse effects**: CNS dampening with *sedation* and cognitive impairment; hypersensitivity with *cutaneous* and *hematological* manifestations. *Osteomalacia*

(vitamin D prophylaxis) and *megaloblastic anemia* (folate supplements) may result from therapy with phenobarbital, primidone and phenytoin. These agents, as well as carbamazepine, cause *induction* of liver *microsomal enzymes* (p. 32).

Phenobarbital is a barbiturate (p. 212) with a long duration of action. **Primidone** is partially converted to phenobarbital in the liver. Both phenobarbital (pK$_a$=7.4) and **phenytoin** (pK$_a$=8.3) can dissociate a proton and are thus present partially in anionic form. Phenytoin also serves as an antiarrhythmic in digitalis intoxication (p. 130). In this instance, it increases membrane potential by reducing Na$^+$-permeability. A peculiar adverse effect is gingival hyperplasia.

Ethosuximide is structurally related to these substances.

Carbamazepine is also used in the treatment of trigeminal neuralgia.

Valproic acid or one of its metabolites elevates brain concentrations of the inhibitory transmitter GABA. Its sedative effect is minor. It is contraindicated in liver and pancreas disease (N.B. alcoholics).

Benzodiazepines (p. 216) are more suitable for acute than for chronic administration because of the development of tolerance.

Clomethiazole can also be used to break through status epilepticus; however, its chief indications are agitated states, particularly alcoholic delirium tremens that may present with seizures. Given intravenously, it can cause respiratory depression and hypotension. Clomethiazole is unsuitable for chronic use due to risk of dependence and loss of effectiveness.

The glucocorticoid **dexamethasone** (p. 234) is used in massive infantile spasm (hypsarrhythmia).

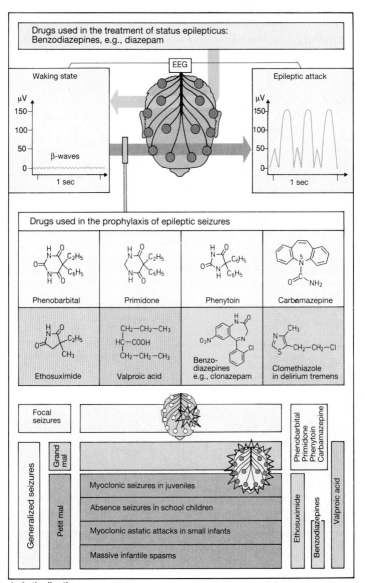

A. Antiepileptics

Pain Mechanisms and Pathways

Pain is a designation for a spectrum of sensations of highly divergent character and intensity ranging from unpleasant to intolerable. Pain stimuli are detected by physiological receptors (sensors, nociceptors) least differentiated morphologically, viz., free nerve endings. The body of the bipolar afferent first-order neuron lies in the dorsal root ganglia. Nociceptive impulses are conducted via unmyelinated (C-fibers, conduction velocity 0.2–2 m/s) and myelinated axons (Aδ-fibers, 5–30 m/s). The free endings of Aδ-fibers respond to intense pressure or heat, those of C-fibers respond to chemical stimuli (H^+, K^+, histamine, bradykinin, etc.) arising from tissue trauma. Such chemical stimuli cause an increase in H^+ and K^+ tissue concentrations and may involve release of histamine, bradykinin, serotonin or acetylcholine. K^+ is of special importance because tissue injury can result in the release of large amounts of intracellular K^+. Pain intensity and extracellular local K^+ concentration are correlated with each other.

The reaction to chemical, mechanical, and thermal stimuli is significantly enhanced in the presence of prostaglandins (p. 188). Chemical stimuli also underlie pain secondary to inflammation or ischemia (angina pectoris, myocardial infarction), or the intense pain that occurs during overdistention or spasmodic excitation of smooth muscle abdominal organs, and that may be maintained by local anoxemia developing in the area of spasm (visceral pain).

Aδ- and C-fibers enter the spinal cord via the dorsal root, ascend in the dorsolateral funiculus, and then synapse in second-order neurons in the dorsal horn. The axons of the second-order neurons cross the midline and ascend to the brain as the anterolateral pathway or spinothalamic tract. Based on phylogenetic age, a neo- and paleospinothalamic tract are distinguished. Thalamic nuclei receiving neospinothalamic input project to circumscribed areas of the postcentral gyrus. Stimuli conveyed via this path are experienced as sharp, clearly localizable pain. The nuclear regions receiving paleospinothalamic input project to the postcentral gyrus as well as the frontal, limbic cortex and most likely represent the pathway subserving pain of a dull, aching, or burning character, i.e., pain that can be localized only poorly.

Impulse traffic in the neo- and paleospinothalamic pathways is subject to modulation by descending projections that originate from the reticular formation and terminate at second-order neurons, at their synapses with first-order neurons, or at spinal segmental interneurons (**descending antinociceptive system**). This system can inhibit impulse transmission from first- to second-order neurons via release of opiopeptides (enkephalins) or monoamines (norepinephrine, serotonin).

Pain sensation can be influenced or modified as follows:
– elimination of the cause of pain
– lowering of the **sensitivity of nociceptors** (antipyretic analgesics, local anesthetics)
– interrupting **nociceptive conduction** in sensory nerves (local anesthetics)
– suppression of **transmission** of **nociceptive impulses** in the spinal medulla (opioids)
– inhibition of **pain perception** (opioids, general anesthetics)
– altering **emotional responses** to pain, i.e. pain behavior (antidepressants as "co-analgesics," p. 220).

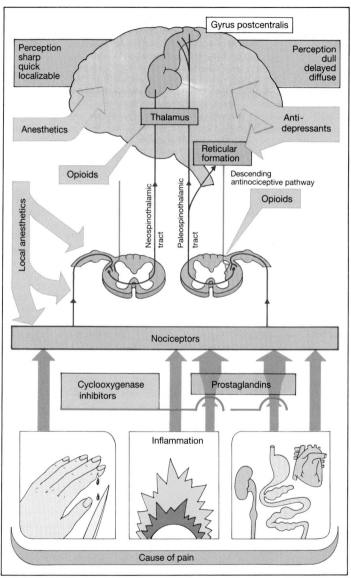

A. Pain mechanisms and pathways

Eicosanoids

Origin and metabolism. The eicosanoids, **prostaglandins**, **thromboxane**, **prostacyclin**, and **leukotrienes** are formed in the body from **arachidonic acid**, a C20 fatty acid with four double bonds (eicosatetraenoic acid). Arachidonic acid is a regular constituent of cell membrane phospholipids; it is released by phospholipase A_2 and forms the substrate of **cyclooxygenases** and **lipoxygenases**.

Synthesis of prostaglandins (PG), prostacyclin, and thromboxane proceeds via intermediary **cyclic endoperoxides**. In the case of PG, a cyclopentane ring forms in the acyl chain. The letters following PG (D, E, F, G, H, or I) indicate differences in substitution with hydroxyl or keto groups; the number subscripts refer to the number of double bonds, and the Greek letter designates the position of the hydroxyl group at C9 (the substance shown is $PGF_{2\alpha}$). PG are primarily inactivated by the enzyme 15-hydroxyprostaglandin-dehydrogenase. Inactivation in plasma is very rapid; during one passage through the lung, 90% of PG circulating in plasma are degraded. PG are **local mediators** that attain biologically effective concentrations only at their site of formation.

Biological effects. The individual PG (PGE, PGF, PGI=prostacyclin) possess different biological effects.

Nociceptors. PG increase the sensitivity of sensory nerve fibers towards ordinary pain stimuli (p. 186), i.e., at a given stimulus strength there is an increased rate of evoked action potentials.

Thermoregulation. PG raise the set point of hypothalamic (preoptic) thermoregulatory neurons; body temperature increases (*fever*).

Vascular smooth muscle. PGE_2 and PGI_2 produce *arteriolar vasodilation;* $PGF_{2\alpha}$ venoconstriction.

Gastric secretion. *PG* promote the production of gastric *mucus* and reduce the formation of *gastric acid* (p. 164).

Menstruation. $PGF_{2\alpha}$ is believed to be responsible for the ischemic necrosis of the endometrium preceding menstruation. The relative proportions of individual PG are said to be altered in dysmenorrhea and excessive menstrual bleeding.

Uterine muscle. PG stimulate *labor contractions*.

Bronchial muscle. PGE_2 and PGI_2 induce *bronchodilatation*; $PGF_{2\alpha}$ *induces constriction*.

Renal blood flow. When renal blood flow is lowered, vasodilating PG are released that act to restore blood flow.

Thromboxane A_2 and **prostacyclin** play a role in regulating the *aggregability of platelets* and *vascular diameter* (p. 148).

Leukotrienes increase capillary permeability and serve as chemotactic factors for neutrophil granulocytes. As "slow-reacting substances of anaphylaxis," they are involved in allergic reactions (p. 298); together with PG, they evoke the spectrum of characteristic inflammatory symptoms: redness, heat, swelling, and pain.

Therapeutic applications. PG derivatives are used to induce labor or to interrupt gestation (p. 126) and in the therapy of peptic ulcer (p. 164) and peripheral arterial disease.

PG are poorly tolerated if they must be given systemically; in this case their effects cannot be confined to the intended site of action.

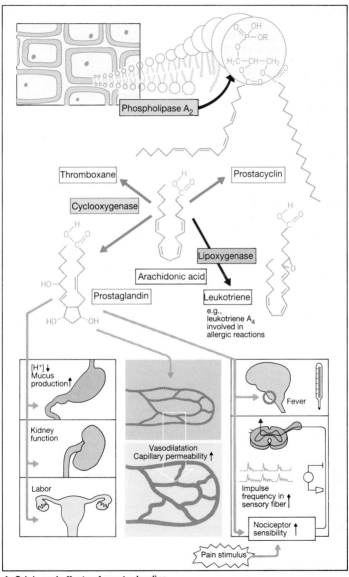

A. Origin and effects of prostaglandins

Antipyretic Analgesics

Acetaminophen, the amphiphilic acids acetylsalicylic acid (ASA), ibuprofen, and others, as well as some pyrazolone derivatives, such as aminopyrine and dipyrone, are grouped under the label **antipyretic analgesics** to distinguish them from opioid analgesics, because they share the ability to reduce fever.

Acetaminophen (paracetamol) has good analgesic efficacy in toothaches and headaches, but is of little use in inflammatory and visceral pain. Its mechanism of action remains unclear. It can be administered orally or in the form of rectal suppositories (single dose 0.5–1 g). The effect develops after about 30 min and lasts for approx. 3 h. Acetaminophen undergoes conjugation to glucuronic acid or sulfate at the phenolic hydroxyl group, with subsequent renal elimination of the conjugate. At therapeutic dosage, a small fraction is oxidized to the highly reactive N-acetyl-p-benzoquinone, which is detoxified by coupling to glutathione. After ingestion of high doses (approx. 10 g), the glutathione reserves of the liver are depleted and the quinone reacts with constituents of liver cells. As a result, the cells are destroyed: liver necrosis. Liver damage can be avoided if the thiol group donor, N-acetylcysteine, is given intravenously within 6–8 h after ingestion of an excessive dose of acetaminophen. Whether chronic regular use leads to impaired renal function remains a matter of debate.

Acetylsalicylic acid (ASA) exerts an anti-inflammatory effect, in addition to its analgesic and antipyretic actions. These can be attributed to inhibition of cyclooxygenase (p. 188). ASA can be given in tablet form, as effervescent powder, or injected systemically as lysinate (analgesic or antipyretic single dose, 0.5–1 g). ASA undergoes rapid ester hydrolysis, first in the gut and subsequently in the blood. The effect outlasts the presence of ASA in plasma ($t^1/_2$ approx. 20 min), because cyclooxygenases are irreversibly inhibited due to covalent binding of the acetyl residue. Hence, the duration of the effect depends on the rate of enzyme re-synthesis. Furthermore, salicylate may contribute to the effect. ASA irritates the gastric mucosa (direct acid effect and inhibition of cytoprotective PG synthesis, p. 188) and can precipitate bronchoconstriction ("aspirin asthma," pseudo-allergy) due to inhibition of PGE_2 synthesis and overproduction of leukotrienes. Because ASA inhibits platelet aggregation and prolongs bleeding time (p. 148), it should not be used in patients with impaired blood coagulability.

Other cyclooxygenase inhibitors (**NSAIDs**, p. 292), such as ibuprofen, act similarly to ASA, but do not covalently bind to the enzyme and do not irreversibly inhibit platelet function.

Among antipyretic analgesics, **dipyrone** (metamizole) displays the highest efficacy. It is also effective in visceral pain. Its mode of action is unclear, but probably differs from that of acetaminophen and ASA. It is rapidly absorbed when given via the oral or rectal route. Because of its water solubility, it is also available for injection. It is eliminated from plasma with a $t^1/_2$ of 4–6 h. Dipyrone is associated with a low incidence of fatal agranulocytosis. In sensitized subjects, cardiovascular collapse can occur, especially after intravenous injection. Therefore, the drug should be restricted to the management of pain refractory to other analgesics.

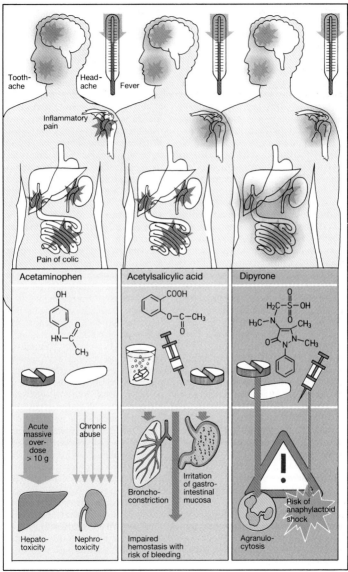

A. Antipyretic analgesics

Thermoregulation and Antipyretics

Body core temperature in the human is about 37 °C and fluctuates within ±1 °C during the 24-h cycle. In the resting state, the metabolic activity of vital organs contributes 60% (liver 25%, brain 20%, heart 8%, kidneys 7%) to total heat production. The absolute contribution to **heat production** from these organs changes little during physical activity, whereas muscle work, which contributes approx. 25% at rest, can generate up to 90% of heat production during strenuous exercise. The set point of the body temperature is programmed in the hypothalamic thermoregulatory center. The actual value is adjusted to the set point by means of various thermoregulatory mechanisms. Blood vessels supplying the skin penetrate the heat-insulating layer of subcutaneous adipose tissue and therefore permit controlled **heat exchange** with the environment as a function of vascular caliber and rate of blood flow. Cutaneous blood flow can range from close to 0% to 30% of cardiac output, depending on requirements. **Heat conduction** via the blood from interior sites of production to the body surface provides a controllable mechanism for heat loss.

Heat dissipation can also be achieved by increased **production of sweat**, because evaporation of sweat on the skin surface consumes heat (**evaporative heat loss**).

Shivering is a mechanism to **generate heat**.

Autonomic neural regulation of cutaneous blood flow and sweat production permit homeostatic control of body temperature (*A*). The sympathetic system can either reduce heat loss via vasoconstriction or promote it by enhancing sweat production.

When sweating is inhibited due to poisoning with **anticholinergics** (e.g., atropine), cutaneous blood flow increases. If insufficient heat is dissipated through this route, overheating occurs (**hyperthermia**).

Thyroid hyperfunction poses a particular challenge to the thermoregulatory system, because the excessive secretion of thyroid hormones causes metabolic heat production to increase. In order to maintain body temperature at its physiological level, excess heat must be dissipated—the patients have a hot skin and are sweating.

The hypothalamic temperature controller (**B1**) can be inactivated by **neuroleptics** (p. 224), without impairment of other centers. Thus, it is possible to lower a patient's body temperature without activating counter-regulatory mechanisms (thermogenic shivering). This can be exploited in the treatment of severe febrile states (hyperpyrexia) or in open-chest surgery with cardiac bypass, during which blood temperature is lowered to 10 °C.

In higher doses, **ethanol** and **barbiturates** also depress the thermoregulatory center (**B1**), thereby permitting cooling of the body to the point of death, given a sufficiently low ambient temperature (freezing to death in drunkeness).

Pyrogens (e.g., bacterial matter) elevate—probably through mediation by interleukin 1 and prostaglandins (p. 188)—the set point of the hypothalamic temperature controller (**B2**). The body responds by restricting heat loss (cutaneous vasoconstriction → chills) and by elevating heat production (shivering), in order to adjust to the new set point (**fever**). **Antipyretics,** such as acetaminophen and ASA (p. 190), return the set point to its normal level (**B2**) and thus bring about a defervescence.

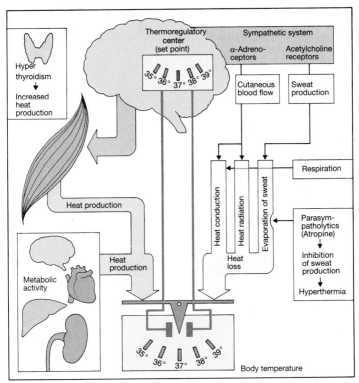

A. Thermoregulation

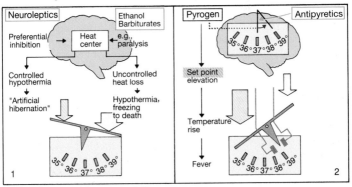

B. Disturbances of thermoregulation

Local Anesthetics

Local anesthetics reversibly inhibit impulse generation and propagation in nerves. In sensory nerves, such an effect is desired when painful procedures must be performed, e.g., surgical or dental operations.

Mechanism of Action

Nerve impulse conduction occurs in the form of an action potential, a sudden reversal in resting transmembrane potential lasting less than 1 ms. The change in potential is triggered by an appropriate stimulus and involves a rapid influx of Na^+ into the interior of the nerve axon (**A**). This inward flow proceeds through a channel, a membrane pore protein, that, upon being opened (activated) (**Aa**), permits rapid movement of Na^+ down a chemical gradient ($[Na^+]_{ext}$ 150 mM, $[Na^+]_{int}$ 7 mM). Local anesthetics are capable of inhibiting this rapid inward flux of Na^+; initiation and propagation of excitation are therefore blocked (**A**).

There are probably two different mechanisms whereby local anesthetics block fast Na^+ influx. From the axoplasmic side, they may react with the channel protein in their amphiphilic cationic form and thus inhibit passage of Na^+ through the opened channel (**Ac**). Drug molecules may also reach the inner mouth of the Na^+-channel by lateral diffusion after having been accumulated in the phospholipid bilayer. Alternatively, Na^+-channel function may be impaired indirectly as a consequence of drug-induced alterations in the characteristics of the phospholipid annulus at the membrane–channel interface (**Ad**). This type of Na^+-channel blockade could also be achieved with drug molecules that are unable to form a cationic amphiphilic species (**Ae**).

Mechanism-Specific Adverse Effects

Since local anesthetics block Na^+ influx not only in sensory nerves but also in other excitable tissues, they are applied locally and measures are taken (p. 196) to impede their distribution into the body, which would lead to such unwanted systemic reactions as

– *blockade of inhibitory CNS neurons*, manifested by restlessness and seizures (countermeasure: injection of a benzodiazepine, p. 216); general paralysis with respiratory arrest after higher concentrations.

– *blockade of cardiac impulse conduction,* as evidenced by impaired AV conduction or cardiac arrest (countermeasure: injection of epinephrine). Depression of excitatory processes in the heart, while undesired during local anesthesia, can be put to therapeutic use in cardiac arrhythmias (p. 134).

Forms of Local Anesthesia

Because of their actions on other tissues, these agents must be used locally. Localization can be achieved by infiltration of the tissue (**infiltration anesthesia**) or injection next to the nerve branch carrying fibers from the region to be anesthetized (**conduction anesthesia** of the nerve, **spinal anesthesia** of segmental dorsal roots), or by drug application to the surface of the skin or mucosa (**surface anesthesia**). In each case, the local anesthetic drug is required to diffuse to the nerves concerned from a depot placed in the tissue or on the skin.

High Sensitivity of Sensory Nerves, Low Sensitivity of Motor Nerves

Impulse conduction in sensory nerves is inhibited at a concentration lower than that needed for motor fibers. This

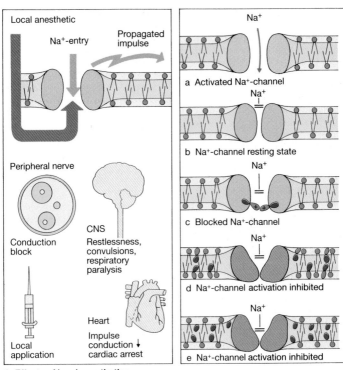

A. Effects of local anesthetics

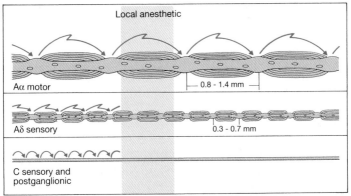

B. Inhibition of impulse conduction in different types of nerve fibers

difference may be due to the higher impulse frequency and the longer duration of the action potential in nociceptive, as opposed to motor, fibers as well as to the smaller distance between nodes of Ranvier in the former. In saltatory impulse conduction, only the nodal membrane is depolarized. Because depolarization can still occur after blockade of three or four nodal rings, the area exposed to a drug concentration sufficient to cause blockade must be larger for motor fibers (p. 195 B).

This relationship explains why sensory stimuli that are conducted via myelinated Aδ-fibers are affected later and to a lesser degree than are stimuli conducted via unmyelinated C-fibers. Since autonomic postganglionic fibers lack a myelin sheath, they are particularly susceptible to blockade by local anesthetics. As a result, vasodilatation ensues in the anesthetized region, because sympathetically driven vasomotor tone decreases. This local vasodilatation is undesirable (see below).

Diffusion and Effect
During diffusion from the injection site (i.e., the interstitial space of connective tissue) to the axon of a sensory nerve, the local anesthetic must traverse the **perineurium**. The multilayered perineurium is formed by connective tissue cells linked by *zonulae occludentes* (p. 22) and therefore constitutes a closed lipophilic barrier.

Local anesthetics in clinical use are usually tertiary amines; at the pH of interstitial fluid these exist partly as the neutral lipophilic base (symbolized by particles marked with two red dots) and partly as the protonated form, i.e., amphiphilic cation (symbolized by particles marked with one blue dot and one red dot). The un-charged form can penetrate the perineurium and enters the **endoneural space**, where a fraction of the drug molecules regains a positive charge in keeping with the local pH. The same process repeats itself when the drug penetrates through the axonal membrane (axolemma) into the **axoplasm** from which it exerts its action on the Na^+-channel; and again when it diffuses out of the endoneural space through the unfenestrated endothelium of capillaries into the blood.

The concentration of local anesthetic at the site of action is, therefore, determined by the speed of penetration into the endoneurium and the speed of diffusion into the capillary blood. In order to ensure a sufficiently fast build-up of drug concentration at the site of action, there must be a correspondingly large concentration gradient between the drug depot in the connective tissue and the endoneural space. Injection of solutions of low concentration will fail to produce an effect; however, too high concentrations must also be avoided because of the danger of intoxication resulting from too rapid systemic absorption into the blood.

To ensure a reasonably long-lasting local effect with minimal systemic action, a **vasoconstrictor** (epinephrine, less frequently norepinephrine or vasopressin derivatives) is often co-administered in an attempt to confine the drug to its site of action. As blood flow is diminished, diffusion from the endoneural space into the capillary blood decreases because the critical concentration gradient between endoneural space and blood quickly becomes small when inflow of drug-free blood is reduced. Addition of a vasoconstrictor, moreover, helps to create a relative ischemia in the surgical field.

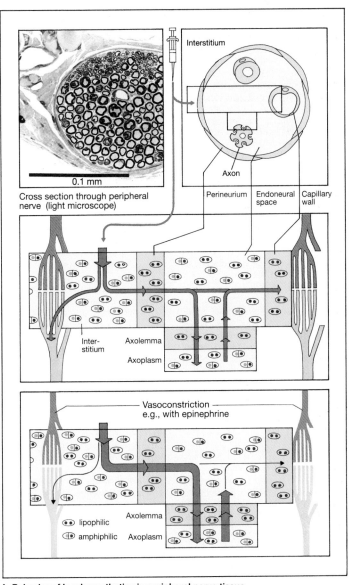

Interstitium

0.1 mm

Cross section through peripheral nerve (light microscope)

Axon

Perineurium   Endoneural space   Capillary wall

Inter-stitium

Axolemma

Axoplasm

Vasoconstriction e.g., with epinephrine

Axolemma

Axoplasm

lipophilic
amphiphilic

A. Behavior of local anesthetics in peripheral nerve tissue

Potential disadvantages of catecholamine–type vasoconstrictors include a reactive hyperemia following washout of the constrictor agent (p. 90) and cardiostimulation when epinephrine enters the systemic circulation. In lieu of epinephrine, the vasopressin analogue felypressin can be used as adjunctive vasoconstrictor (less pronounced reactive hyperemia, no arrhythmogenic action, but danger of coronary constriction). Vasoconstrictors must not be applied in local anesthesia involving the appendages (e.g., fingers, toes).

Characteristics of Chemical Structure

Local anesthetics possess a uniform structure. Generally they are secondary or tertiary amines. The nitrogen is linked through an intermediary chain to a lipophilic moiety—most often an aromatic ring system.

The amine function means that local anesthetics exist either as the neutral amine or positively charged ammonium cation, depending upon their dissociation constant (pK_a value) and the actual pH value. The pK_a of typical local anesthetics lies between 7.5 and 9. The pK_a indicates the pH value at which 50% of molecules carry a proton. In its protonated form, the molecule possesses both a polar hydrophilic moiety (protonated nitrogen) and an apolar lipophilic moiety (ring system). As regards solubility the molecule is a "zwitterion"—it is amphiphilic. Depending on the pK_a, between 50% and 5% of the drug may be present at physiological pH in the uncharged lipophilic form. This fraction is important, because it represents the lipid-membrane-permeable form of the local anesthetic (p. 26), which must take on its cationic amphiphilic form in order to exert its action (p. 194).

Clinically used local anesthetics are either esters or amides. This structural element is unimportant for efficacy; even drugs containing a methylene bridge, such as chlorpromazine (p. 225) or imipramine (p. 221), would exert a local anesthetic effect with appropriate application. Ester-type local anesthetics are subject to inactivation by tissue esterases. This is advantageous because of the diminished danger of systemic intoxication. On the other hand, the high rate of bio-inactivation and, therefore, shortened duration of action is a disadvantage.

Procaine cannot be used as a surface anesthetic because it is inactivated faster than it can penetrate the dermis or mucosa.

Lidocaine is broken down primarily in the liver by oxidative N-dealkylation. This step can occur only to a restricted extent in *prilocaine* and *articaine*, because both carry a substituent on the C-atom adjacent to the nitrogen group. Articaine possesses a carboxymethyl group on its thiophen ring. At this position, ester cleavage can occur, resulting in the formation of a polar $-COO^-$ group, loss of the amphiphilic character, and conversion to an inactive metabolite.

Benzocaine is a member of the group of local anesthetics lacking a nitrogen that can be protonated at physiological pH. It is used exclusively as a surface anesthetic.

Other agents employed for surface anesthesia include cocaine, tetracaine, and lidocaine.

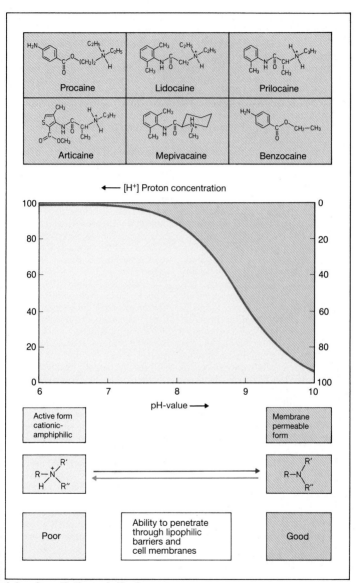

A. Local anesthetics and pH-value

Opioid Analgesics –
Morphine Type

Source of opioids. *Morphine* is an opium alkaloid (p. 4). It has much stronger analgesic activity than do the antipyretic analgesics. Besides morphine, opium contains alkaloids devoid of analgesic activity, e.g., the spasmolytic papaverine, that are also classified as opium alkaloids. In contradistinction, morphine, semisynthetic derivatives such as *hydromorphone* and *pentazocine*, and fully synthetic derivatives, such as *meperidine* (*pethidine*), *l-methadone*, and *fentanyl*, are collectively referred to as *opiates* or *opioids*. The high analgesic efficacy of opioids derives from their affinity for receptors normally acted upon by endogenous ligands. These are termed endogenous opioids because, after their discovery, they were found to act like the exogenous (xenobiotic) opioids (**A**).

Endogenous opioids. The physiological ligands at opioid receptors are the **opiopeptides**, such as the **enkephalins**, **β-endorphin**, and **dynorphins**. Their respective precursors are proenkephalin, pro-opiomelanocortin, and prodynorphin. These substances are peptides, all of which contain the amino acid sequence of the pentapeptides [Met]- or [Leu]-enkephalin. Morphine and other opioid agonists mimic endorphin, the enkephalins and dynorphins at opioid receptors. β-Endorphin may be more hormone-like in character, whereas enkephalins and dynorphins are stored in certain neurons and released upon excitation (e.g., at spinal synapses of the descending antinociceptive system, p. 186).

Opioid receptors are found on neurons in various areas of the brain and spinal cord, as well as in intramural nerve plexuses that regulate the motility of the gastrointestinal and urogenital tracts. There are several subtypes of opioid receptors, designated μ, δ, κ, that mediate the various opioid effects. Opioids can differ in their affinities and their intrinsic activities at the subtypes and, correspondingly, in the pattern of therapeutic actions.

Mode of action of opioids. Most neurons react to opioids with a hyperpolarization, possibly due to an increase in K^+ conductance (μ and δ). Ca^{2+} influx into nerve terminals during excitation is thought to be decreased (κ-mediated), leading to a decreased release of excitatory transmitters and decreased synaptic activity (**A**). Depending on the cell population affected, this synaptic inhibition translates into a depressant or excitant effect (**B**).

Effects of opioids (B). The **analgesic** effect results from actions at the level of the spinal cord and the brain (attenuation of impulse spread, inhibition of pain perception). Attention and ability to concentrate are impaired. Tranquilization and hypnotic effects can be prominent. There is a **mood change**, the direction of which depends on the initial condition. Aside from the relief associated with the abatement of strong pain, there is a feeling of detachment (floating sensation) and sense of well-being (**euphoria**), particularly after intravenous injection. During chronic intake, the sensitivity of the body can decrease, necessitating an increase in dose in order to elicit an effect of equal intensity (**tolerance**). If an attempt is then made to stop repeated use, an **abstinence syndrome** will occur, characterized by **physical** (e.g., circulatory failure) and **psychic symptoms** (e.g., agitation, anxiety, depression). In order to prevent abstinence symptoms, continuous drug in-

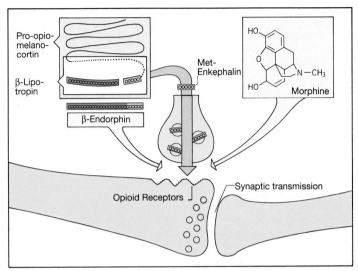

A. Action of endogenous and exogenous opioids at opioid receptors

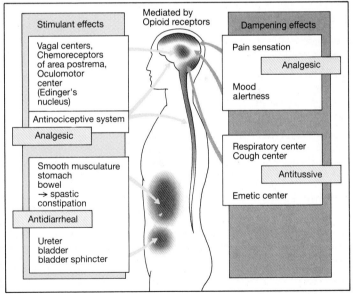

B. Effects of opioids

take becomes necessary (**physical dependence**). Opioids are prototypical addictive agents. Because of their significant abuse potential in **nontherapeutic situations**, most opioids are subject to special rules (schedules) regarding their prescription (Controlled Substances Act, FDA, USA, etc.). Regulations specify, among other things, the maximum dosage (permissible single dose, daily maximal dose, maximum amount per single prescription).

Prescriptions need to be issued on special forms that must be completed rigorously. Less potent opioid analgesics, such as *codeine,* can be prescribed in the usual manner because of their lesser abuse potential. The different abuse potential of opioids probably reflects differing affinity spectra for the individual receptor subtypes.

With any of the high-efficacy opioid analgesics, overdosage is likely to result in **respiratory paralysis** (impaired sensitivity of medullary chemoreceptors to CO_2). The maximally possible extent of respiratory depression is thought to be less in partial agonist/antagonists at opioid receptors (*pentazocine, nalbuphine*).

The cough-suppressant (antitussive) effect produced by **inhibition of the cough reflex** is independent of the effects on nociception or respiration. Thus, some substances exert an antitussive effect at subanalgesic dosages (*antitussives: codeine, noscapine).*

Stimulation of **chemoreceptors** in the area postrema (p. 300), rather than a direct action on the emetic center, results in **vomiting** particularly after first-time administration or in the ambulant patient. The emetic effect disappears with repeated use because a direct **inhibition of the emetic center** then predominates, which overrides the stimulation of area postrema chemoreceptors.

Opioids elicit pupillary narrowing (**miosis**) by stimulating the parasympathetic portion (Edinger–Westphal nucleus) of the oculomotor nucleus.

The peripheral effects concern the motility and tonus of gastrointestinal smooth muscle; **segmentation** is enhanced, but **propulsive peristalsis** is inhibited. The tonus of sphincter muscles is raised markedly. In this fashion, morphine elicits the picture of **spastic constipation** (p. 201 B; *antidiarrheal loperamide*, p. 174). Gastric emptying is delayed (pyloric spasm) and drainage of bile and pancreatic juice is impeded, because the sphincter of Oddi contracts. Likewise, bladder function is affected; specifically **bladder emptying** is impaired due to an increased tone of the vesicular sphincter. *Meperidine* (pethidine) and buprenorphine are believed to possess less spasmogenic activity and are, therefore, given parenterally in biliary or renal colic. With chronic use of opioids, **tolerance** develops to the central depressant effects. In the course of prolonged treatment, increasingly larger doses are needed to produce an equally strong effect. Peripheral agonist effects are less prone to develop tolerance. Thus, constipation during prolonged opiate use may call for administration of purgatives.

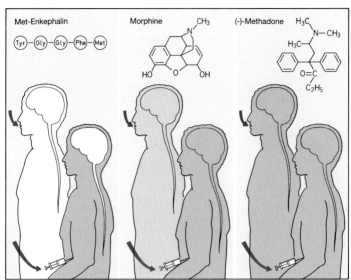

A. Bioavailability of opioids with different routes of administration

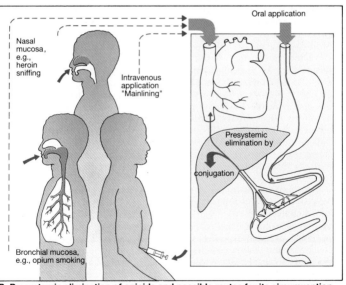

B. Presystemic elimination of opioids and possible routes for its circumvention

Uses and Pharmacokinetics of Opioids

The endogenous opioids (met-enkephalin, leu-enkephalin, β-endorphin) cannot be used therapeutically because, due to their peptide nature, they are either rapidly degraded or excluded from passage through the blood–brain barrier, thus preventing access to their sites of action even after parenteral administration (p. 203).

Morphine can be given orally or parenterally, as well as epidurally or intrathecally in the spinal cord. Given orally, it is less bioavailable (p. 203 A) because, like most opioids (e.g., meperidine, pentazocine), it is subject to **presystemic elimination** (p. 203). However, there is evidence that morphine gives rise to an active metabolite with greater analgesic efficacy (morphine 6-glucuronide). *l-Methadone* does not undergo presystemic elimination and can be employed either orally or parenterally with equal success (p. 203 A).

In opiate abuse, *heroin* (known by assorted street names) is self-administered by i.v. injection ("mainlining") to avoid first-pass metabolism and to achieve a faster rise in brain concentration. Evidently, psychic effects ("kick," buzz," "rush") are especially intense with this route of administration. The addict may also resort to other more unusual routes: opium can be **smoked**, and heroin can be taken as **snuff**.

Opioid antagonists. The effects of opioids can be abolished by the antagonist **naloxone** (A). In normal individuals, naloxone by itself has little or no effect; in opioid-dependent subjects, it precipitates acute withdrawal signs. This antagonist is used as an **antidote** in the treatment of opioid poisoning, where it effectively reverses the depression of the respiratory center. With *buprenorphine* (partial μ-agonist), however, naloxone fails to overcome respiratory depression, because this agonist dissociates too slowly from the receptors to permit its competitive displacement by the antagonist.

Treatment of Chronic Pain with Opioids

In treating patients with severe chronic pain, it is important to maintain a steady plasma level of opioid within the effective range, because the patient will experience pain when the plasma level falls below a critical level and will require larger doses when break-through pain occurs. The therapeutic goal, therefore, is not to treat but to prevent pain.

Like some other opioids (*hydromorphone, meperidine, pentazocine, codeine*), *morphine* is quickly eliminated; its duration of action is approx. 4 h. In order to safeguard a steady analgesic effect, these substances need to be given every 4 h. For the patient with chronic pain, frequent dosing, e.g., during the night, is a major inconvenience. Although dose intervals can be lengthened by increasing the individual dose, this would entail a temporary increase in plasma level beyond the therapeutically needed concentration and enhance the risk of unwanted toxic effects.

Oral use of *sustained-release morphine preparations* or use of long-acting opioids, e.g., l-methadone, offer better alternatives to frequent dosing. The kinetics of l-methadone, however, necessitate dose adjustments during treatment, because pain relief cannot be achieved with low doses during the initial phase of treatment, whereas accumulation into the toxic concentration range would occur with high doses later in the course of treatment (**B**).

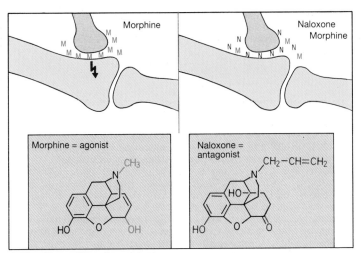

A. Morphine and its antagonist naloxone

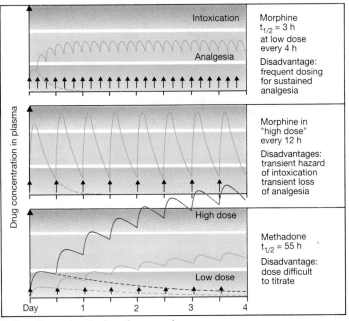

B. Morphine and methadone dosage regimens

General Anesthesia and General Anesthetic Drugs

General anesthesia is a state of drug-induced reversible inhibition of central nervous function, during which surgical procedures can be carried out in the absence of consciousness, responsiveness to pain, defensive or involuntary movements, and significant autonomic reflex responses (**A**).

The required level of anesthesia depends on the intensity of the pain-producing stimuli, i.e., the degree of nociceptive stimulation. The skillful anesthetist, therefore, dynamically adapts the plane of anesthesia to the demands of the surgical situation. Originally, anesthetization was achieved with a single anesthetic agent (e.g., diethylether—first successfully demonstrated in 1864 by W.T.G. Morton, Boston). To suppress defensive reflexes, such a "mono-anesthesia" necessitate a dosage in excess of that needed to cause unconsciousness, thereby increasing the risk of paralyzing vital functions, such as cardiovascular homeostasis (**B**). Modern anesthesia employs a combination of different drugs to achieve the goals of surgical anesthesia (**balanced anesthesia**). This approach reduces the hazards of anesthesia. In **C**, examples of drugs are listed that are used concurrently or sequentially as anesthesia adjuncts. In the case of the inhalational anesthetics, the choice of adjuncts relates to the specific property to be exploited (see below). Muscle relaxants, opioid analgesics such as fentanyl, and the parasympatholytic atropine are covered elsewhere in more detail.

Neuroleptanalgesia can be considered a special form of combination anesthesia, in which the short-acting **opioid analgesic** fentanyl is combined with the strongly sedating and affect-blunting **neuroleptic** droperidol.

Neuroleptanesthesia refers to the combined use of a short-acting analgesic, an injectable anesthetic, a short-acting muscle relaxant, and a low dose of a neuroleptic.

In **regional anesthesia** (spinal anesthesia) with a local anesthetic, nociception is eliminated, while consciousness is preserved. This procedure, therefore, does not fall under the definition of anesthesia.

According to their mode of application, general anesthetics are divided into inhalational (gaseous, volatile) and injectable agents.

Injectable anesthetics are frequently employed for induction. Intravenous injection and rapid onset of action are clearly more agreeable to the patient than is breathing a stupefying gas. The effect of most injectable anesthetics is limited to a few minutes. This allows brief procedures to be carried out or to prepare the patient for inhalational anesthesia (intubation). Administration of the volatile anesthetic must then be titrated in such a manner as to counterbalance the waning effect of the injectable agent.

Increasing use is now being made of injectable instead of inhalational anesthetics during prolonged combined anesthesia (total intravenous anesthesia—TIVA).

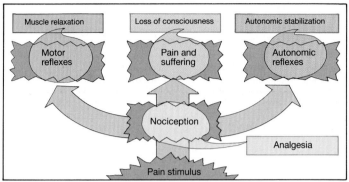

A. Goals of a surgical anesthesia

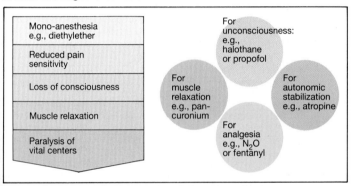

B. Formerly: monoanesthesia, nowadays: balanced anesthesia

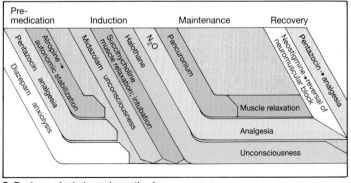

C. Regimens for balanced anesthesia

Inhalational Anesthetics

The mechanism of action of inhalational anesthetics is unknown. The diversity of chemical structures (inert gas xenon; hydrocarbons; halogenated hydrocarbons) possessing anesthetic activity appears to rule out involvement of specific receptors. According to one hypothesis, uptake into the hydrophobic interior of the plasmalemma of neurons results in inhibition of electrical excitability and impulse propagation in the brain. This concept would explain the *correlation between anesthetic potency and lipophilicity* of anesthetic drugs (**A**). Anesthetic potency can be expressed in terms of the minimal alveolar concentration (**MAC**) at which 50% of patients remain immobile following a defined painful stimulus (skin incision). Whereas the poorly lipophilic N_2O must be inhaled in high concentrations (>70% of inspired air has to be replaced), much smaller concentrations (< 5%) are required in the case of the more lipophilic halothane.

The *rates of onset and cessation of action* vary widely between different inhalational anesthetics and also depend on the degree of lipophilicity. In the case of N_2O, there is rapid elimination from the body when the patient is ventilated with normal air. Due to the high partial pressure in blood, the driving force for transfer of the drug into expired air is large and, since tissue uptake is minor, the body can be quickly cleared of N_2O. In contrast, with halothane, partial pressure in blood is low and tissue uptake is high, resulting in a much slower elimination.

Given alone, N_2O (*nitrous oxide,* "laughing gas") is incapable of producing anesthesia of sufficient depth for surgery. It has good analgesic efficacy that can be exploited when it is used in conjunction with other anesthetics. As a gas, N_2O can be administered directly. Although it irreversibly oxidizes Vitamin B_{12}, N_2O is not metabolized appreciably and is cleared entirely by exhalation (**B**).

Halothane (boiling point [BP] 50 °C), like *enflurane* (BP 56 °C), *isoflurane* (BP 48 °C), and the obsolete *methoxyflurane* (BP 104 °C), has to be vaporized by special devices. Part of the administered halothane is converted into hepatotoxic metabolites (**B**). Liver damage may result from halothane anesthesia. With a single exposure, the risk involved is unpredictable; however, there is a correlation with the frequency of exposure and the shortness of the interval between successive exposures.

Up to 70% of inhaled methoxyflurane is converted to potentially nephrotoxic metabolites.

Degradation products of enflurane or isoflurane (fraction biotransformed <2%) are of no concern.

Halothane exerts a pronounced hypotensive effect, to which a negative inotropic effect contributes. Enflurane and isoflurane cause less circulatory depression. Halothane sensitizes the myocardium to catecholamines (caution: serious tachyarrhythmias or ventricular fibrillation may accompany use of catecholamines as antihypotensives or tocolytics). This effect is much less pronounced with enflurane and isoflurane. Unlike halothane, enflurane and isoflurane have a muscle-relaxant effect that is additive with that of nondepolarizing neuromuscular blockers.

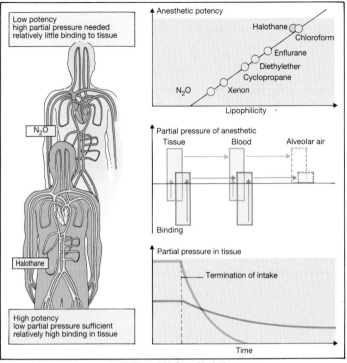

A. Lipophilicity, potency, elimination of N_2O and halothane

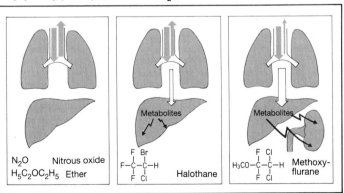

B. Elimination routes of different volatile anesthetics

Injectable Anesthetics

Substances from different chemical classes suspend consciousness when given intravenously and can be used as injectable anesthetics (**B**). Unlike inhalational agents, most of these drugs affect consciousness only and are devoid of analgesic activity (exception: ketamine). The effect cannot be ascribed to nonselective binding to neuronal cell membranes, although this may hold for propofol.

Most injectable anesthetics are characterized by a short duration of action. The rapid cessation of action is largely due to redistribution: after intravenous injection, brain concentration climbs rapidly to anesthetic levels because of high cerebral blood flow; the drug then distributes evenly in the body, i.e., concentration rises in the periphery, but falls in the brain → redistribution and cessation of anesthesia (**A**). Thus, the effect subsides before the drug has left the body. A second injection of the same dose, given immediately after recovery from the preceding dose, can therefore produce a more intense and longer effect. Usually, a single injection is administered. However, etomidate and propofol may be given by infusion over a longer time period to maintain unconsciousness.

Thiopental and *methohexital* belong to the barbiturates which, depending on dose, produce sedation, sleepiness, or anesthesia. Barbiturates lower the pain threshold and thereby facilitate defensive reflex movements; they also depress the respiratory center. Barbiturates are frequently used for induction of anesthesia.

Ketamine has analgesic activity that persists beyond the period of unconsciousness up to 1 h after injection. On regaining consciousness, the patient may experience a disconnection between outside reality and inner mental state (*dissociative anesthesia*). Frequently there is memory loss for the duration of the recovery period; however, adults in particular complain about distressing dream-like experiences. These can be counteracted by administration of a benzodiazepine (e.g., midazolam). Ketamine can increase heart rate and blood pressure by releasing catecholamines.

Propofol has a remarkably simple structure. Its effect has a rapid onset and decays quickly, being experienced by the patient as fairly pleasant. The intensity of the effect can be well controlled during prolonged administration. *Etomidate* hardly affects the autonomic nervous system. Since it inhibits cortisol synthesis, it can be used in the treatment of adrenocortical overactivity (Cushing's disease).

Midazolam is a rapidly metabolized benzodiazepine (p. 216) that is used for induction of anesthesia.

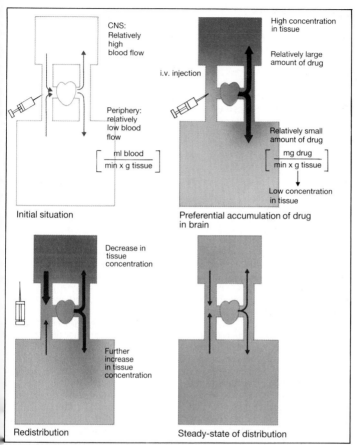

A. Termination of drug effect by redistribution

B. Intravenous anesthetics

Soporifics, Hypnotics

Sleep is a patterned rhythmic activity of the brain that can be monitored by means of the electroencephalogram (EEG). Internal sleep cycles recur four to five times per night, each cycle being interrupted by a rapid eye movement (REM) sleep phase (A). The REM stage is characterized by EEG activity similar to that seen in the waking state: rapid eye movements, vivid dreams, and occasional twitches of individual muscle groups against a background of generalized atonia of skeletal musculature. Normally, the REM stage is entered only after a preceding non-REM cycle. Frequent interruption of sleep will, therefore, decrease the REM portion. Shortening of REM sleep (normally approx. 25% of total sleep duration) results in increased irritability and restlessness during the daytime. With undisturbed night rest, REM deficits are compensated by increased REM sleep on subsequent nights (B).

Hypnotics fall into different categories, including the **benzodiazepines** (e.g., triazolam, temazepam, clotiazepam, nitrazepam), **barbiturates** (e.g., hexobarbital, pentobarbital), chloral hydrate, and H_1-antihistamines with sedative activity. Benzodiazepines act on specific binding sites (p. 216). The site and mechanism of action of barbiturates, antihistamines, and chloral hydrate are incompletely understood.

All hypnotics shorten the REM stage (B). With repeated ingestion of a hypnotic on several successive days, the proportion of time spent in REM vs. non-REM sleep returns to normal despite continued drug intake. Withdrawal of the hypnotic drug results in REM rebound, which tapers off only over many days (B). Since REM stages are associated with vivid dreaming, sleep with excessively long REM episodes is experienced as unrefreshing. Thus, the attempt to discontinue use of hypnotics may result in the impression that refreshing sleep calls for a hypnotic, probably promoting **hypnotic drug dependence**.

Depending on their blood levels, both benzodiazepines and barbiturates produce **calming** and **sedative** effects, the former also being **anxiolytic**. At higher dosage, both groups **promote the onset of sleep** or **induce** it (C).

Unlike barbiturates, **benzodiazepine derivatives** administered orally lack a general anesthetic action in that cerebral activity is not globally inhibited (respiratory paralysis is virtually impossible) and autonomic functions, such as blood pressure, heart rate, or body temperature, are unimpaired. Thus, benzodiazepines possess a therapeutic margin considerably wider than that of barbiturates.

Due to their narrower margin of safety (risk of misuse for suicide) and their potential to produce physical dependence, **barbiturates** are no longer or only rarely used as hypnotics. Dependence on them has all the characteristics of an addiction.

Because of rapidly developing tolerance, **chloral hydrate** is suitable only for short-term use.

Antihistaminics enjoy use as over-the-counter (nonprescription) sleep remedies (e.g., diphenhydramine, doxylamine, p. 114), in which case their sedative side effect is used as the principal effect.

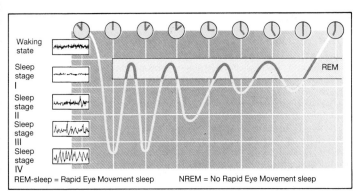

A. Succession of different sleep phases during night rest

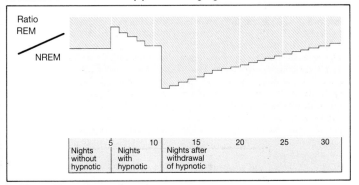

B. Effect of hypnotics on sleep phases

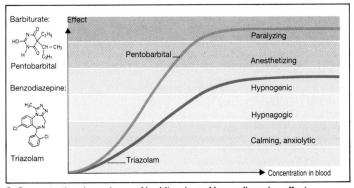

C. Concentration dependence of barbiturate and benzodiazepine effects

Sleep Threshold—
Sleep Propensity

Hypnotic drugs **promote a propensity for sleep** so that a condition **(sleep threshold)** is reached in which the subject goes to sleep and stays asleep. **Sleep disturbances** can be viewed as resulting from a pathologically high sleep threshold; they may involve either difficulty **falling asleep** (increased latency for onset of sleep) or **staying asleep** (frequent awakenings per night and reduced total sleep duration). Depending on the type of disturbance, a hypnotic drug may be indicated to increase sleep propensity, either briefly (about 1 h) or for 6–8 h maximally.

When substances with half-lives >8 h are used, plasma concentrations will remain high even after the completion of a night's rest (6–8 h). A "hangover" effect would be expected to be evident the next day in the form of fatigue, inability to concentrate, and prolonged reaction time. Because **propensity for sleep** follows a **circadian rhythm**, these effects are not normally evident. Sleep propensity is low in the morning, rises slowly until early afternoon, and declines again towards early evening. By about midnight, it reaches a maximum and then gradually returns to morning levels. Hypnotics diminish the gap between sleep propensity and sleep threshold; however, with therapeutic dosage, the sleep threshold will be reached only during the physiological peak of sleep proneness (hypnotic effect at 12 p. m., subliminal effect at 6 a.m., despite similar plasma levels of nitrazepam [$t_{1/2} \geq 20$ h]).

A pharmacologically induced increase in sleep proneness may, however, become unmasked at daytime when other substances having a sedative action (e.g., ethanol) are ingested. Because of additive effects, the capacity to concentrate or react will be impaired.

Treatment of Insomnia
Causes of insomnia include **emotional stress** (anxiety), **physical complaints** (cough, pain), and **ingestion of substances** possessing a centrally stimulant action (caffeinated beverages, sympathomimetics, theophylline, or antidepressants). Pharmacological intervention is not indicated unless causal therapy fails. Depending on the type of insomnia, sleep remedies with a short (oxazepam, brotizolam, $t_{1/2} \sim 4$–6 h) or an intermediate (nitrazepam, lormetazepam) duration of action may be considered.

Use of a hypnotic drug should not be extended beyond 4 weeks, because tolerance may develop. The risk of a rebound decrease in sleep propensity after drug withdrawal is said to be avoidable by tapering off the dose over 2 to 3 weeks.

With any hypnotic, the risk of suicidal overdosage cannot be ignored. Compared with benzodiazepines, poisoning by barbiturates occurs more readily and is harder to treat. Thus, benzodiazepines have all but replaced barbiturates as hypnotics.

Hypnotics may exert "paradoxical" effects (restlessness, more excitement) and mental confusion, particularly in elderly individuals.

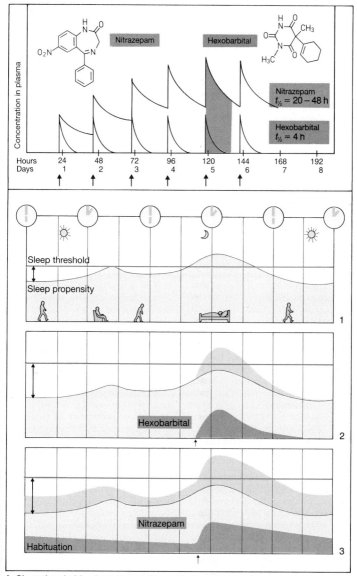

A. Sleep threshold - sleep propensity and action of hypnotics

Benzodiazepines

Benzodiazepines modify affective responses to sensory perceptions; specifically, they render a subject indifferent towards anxiogenic stimuli, i.e., **anxiolytic** action. Furthermore, benzodiazepines exert **sedating, anticonvulsant**, and **muscle–relaxant** effects at the level of the spinal cord (p. 176). All these actions result from augmenting the activity of **inhibitory neurons** and are mediated by specific **benzodiazepine receptors** that form an integral part of the GABA$_A$ receptor-chloride channel complex. The inhibitory transmitter GABA acts to open the membrane **chloride channels**. Increased chloride conductance of the neuronal membrane effectively short-circuits responses to depolarizing inputs. Benzodiazepine receptor agonists increase the affinity of GABA to its receptor. At a given concentration of GABA, binding to the receptors will, therefore, be increased, resulting in an augmented response. Excitability of the neurons is diminished.

Therapeutic indications for benzodiazepines include: **anxiety states** associated with **neurotic, phobic, and depressive** disorders, or **myocardial infarction** (decrease in cardiac stimulation due to anxiety); **insomnia; preanesthetic** (preoperative) medication; **epileptic seizures**; and hypertonia of **skeletal musculature** (**spasticity**, rigidity).

Since GABA-ergic synapses are confined to neural tissues, specific inhibition of central nervous functions can be achieved for instance, there is little change in blood pressure, heart rate, and body temperature. The therapeutic index of benzodiazepines, calculated with reference to the toxic dose producing respiratory depression, is greater than 100 and thus exceeds that of barbiturates and other sedative-hypnotics by more than tenfold.

Since benzodiazepines depress responsivity to external stimuli, automotile driving skills and other tasks requiring precise sensorimotor coordination will be impaired. *Triazolam* (t$^1/_2$ of elimination 1.5 to 5.5 h) is especially prone to impair memory (anterograde amnesia) and to cause rebound anxiety or insomnia and daytime confusion. Because of the severity of these and other adverse reactions (e.g., rage, violent hostility, hallucinations), and their increased frequency in the elderly, use of triazolam has been curtailed or suspended in some countries (UK).

Although benzodiazepines are well tolerated, the possibility of personality changes (nonchalance) and the risk of physical dependence with chronic use must not be overlooked. Conceivably, benzodiazepine dependence results from a kind of habituation, the functional counterparts of which become manifest during abstinence as restlessness and anxiety; even seizures may occur.

Benzodiazepine antagonists, such as *flumazenil*, possess affinity for benzodiazepine receptors, but they lack intrinsic activity. Flumazenil is an effective antidote in the treatment of benzodiazepine overdosage or can be used postoperatively to arouse patients sedated with a benzodiazepine.

Whereas benzodiazepines possessing agonist activity indirectly augment chloride permeability, **inverse agonists** exert an opposite action. These substances give rise to pronounced restlessness, excitement, anxiety, and convulsive seizures. There is, as yet, no therapeutic indication for their use.

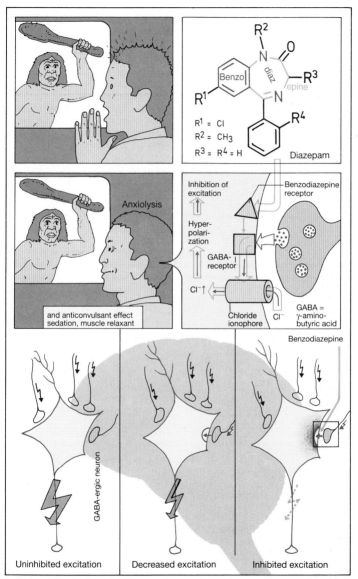

A. Action of benzodiazepines

Pharmacokinetics
of Benzodiazepines

All benzodiazepines exert their actions at specific receptors (p. 216). The choice between different agents is dictated by the speed of action, its intensity, and duration. These, in turn, reflect their physicochemical and pharmacokinetic properties. Individual benzodiazepines remain in the body for very different lengths of time and are chiefly eliminated through biotransformation. Inactivation may entail a single chemical reaction or several steps (e.g., diazepam) before an inactive metabolite suitable for renal elimination is formed. Since the intermediary products may, in part, be pharmacologically active and, in part, be excreted much more slowly than the parent substance, metabolites will accumulate with continued regular dosing and contribute significantly to the final effect.

Biotransformation begins either at substituents on the diazepine ring (diazepam: N-dealkylation at position 1; midazolam: hydroxylation of the methyl group on the imidazole ring) or at the diazepine ring itself. Hydroxylated midazolam is quickly eliminated following glucuronidation ($t_{1/2} \sim 2$ hr). N-Demethyldiazepam (nordiazepam, or nordazepam) is biologically active and undergoes hydroxylation at position 3 on the diazepine ring. The hydroxylated product (oxazepam) again is pharmacologically active. By virtue of their long half-lives, diazepam ($t_{1/2} \sim 32$ h) and, still more so, its metabolite, nordazepam ($t_{1/2} = 50$–90 h), are eliminated slowly and accumulate during repeated intake. Oxazepam undergoes conjugation to glucuronic acid via its hydroxyl group ($t_{1/2} = 8$ h) and renal excretion (**A**).

The range of elimination half-lives for different benzodiazepines or their active metabolites is represented by the shaded areas (**B**). Substances with a short half-life that are not converted to active metabolites can be used for induction or maintenance of sleep (light blue area in **B**). Substances with a long half-life are preferable for long-term anxiolytic treatment (light green area) because they permit maintenance of steady plasma levels with single daily dosing. Midazolam enjoys use by the i.v. route in preanesthetic medication and anesthetic combination regimens.

Benzodiazepine Dependence
Prolonged regular use of benzodiazepines can lead to physical dependence. With the long-acting substances marketed initially, this problem was less obvious in comparison with other dependence-producing drugs, because of the delayed appearance of withdrawal symptoms. The severity of the abstinence syndrome is inversely related to the elimination $t_{1/2}$, ranging from mild to moderate (restlessness, irritability, sensitivity to sound and light, insomnia, and shaking) to dramatic (depression, panic, delirium, grand mal seizures). Some of these symptoms pose diagnostic difficulties, being indistinguishable from the ones originally treated. Administration of a benzodiazepine antagonist would abruptly provoke abstinence signs. There are indications that substances with intermediate elimination half-lives are most frequently abused (violet area in **B**).

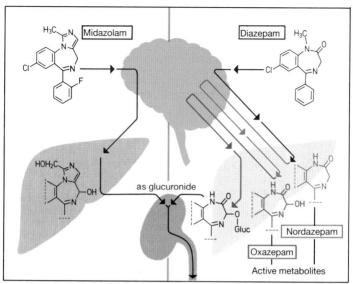

A. Biotransformation of benzodiazepines

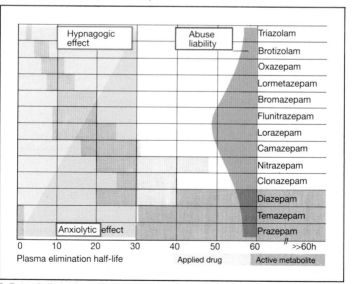

B. Rate of elimination of benzodiazepines

Therapy of Manic-Depressive Illnesses

Manic-depressive illness connotes a psychotic disorder of affect that occurs episodically without external cause. In *endogenous depression* (melancholia), mood is persistently low. *Mania* refers to the opposite condition (p. 222). Patients may oscillate between these two extremes with interludes of normal mood. Depending on the type of disorder, mood swings may alternate between both directions (bipolar depression, cyclothymia) or move only in one direction (unipolar depression).

I. Endogenous Depression

In this condition, the patient experiences profound misery (beyond the observer's empathy) and feelings of severe guilt because of imaginary misconduct. The drive to act or move is inhibited. In addition, there are disturbances mostly of a somatic nature (insomnia, loss of appetite, constipation, palpitations, loss of libido, impotence, etc.). Although the patient may have suicidal thoughts, psychomotor retardation prevents suicidal impulses from being carried out. In **A**, endogenous depression is illustrated by the layers of somber colors; psychomotor drive, symbolized by a sine oscillation, is strongly reduced.

Tricyclic antidepressants (thymoleptics). The **therapy of endogenous depression** aims at reelevating mood from a pathological low level. In many cases, this may be accomplished with a tricyclic antidepressant, such as imipramine. With chronic administration of substances belonging to this group, mood improves slowly *in the course of weeks*, and drive increases. Dosage must be adjusted individually. The ultimate mode of action of thymoleptics is yet

to be elucidated. Most probably, these agents act by interfering with the metabolism of brain biogenic amines (norepinephrine, serotonin) that are thought to serve as neurotransmitters or modulators.

It would be improper to administer drive-enhancing drugs, such as amphetamines, to a patient with endogenous depression. Because this therapy fails to elevate mood but removes psychomotor inhibition, the danger of suicide increases.

Apart from their slowly developing antipsychotic and mood-elevating effect, antidepressants elicit acute effects that also occur in healthy subjects, viz., sedation and dampening of intellectual and physical activity. In nondepressive patients whose complaints are predominantly of psychogenic origin, this effect may be useful in efforts to bring about a temporary "psychosomatic uncoupling." In this connection, clinical use of "co-analgesics" (p. 186) may be noted.

The **side effects** of tricyclic antidepressants are largely attributable to the ability of these compounds to bind to and block receptors for endogenous transmitter substances. These effects appear immediately after therapy has been started. Antagonism at muscarinic cholinoceptors leads to *atropine-like* effects, such as tachycardia, inhibition of exocrine glands, constipation, and disturbances of micturition and of vision. Furthermore, re-uptake of biogenic amines is inhibited, giving rise to superimposed indirect sympathomimetic stimulation. Patients are supersensitive to catecholamines (e.g. epinephrine in local anesthetic injections must be avoided).

Only a few of the large number of antidepressants will be mentioned, viz., **imipramine**, which combines psychomotor dampening and stimu-

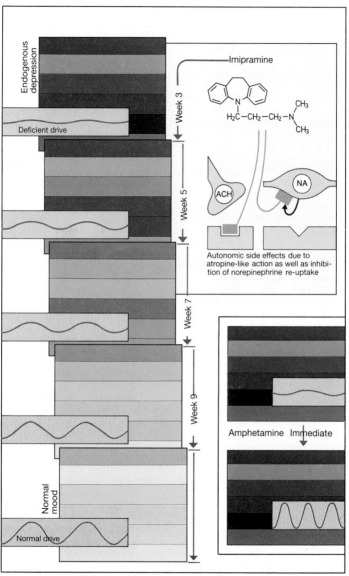

Imipramine

Autonomic side effects due to atropine-like action as well as inhibition of norepinephrine re-uptake

Amphetamine   Immediate

A. Effect of antidepressants

lant actions; **desipramine**, exhibiting stronger stimulant activity, and **amitriptyline**, having predominantly dampening properties. Therapeutic choice between these drugs takes into account the individual quality ("coloration") of a depressive phase. In special cases, use of **MAO-inhibitors**, e.g., **tranylcypromine** or **moclobemide**.

II. Therapy of Mania

The manic phase is characterized by exaggerated elation, flight of ideas, and a pathologically increased psychomotor drive. This is symbolically illustrated in **A** by a disjointed structure and aggressive color tones. The patients are overconfident, continuously active, show progressive incoherence of thought and loosening of associations, and act irresponsibly (financially, sexually).

Lithium ions. Lithium salts (e.g., acetate, carbonate) are effective in **controlling the manic phase**. The effect becomes evident approx. 10 days after the start of therapy. The small therapeutic index necessitates frequent monitoring of Li^+ serum levels. Therapeutic levels should be kept between 0.8–1.0 mM in fasting morning blood samples. At higher values there is a risk of *adverse effects*. CNS symptoms include fine tremor, ataxia, or seizures. Inhibition of the renal actions of vasopressin (p. 160) leads to polyuria and thirst. Thyroid function is impaired (p. 232) with development of euthyroid goiter.

The *mechanism of action* of Li ions remains to be fully elucidated. Chemically, lithium is the lightest of the alkali metals, which include biologically important elements such as sodium and potassium. Apart from interference with transmembrane cation fluxes (via ion channels and pumps), a lithium effect of major significance appears to be membrane depletion of phosphatidylinositol biphosphates, the principal lipid substrate used by various receptors in transmembrane signalling. Blockade of this important signal transduction pathway leads to impaired ability of neurons to respond to activation of membrane receptors for transmitters or other chemical signals. Another site of action of lithium may be GTP-binding proteins responsible for signal transduction initiated by formation of the agonist–receptor complex.

Rapid control of an acute attack of mania may require the use of a **neuroleptic** (see below).

III. Prophylaxis of Manic Depression

With continued treatment for 6 to 12 months, **lithium salts** prevent the recurrence of either manic or depressive states, effectively stabilizing mood at a normal level.

Therapy of Schizophrenia

Schizophrenia is an endogenous psychosis of episodic character. Basic symptoms reflect a thought disorder (e.g., distracted, incoherent, illogical thinking; poverty of intellectual content; blockage of ideation; abrupt breaking off of a train of thought: the patient claims being subject to outside agencies that control his or her thoughts) and disturbance of affect (mood inappropriate to the situation) and of psychomotor drive. Additional symptoms are delusional paranoia (persecution mania) or hallucinations (fearful, hearing of voices). The disruption and incoherence of ideation is symbolically represented at the top left on p. 225, and the normal psychic state is illustrated at the bottom left on p. 223.

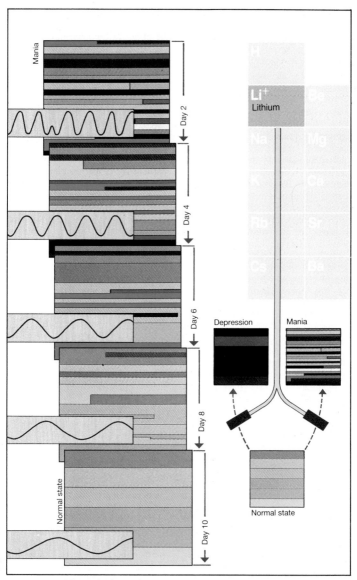

A. Effect of lithium salts in mania

Neuroleptics

After administration of a neuroleptic, there is at first only psychomotor dampening. This sedating effect would also be experienced by a healthy individual. In the schizophrenic patient, psychotic processes still persist but lose their subjective importance. In the course of weeks, psychic processes gradually normalize; the psychotic episode wanes. Complete normalization can, however, not be achieved. Nonetheless, these changes amount to therapeutic success because the patient experiences relief from the torment of psychotic personality changes, care of the patient is made easier, and return into a familiar environment is accelerated.

For neuroleptic antipsychotic therapy, compounds from two different chemical series are available: (1) the **phenothiazines** (prototype: chlorpromazine), and (2) the **butyrophenones** (prototype: *haloperidol*).

The antipsychotic effect is probably due to an antagonistic action at receptors for CNS neurotransmitters. Both series possess other variably pronounced actions, as illustrated graphically (p. 225). These are also evident in healthy subjects. Acutely, there is sedation with anxiolytic effect after neuroleptization has been started. This effect can be exploited in other medical areas; for "psychosomatic uncoupling" in disorders with a prominent psychogenic component; neuroleptanalgesia (p. 206) by means of the butyrophenone *droperidol* in combination with an opioid; tranquilization of overexcited, agitated patients; treatment of delirium tremens with haloperidol.

It should be pointed out that neuroleptics do *not* exert an anticonvulsant action. The *antiemetic effect* is also exploited (p. 300). Because they *inhibit the thermoregulatory center*, neuroleptics can be employed for controlled hypothermia (p. 192).

The autonomic side effects of neuroleptics result from blockade of receptors, e.g., muscarinic cholinoceptors → atropine-like effects, or α-adrenoceptors → hypotension.

Blockade of dopamine (D_2) receptors can cause *extrapyramidal disturbances* with impaired motor function. *Acute dystonias* occur immediately after neuroleptization and are manifested by motor impairments, particularly in the head and neck region. After several days to months, a *parkinsonian syndrome* (pseudoparkinsonism) or *akathisia* (motor restlessness) may develop. During acute administration of neuroleptics to experimental animals, nigrostriatal dopaminergic neurons become hyperactive; however, during chronic exposure, a membrane depolarization and neuronal inactivity ("depolarization blockade") may develop.

All these disturbances can be treated by administration of antiparkinsonian drugs of the anticholinergic type, such as *biperiden* (i.e., in acute dystonia). As a rule, these disturbances disappear after withdrawal of neuroleptic medication.

Tardive dyskinesia may become evident after chronic neuroleptization for several years, particularly when the drug is discontinued. It is due to hypersensitivity of the dopamine receptor system and can be exacerbated by administration of anticholinergics.

Chronic use of neuroleptics can on occasion give rise to *hepatic damage* associated *with cholestasis*. A very rare, but dramatic, adverse effect is the *malignant neuroleptic syndrome* (skeletal muscle rigidity, hyperthermia, stupor) that can end fatally in the absence of intensive countermeasures (including treatment with dantrolene, p. 176).

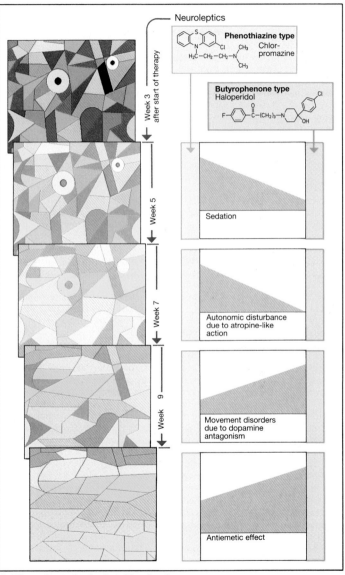

A. Effect of neuroleptics in schizophrenia

Psychotomimetics
(Psychedelics, Hallucinogens)

Psychotomimetics are able to elicit psychic changes like those manifested in the course of a psychosis, such as **illusionary distortion of perception** and **hallucinations**. This experience may be of dreamlike character; its emotional or intellectual transposition appears inadequate to the outsider.

A psychotomimetic effect is pictorially recorded in the series of portraits drawn by an artist under the influence of *lysergic acid diethylamide* (LSD). During the wavelike waxing and waning of the intoxication, he reports seeing the face of the portrayed subject turn into a grimace, phosphoresce bluish purple, and decrease or increase in size as if viewed through a moving zoom lens, giving the illusion of abstruse changes in proportion and grotesque motion sequences. The diabolic caricature is perceived as threatening.

Illusions also affect the senses of hearing and smell; sounds (tones) are "experienced" as floating beams and visual impressions as odors (e.g., ozone). Intoxicated individuals see themselves temporarily from the outside and pass judgement on themselves and their condition. On the other hand, the boundary between self and the environment becomes blurred. An elating sense of being one with the other and the cosmos sets in. The sense of time is suspended; time is neither present nor past. Objects are seen that do not exist, and experiences felt that transcend explanation, hence the term "psychedelic" (Greek *delosis* = revelation) implying expansion of consciousness.

The contents of such illusions and hallucinations can occasionally become extremely threatening ("bad trip"); the individual may feel provoked to turn violent or to commit suicide.

The LSD intoxication is followed by a phase of intense fatigue, feelings of shame, and humiliating emptiness.

The mechanism of the psychotogenic effect is unknown. Since some hallucinogens, such as LSD (chemically synthesized), *psilocin, psilocybin* (from Fungi), *bufotenine* (the cutaneous gland secretion of a toad), and *mescaline* (from the Mexican cactus *Anhalonium lewinii*—peyote) exhibit structural resemblance to 5-HT (p. 116) and epinephrine, an interaction in the CNS with these biogenic amines has been inferred. The structure of other agents, such as *tetrahydrocannabinol* (from *Cannabis sativa*, the hemp plant—hashish, marihuana), *muscimol* (from the fly agaric, *Amanita muscaria*), or *phencyclidine* (formerly used as injectable general anesthetic) does not reveal a similar connection. Hallucinations may also occur as adverse effects after intake of other substances, e.g., *scopolamine* (pp. 106, 301; ingredient of medieval witch's ointments) and other centrally active parasympatholytics.

Naturally occurring hallucinations were employed by priests (shamans, medicine men) in indigenous religions to achieve a **trance state**. Synthetic LSD was popular in the 1960s, especially among artists: psychedelic art, i.e., pictorial representation of experiential spaces and hallucinatory imagery beyond the reach of reason.

Although development of psychological dependence and permanent psychic damage cannot be considered established sequelae of chronic use of psychotomimetics, the manufacture and commercial distribution of these drugs is prohibited (Schedule I, Controlled Drugs).

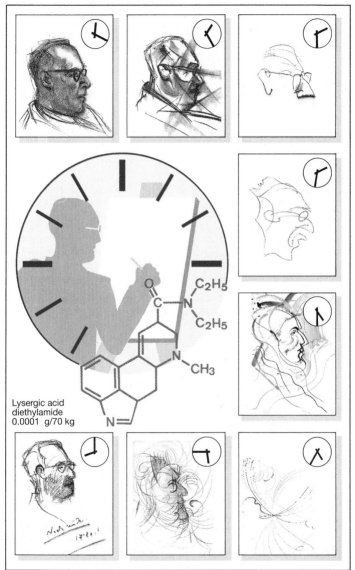

Lysergic acid
diethylamide
0.0001 g/70 kg

A. Psychotomimetic effect of LSD in a portrait artist

Hypothalamic and Hypophyseal Hormones

The endocrine system is controlled by the brain. **Nerve cells of the hypothalamus** synthesize and release messenger substances that regulate adenohypophyseal (AH) hormone release or that are themselves secreted into the body as hormones. The latter comprise the so-called **neurohypophyseal (NH) hormones**.

The axonal processes of hypothalamic neurons project to the neurohypophysis, where they store the *nonapeptides vasopressin* (= antidiuretic hormone, ADH) and *oxytocin* and release them on demand into the blood. Therapeutically, these peptide hormones are given parenterally or via the nasal mucosa.

The **hypothalamic releasing hormones** are *peptides*. They reach their target cells in the AH lobe by way of a portal vascular route consisting of two serially connected capillary beds. The first of these lies in the hypophyseal stalk, the second corresponds to the capillary bed of the AH lobe. Here, the hypothalamic hormones diffuse from the blood to their target cells, whose activity they control. Hormones released from the AH cells enter the blood, in which they are distributed to peripheral organs (**1**).

Nomenclature of releasing hormones:

RH—releasing hormone; RIH—release inhibiting hormone.

GnRH: gonadotropin RH = gonadorelin—stimulates the release of FSH (follicle-stimulating hormone) and LH (luteinizing hormone).

TRH: thyrotropin RH (protirelin) stimulates the release of TSH (thyroid-stimulating hormone = thyrotropin).

CRH: corticotropin RH—stimulates the release of ACTH (adrenocorticotropic hormone = corticotropin).

GRH: growth hormone RH (somatocrinin)—stimulates the release of GH (growth hormone = STH, somatotropic hormone). **GRIH** = somatostatin—inhibits release of STH (and also other peptide hormones including insulin, glucagon, and gastrin).

PRH: prolactin RH—remains to be characterized or established.

PRIH inhibits the release of prolactin and could be identical with dopamine.

Hypothalamic releasing hormones are mostly administered (parenterally) for diagnostic reasons to test AH function.

Therapeutic control of AH cells. GnRH is used in *hypothalamic infertility in women* to stimulate FSH and LH secretion and to induce ovulation. For this purpose, it is necessary to mimic the physiologic intermittent "pulsatile" release (approx. every 90 min) by use of a programmed infusion pump.

Gonadorelin superagonists are analogs that bind with very high affinity to GnRH receptors of AH cells. As a result of the nonphysiologic uninterrupted receptor stimulation, initial augmentation of FSH and LH output is followed by a prolonged decrease. *Buserelin, leuprorelin,* and *goserelin* are used in patients with *prostatic carcinoma* to reduce production of testosterone, which promotes tumor growth. Testosterone levels fall as much as after orchidectomy (**2**).

The **dopamine D_2-agonist** bromocriptine (pp. 114, 301) inhibits prolactin-releasing AH cells (indications: suppression of lactation, prolactin-producing tumors). Excessive, but not normal, growth hormone release can also be inhibited (indication: acromegaly) (**3**).

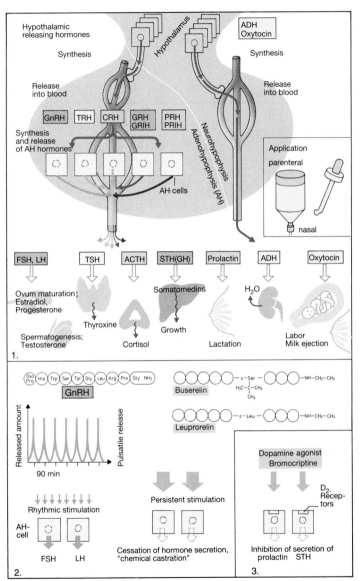

1.

2.

3.

A. Hypothalamic and hypophyseal hormones

Thyroid Hormone Therapy

Thyroid hormones accelerate metabolism. Their release (**A**) is regulated by the hypophyseal glycoprotein TSH, whose release, in turn, is controlled by the hypothalamic tripeptide TRH. Secretion of TSH declines as the blood level of thyroid hormones rises; by means of this negative feedback mechanism, hormone production is "automatically" adjusted to demand.

The thyroid releases predominantly thyroxine (T_4). However, the active form appears to be triiodothyronine (T_3); T_4 is converted in part to T_3, receptor affinity in target organs being 10-fold higher for T_3. The effect of T_3 develops more rapidly and has a shorter duration than does that of T_4. Plasma elimination $t^{1/2}$ for T_4 is about 7 days; that for T_3, however, is only 1.5 days. Conversion of T_4 to T_3 releases iodide; 150 μg of T_4 contains 100 μg of iodine.

For therapeutic purposes, T_4 is chosen, although T_3 is the active form and better absorbed from the gut. However, with T_4 administration, more constant blood levels can be achieved because degradation of T_4 is so slow. Since T_4 absorption is maximal from an empty stomach, T_4 is taken about $^{1/2}$ h before breakfast.

Replacement therapy of hypothyroidism. Whether primary, i.e., caused by thyroid disease, or secondary, i.e., resulting from TSH deficiency, hypothyroidism is treated by oral administration of T_4. Since too rapid activation of metabolism entails the hazard of cardiac overload (angina pectoris, myocardial infarction), therapy is usually started with low doses and gradually increased. The final maintenance dose required to restore a euthyroid state depends on individual needs (approx. 150 μg/day).

Thyroid suppression therapy of euthyroid goiter (B). The cause of goiter (struma) is usually a dietary deficiency of iodine. Due to an increased TSH action, the thyroid is activated to raise utilization of the little iodine available to a level at which hypothyroidism is averted. Therefore, the thyroid increases in size.

Because of the negative feedback regulation of thyroid function, thyroid activation can be inhibited by administration of T_4 doses equivalent to the endogenous daily output (approx. 150 μg/d). Deprived of stimulation, the inactive thyroid regresses in size.

If a euthyroid goiter has not persisted for too long, increasing the iodine supply (potassium iodide tablets) can also be effective in reversing overgrowth of the gland.

In older patients with goiter due to iodine deficiency there is a risk of provoking hyperthyroidism by increasing iodine intake (p. 233 B). During chronic maximal stimulation, thyroid follicles can become independent of TSH stimulation ("autonomic tissue"). If the iodine supply is increased, thyroid hormone production increases while TSH secretion decreases due to feedback inhibition. The activity of autonomic tissue, however, persists at a high level; thyroxine is released in excess, resulting in iodine-induced hyperthyroidism.

Iodized salt prophylaxis. Goiter is endemic in regions where soils are deficient in iodine. Use of iodized table salt allows iodine requirements (150–300 μg/day) to be met and effectively prevents goiter.

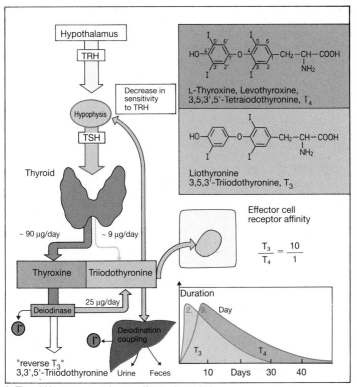

A. Thyroid hormones - release, effects, degradation

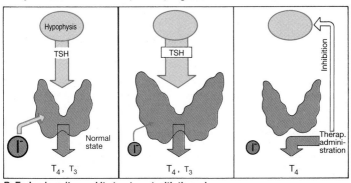

B. Endemic goiter and its treatment with thyroxine

Hyperthyroidism and Antithyroid Drugs

Thyroid overactivity in Graves' disease (**A**) results from formation of IgG antibodies that bind to and activate TSH receptors. Consequently, there is overproduction of hormone with cessation of TSH secretion. Graves' disease can abate spontaneously after 1–2 years. Therefore, initial therapy consists in reversible suppression of thyroid activity by means of antithyroid drugs. In other forms of hyperthyroidism, such as hormone-producing (morphologically benign) thyroid adenoma, the preferred therapeutic method is removal of tissue, either by surgery or by administration of ^{131}I in sufficient dosage. Radioiodine is taken up into thyroid cells and destroys tissue within a sphere of a few millimeters by emitting β-(electron) particles during its radioactive decay.

Concerning iodine-induced hyperthyroidism, see p. 230.

Antithyroid drugs inhibit thyroid function. Release of thyroid hormone (**C**) is preceded by a chain of events. A membrane transporter actively accumulates iodide in thyroid cells; this is followed by: oxidation to iodine, iodination of tyrosine residues in thyroglobulin, conjugation of two diiodotyrosine groups, and formation of T_4 and T_3 moieties. These reactions are catalyzed by thyroid peroxidase. T_4-containing thyroglobulin is stored inside the thyroid follicles in the form of thyrocolloid. Upon endocytotic uptake, colloid undergoes lysosomal enzymatic hydrolysis, enabling thyroid hormone to be released as required. A "thyrostatic" effect can result from inhibition of synthesis or release. When synthesis is arrested, the antithyroid effect develops after a delay, as stored colloid continues to be utilized.

Antithyroid drugs for long-term therapy (C). Thiourea derivatives (thioureylenes, **thioamides**) inhibit peroxidase and, hence, hormone synthesis. In order to restore a euthyroid state, two therapeutic principles can be applied in Graves' disease: a) monotherapy with a thioamide with gradual dose reduction as the disease abates; b) administration of high doses of a thioamide with concurrent administration of thyroxine to offset diminished hormone synthesis. Adverse effects of thioamides are rare; however, the possibility of agranulocytosis has to be kept in mind.

Perchlorate, given orally as the sodium salt, inhibits the iodide pump. Adverse reactions include aplastic anemia. Compared with thioamides, its therapeutic importance is low.

Short-term thyroid suppression (C). Iodine in high dosage (> 6000 µg/day) exerts a **transient** "thyrostatic" effect in hyperthyroid, but usually not in euthyroid, individuals. Since release is also blocked, the effect develops more rapidly than does that of thioamides.

Clinical applications include: preoperative suppression of thyroid secretion according to Plummer with Lugol's solution (5% iodine + 10% potassium iodide, 50–100 mg iodine/day for a maximum of 10 days). In thyrotoxic crisis, Lugol's solution is given together with thioamides and β-blockers. Adverse effects: allergies; contraindications: iodine-induced thyrotoxicosis.

Lithium ions inhibit thyroxine release. Lithium salts can be used instead of iodine for rapid thyroid suppression in iodine-induced thyrotoxicosis. Regarding administration of lithium in endogenous manic-depressive illness, see p. 222.

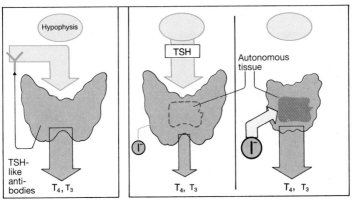

A. Graves' disease

B. Iodine hyperthyroidosis in endemic goiter

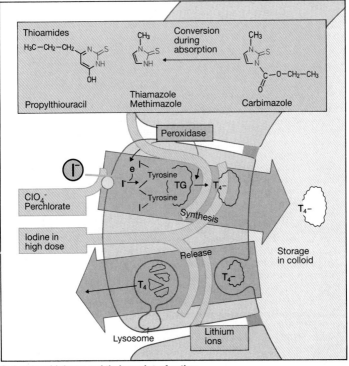

C. Antithyroid drugs and their modes of action

Glucocorticoid Therapy

I. Replacement therapy. The adrenal cortex (AC) produces the *glucocorticoid cortisol* (hydrocortisone) and the *mineralocorticoid aldosterone*. Both steroid hormones are vitally important in adaptation responses to stress situations, such as disease, trauma, or surgery. Cortisol secretion is stimulated by hypophyseal ACTH; aldosterone secretion by angiotensin II in particular (p. 124). In AC failure (*primary AC insufficiency*; Addison's disease), both *cortisol* and *aldosterone* must be replaced; when ACTH production is deficient (*secondary AC insufficiency*), *cortisol alone* needs to be replaced. Cortisol is effective when given orally (30 mg/day, 2/3 a.m., 1/3 p.m.). In stress situations, the dose is raised by 5- to 10-fold. Aldosterone is poorly effective via the oral route; instead, the mineralocorticoid fludrocortisone (0.1 mg/day) is given.

II. Pharmacodynamic therapy with glucocorticoids (A). In unphysiologically high concentrations, cortisol or other glucocorticoids suppress all phases (exudation, proliferation, scar formation) of the inflammatory reaction, i.e., the body's defensive measures against foreign or noxious matter. In this process, the protein lipocortin (macrocortin), synthesis of which is stimulated by glucocorticoids, probably plays a role. Lipocortin inhibits the enzyme phospholipase A_2. Consequently, release of arachidonic acid is diminished, as is the formation of inflammatory mediators of the prostaglandin and leukotriene series (p. 188).

Desired effects. As *antiallergics*, *immunosuppressants*, or *anti-inflammatory* drugs, glucocorticoids display excellent efficacy against "undesired" inflammatory reactions.

Unwanted effects. With *short-term use*, glucocorticoids are practi-

cally *free of adverse effects*, even at the highest dosage. **Long-term use** is likely to cause changes mimicking the signs of **Cushing's syndrome** (endogenous overproduction of cortisol). Sequelae of the anti-inflammatory action: lowered resistance to infection, delayed wound healing, impaired healing of peptic ulcers. Sequelae of exacerbated glucocorticoid action: a) increased gluconeogenesis and release of glucose; insulin-dependent conversion of glucose to triglycerides (adiposity mainly noticeable in the face, neck, and trunk); "steroid-diabetes," if insulin release is insufficient; b) increased protein catabolism with atrophy of skeletal musculature (thin extremities), osteoporosis, growth retardation in infants, skin atrophy. Sequelae of the intrinsically weak, but now manifest, mineralocorticoid action of cortisol: salt and fluid retention, hypertension, edema; KCl loss with danger of hypokalemia.

Measures for Attenuating or Preventing Drug-Induced Cushing's Syndrome

a) *Use of cortisol derivatives with less* (e.g., prednisolone) or *negligible mineralocorticoid activity* (e.g., triamcinolone, dexamethasone). Glucocorticoid activity of these congeners is more pronounced. Glucorticoid, anti-inflammatory, and feedback inhibitory (p. 236) actions on the hypophysis are correlated. An exclusively anti-inflammatory congener does not exist. The "glucocorticoid"-related Cushingoid symptoms cannot be avoided. The table lists relative activity (potency) with reference to cortisol, whose mineralo- and glucocorticoid activities are assigned a value of 1.0. All listed glucocorticoids are effective orally.

b) *Local application.* Typical adverse effects, however, also occur locally, e.g., skin atrophy or mucosal

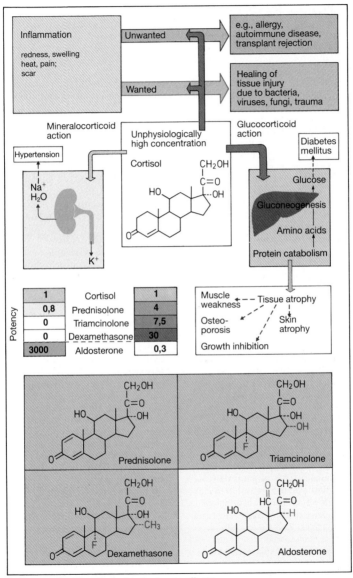

A. Glucocorticoids: principal and adverse effects

colonization with candidal fungi. To minimize systemic absorption after inhalation, derivatives should be used that have a high rate of presystemic elimination, such as beclomethasone or budesonide (p. 14).

c) *Lowest dosage possible*. For long-term medication, a just sufficient dose should be given. However, in attempting to lower the dose to the minimal effective level, it is necessary to take into account that administration of exogenous glucocorticoids will suppress production of endogenous cortisol due to activation of an inhibitory feedback mechanism. In this manner, a very low dose could be "buffered" so that unphysiologically high glucocorticoid activity is prevented, as is the anti-inflammatory effect.

Effect of Glucocorticoid Administration on Adrenocortical Cortisol Production (A)

Release of cortisol depends on stimulation by hypophyseal ACTH, which in turn is controlled by hypothalamic corticotropin releasing hormone (CRH=CRF, factor). Both in the hypophysis and the hypothalamus there are cortisol receptors through which cortisol can exert a feedback inhibition of ACTH or CRH release. By means of these cortisol "sensors," the regulatory centers can monitor whether the actual blood level of the hormone corresponds to the "set point." If the blood level exceeds the set point, ACTH output is decreased, and thus also the cortisol production. In this way cortisol level is maintained within the required range. The regulatory centers respond to synthetic glucocorticoids as they do to cortisol. Administration of exogenous cortisol or any other glucocorticoid reduces the amount of endogenous cortisol needed to maintain homeostasis. Release

of CRH and ACTH declines ("inhibition of higher centers by exogenous glucocorticoid") and thus cortisol secretion ("adrenocortical suppression"). After weeks of exposure to unphysiologically high glucocorticoid doses, the cortisol-producing portions of the adrenal cortex shrink ("adrenocortical atrophy"). Aldosterone-synthezising capacity, however, remains unaffected. When glucocorticoid medication is suddenly withheld, the atrophic cortex is unable to produce sufficient cortisol and a potentially life-threatening cortisol deficiency may develop. Therefore, glucocorticoid therapy should always be tapered off by gradual reduction of the dosage.

Regimens for Prevention of Adrenocortical Atrophy

Cortisol secretion is high in the early morning and low in the late evening (circadian rhythm). This implies that the regulatory centers continue to release CRH or ACTH in the face of high morning blood levels of cortisol; accordingly, sensitivity to feedback inhibition must be low in the morning, whereas the opposite holds true in the late evening.

a) *Circadian administration*: The daily dose of glucocorticoid is given in the morning. Endogenous cortisol production will have already begun, the regulatory centers being relatively insensitive to inhibition. In the early morning hours of the next day, CRF/ACTH release and adrenocortical stimulation will resume.

b) *Alternate-day therapy*: Twice the daily dose is given on alternate mornings. On the "off" day, endogenous cortisol production is allowed to occur.

The disadvantage with either regimen is a recrudescence of disease symptoms during the glucocorticoid-free interval.

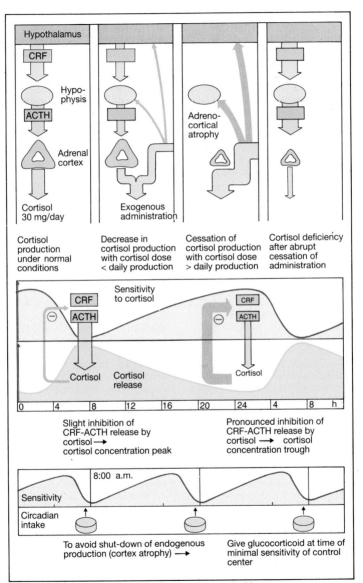

A. Cortisol release and its modification by glucocorticoids

Androgens, Anabolic Steroids, Antiandrogens

Androgens are masculinizing substances. The endogenous male gonadal hormone is the steroid **testosterone** from the interstitial Leydig cells of the testis. Testosterone secretion is stimulated by hypophyseal luteinizing hormone (LH), whose release is controlled by hypothalamic GnRH (gonadorelin, p. 228). Release of both hormones is subject to feedback inhibition by circulating testosterone. Reduction of testosterone to dihydrotestosterone occurs in most target organs; the latter possesses higher affinity for androgen receptors. Rapid intrahepatic degradation (plasma $t^{1/2} \sim$ 15 min) yields androsterone among other metabolites (17-ketosteroids) that are eliminated as conjugates in the urine. Because of rapid hepatic metabolism, testosterone is unsuitable for oral use. Although it is well absorbed, it undergoes virtually complete presystemic elimination.

Testosterone (T.) derivatives for clinical use. *T. esters for i.m. depot injection are T. propionate* and *enanthate (T.heptanoate).* These are given in oily solution by deep intramuscular injection. Upon diffusion of the ester from the depot, esterases quickly split off the acyl residue, to yield free T. With increasing lipophilicity, esters will tend to remain in the depot, and the duration of action therefore lengthens. A *T. ester for oral use* is the *undecanoate.* Because of the fatty acid nature of undecanoic acid, this ester is absorbed into the lymph, enabling it to bypass the liver and enter, via the thoracic duct, the general circulation. *17-α Methyltestosterone* is effective by the oral route due to its increased metabolic stability. On account of the hepatotoxicity of C17-alkylated androgens (cholestasis, tumors), its use should, however, be avoided. Orally active *mesterolone* is 1-α-methyl-dihydrotestosterone.

Indications. For hormone replacement in deficiency of endogenous T. production, T. esters for depot injection are optimally suited. Secondary sex characteristics and libido are maintained; however, fertility is not promoted. On the contrary, spermatogenesis may be suppressed because of feedback inhibition of hypothalamo-hypophyseal gonadotropin secretion.

Stimulation of spermatogenesis in gonadotropin (FSH, LH) deficiency can be achieved by injection of HMG and HCG. HMG or *human menopausal gonadotropin* is obtained from the urine of postmenopausal women and is rich in FSH activity. HCG, *human chorionic gonadotropin* from the urine of pregnant women, acts like LH.

Anabolics are testosterone derivatives (e.g., clostebol, metenolone, nandrolone, stanozolol) that are used in debilitated patients, and misused by athletes, because of their protein anabolic effect. They act via stimulation of androgen receptors and thus also display androgenic actions (e.g., virilization in females, suppression of spermatogenesis).

The **antiandrogen cyproterone** acts as a competitive antagonist of T. In addition, it has progestin activity whereby it inhibits gonadotropin secretion (p. 242). **Indications**: in men, inhibition of sex drive in hypersexuality; prostatic cancer. In women: treatment of virilization.

Finasteride inhibits 5 α-reductase, the enzyme converting T. to dihydro-T. in many target tissues. In benign prostatic hyperplasia the drug may reduce the size of the gland.

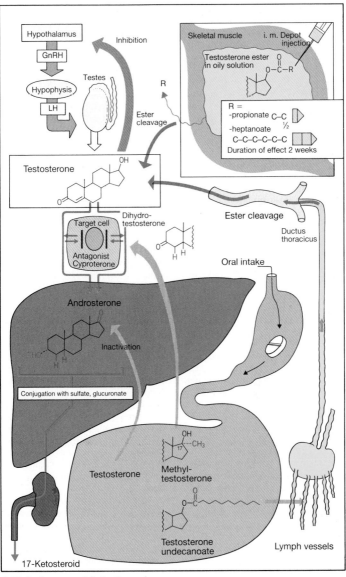

A. Testosterone and derivatives

Follicular Growth and Ovulation, Estrogen and Progestin Production

Follicular maturation and ovulation, as well as the associated production of female gonadal hormones, are controlled by the hypophyseal gonadotropins FSH (follicle stimulating hormone) and LH (luteinizing hormone). In the first half of the menstrual cycle, FSH promotes growth and maturation of ovarian follicles that respond with accelerating synthesis of estradiol. Estradiol stimulates endometrial growth and increases the permeability of cervical mucus for sperm cells. When the estradiol blood level approaches a predetermined set point, FSH release is inhibited due to feedback action on the anterior hypophysis. Since follicle growth and estrogen production are correlated, hypophysis and hypothalamus can "monitor" the follicular phase of ovarian cycle through their estrogen receptors. Within hours after ovulation, the tertiary follicle develops into the corpus luteum, which then also releases progesterone in response to LH. The former initiates the secretory phase of the endometrial cycle and lowers the permeability of cervical mucus. Nonruptured follicles continue to release estradiol under the influence of FSH. After 2 weeks, production of progesterone and estradiol subsides, causing the secretory endometrial layer to be shed (menstruation).

The natural hormones are unsuitable for oral application because they are subject to presystemic hepatic elimination. Estradiol is converted via estrone to estriol; by conjugation, all three can be rendered water-soluble and amenable to renal excretion. The major metabolite of progesterone is pregnanediol, which is also conjugated and eliminated renally.

Estrogen preparations. Depot preparations for i.m. injection are oily solutions of esters of estradiol (3- or 17-OH group). The hydrophobicity of the acyl moiety determines the rate of absorption, hence the duration of effect (p. 238). Released ester is hydrolyzed to yield free estradiol. **Orally used preparations.** *Ethinyl estradiol (EE)* is more stable metabolically, passes the liver after oral intake and mimics estradiol at estrogen receptors. *Mestranol* itself is inactive; however, cleavage of the C-3 methoxy group again yields EE. In oral contraceptives, one of the two agents forms the estrogen component (p. 242). *Conjugated estrogens* can be extracted from equine urine and are used for the prevention of postmenopausal osteoporosis and in the therapy of climacteric complaints. Because of their high polarity (sulfate, glucuronide), they would hardly appear suitable for oral administration. For **transdermal delivery**, an adhesive patch is available that releases estradiol transcutaneously into the body.

Progestin preparations. Depot formulations for i.m. injection are *17-α-hydroxyprogesterone caproate* and *medroxyprogesterone acetate*. Preparations for oral use are derivatives of ethisterone (= 17-α-ethinyltestosterone, e. g., norethindrone [= norethisterone], desogestrel) or 17-α-hydroxyprogesterone acetate (e. g., chlormadinone acetate or cyproterone acetate). These agents are mainly used for the progestin component in oral contraceptives.

Indications for estrogens and progestins include: hormonal contraception (p. 242), hormone replacement, as in postmenopausal women for prophylaxis of osteoporosis; bleeding anomalies, menstrual complaints. Concerning adverse effects, see p. 242.

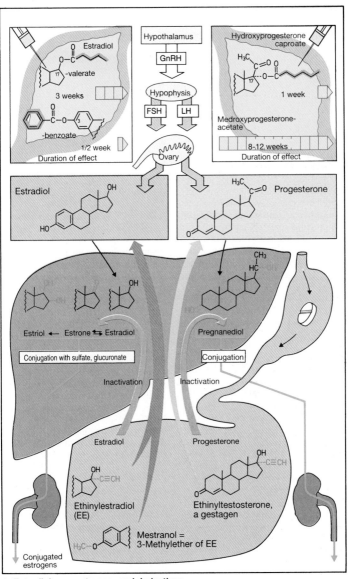

A. Estradiol, progesterone, and derivatives

Oral Contraceptives

Inhibitors of ovulation. Negative feedback control of gonadotropin release can be utilized to inhibit the ovarian cycle. **Administration of exogenous estrogens** (ethinylestradiol or mestranol) during the first half of the cycle permits **FSH production to be suppressed** (also by administration of progestins). Due to the reduced FSH stimulation of tertiary follicles, **maturation of follicles and hence ovulation are prevented**. In effect, the regulatory brain centers are deceived, as it were, by the elevated estrogen blood level, which signals normal follicular growth and a decreased requirement for FSH stimulation. If estrogens alone are given during the first half of the cycle, endometrial and cervical responses, as well as other functional changes, would occur in the normal fashion. By adding a progestin (p. 240) during the second half of the cycle, the secretory phase of the endometrium and associated effects can be elicited. Discontinuance of hormone administration would be followed by menstruation.

The physiological time course of estrogen–progesterone release is simulated in the so-called **biphasic (sequential) preparations (A)**. In **monophasic preparations**, estrogen and progestin are taken concurrently. Early administration of progestin reinforces the inhibition of CNS regulatory mechanisms, prevents both normal endometrial growth and conditions for ovum implantation, and decreases penetrability of cervical mucus for sperm cells. The two latter effects also act to prevent pregnancy. According to the staging of progestin administration, one distinguishes (**A**): one-, two-, and three-stage preparations. In all cases, "withdrawal bleeding" occurs when hormone intake is discontinued (if necessary, by substituting dummy tablets).

Unwanted effects. An increased incidence of thrombosis and embolism is attributed to the estrogen component in particular. Hypertension, fluid retention, cholestasis, benign liver tumors, nausea, chest pain, etc. may occur. Apparently there is no increased overall risk of malignant tumors.

Minipill. Continuous low-dose administration of progestin alone can prevent pregnancy. Ovulations are not suppressed regularly; the effect is then due to progestin-induced alterations in cervical and endometrial function. Because of the need for constant intake at the same time of day, a lower success rate, and relatively frequent bleeding anomalies, these preparations are rarely employed.

"Morning-after" pill. This refers to administration of a high dose of estrogen and progestin, preferably within 12–24 h, but no later than 72 h, after coitus. Menstrual bleeding ensues, which prevents implantation of the fertilized ovum (normally on the 7th day after fertilization, p. 74). Similarly, implantation could be inhibited by **mifepristone**, which is an antagonist at progesteron receptors. Mifeproston is currently under investigation as an agent to induce therapeutic abortion in early pregnancy.

Stimulation of ovulation. Gonadotropin secretion can be increased by *pulsatile delivery of GnRH* (p. 228). The *estrogen antagonists clomiphene* and *cyclofenil* block receptors mediating feedback inhibition of central neuroendocrine circuits and thereby disinhibit gonadotropin release. **Gonadotropins can be given** in the form of HMG and HCG (p. 238).

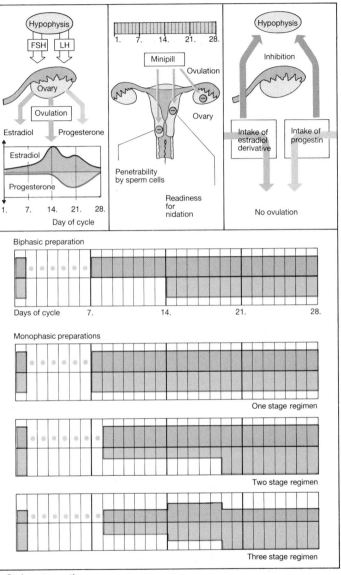

A. Oral contraceptives

Insulin Therapy

Insulin is synthesized in the B-(or β-) cells of the pancreatic islets of Langerhans. It is a protein (MW 5800) consisting of two peptide chains linked by two disulfide bridges; the A chain has 21 and the B chain 30 amino acids. Insulin is the "blood-sugar lowering" hormone. Upon ingestion of dietary carbohydrates, it is released into the blood and acts to prevent a significant rise in blood glucose concentration by promoting uptake and utilization of glucose in various organs, including the liver, adipose tissue, and skeletal muscle.

Insulin is used in the **replacement therapy** of **diabetes mellitus** to supplement a deficient secretion of endogenous hormone.

Sources of therapeutic insulin preparations (A). Insulin can be obtained from pancreatic tissue of slaughtered animals. *Porcine insulin* differs from human insulin merely by one B-chain amino acid, *bovine insulin* by two amino acids in the A chain and one in the B chain. With these slight differences, animal and human hormone display similar biological activity. Compared with human hormone, porcine insulin is barely antigenic and bovine insulin has a little higher antigenicity.

Human insulin is produced by two methods: biosynthetically, by substituting threonine for the C-terminal alanine in the B chain of porcine insulin; or by gene technology involving insertion of the appropriate human DNA into *E. coli* bacteria.

Types of preparations (B). As a peptide, insulin is unsuitable for oral administration (destruction by gastrointestinal proteases) and thus needs to be given parenterally. Usually, insulin preparations contain 100 U/mL (22 U = 1 mg) and are injected subcutaneously. The duration of action depends on the rate of absorption from the injection site.

Short-acting insulin is dispensed as a clear neutral **solution** known as **regular insulin.** In emergencies, such as hyperglycemic coma, it can be given intravenously (mostly by infusion because i.v. injections have too short an action). With the usual subcutaneous application, the effect is evident within 15 to 20 min, reaches a peak after approx. 3 h, and lasts for approx. 6 h.

Insulin suspensions. When injected as a suspension of insulin-containing particles, dissolution and release of the hormone in subcutaneous tissue is retarded (**rapid, intermediate,** and **slow insulins**). Suitable particles can be obtained by precipitation of apolar, poorly water-soluble complexes consisting of anionic insulin and cationic partners, e.g., the polycationic protein protamine or the compound aminoquinuride (Surfen). In the presence of zinc and acetate ions, insulin crystallizes; crystal size determines the rate of dissolution.

Combination preparations contain insulin mixtures in solution and in suspension; the plasma concentration–time curve represents the sum of the two components.

Unwanted effects. *Hypoglycemia* results from absolute or relative overdosage (see p. 246). *Allergic reactions* are rare—locally: redness at injection site, atrophy of adipose tissue *(lipodystrophy)*; systemically: uricaria, skin rash, anaphylaxis.

Insulin resistance can result from binding to inactivating antibodies. A possible local *lipohypertrophy* can be avoided by alternating injection sites.

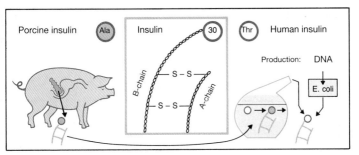

A. Insulin production

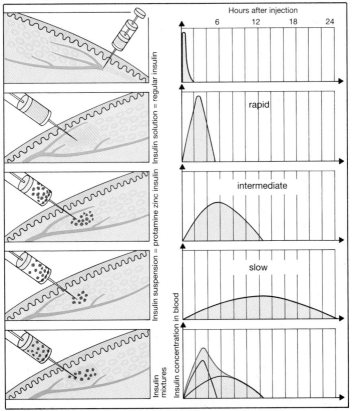

B. Insulin: preparations and blood level - time curves

Treatment of Insulin-Dependent Diabetes Mellitus

"Juvenile-onset" (type I) diabetes mellitus is caused by the destruction of insulin-producing B cells in the pancreas, necessitating replacement of insulin (daily dose approx. 40 U, equivalent to approx. 1.6 mg).

Therapeutic objectives are: (1) prevention of life-threatening hyperglycemic (diabetic) coma; (2) prevention of diabetic sequelae (angiopathy with blindness, myocardial infarction, renal failure), with precise "titration" of the patient being essential to avoid even short-term spells of pathological hyperglycemia; (3) prevention of insulin overdosage leading to life-threatening hypoglycemic shock (CNS disturbance due to lack of glucose).

Therapeutic principles. In healthy subjects, the amount of insulin is "automatically" matched to carbohydrate intake, hence to blood glucose concentration. The critical secretory stimulus is the rise in plasma glucose level. Food intake and physical activity (increased glucose uptake into musculature, decreased insulin demand) are accompanied by corresponding changes in insulin secretion (**A**, left track).

In the diabetic, insulin could be administered as it is normally secreted; that is, injection of short-acting insulin before each main meal plus bedtime administration of a lente preparation to avoid a nocturnal shortfall of insulin. This regimen requires a well-educated, cooperative, and competent patient. In other cases, a fixed-dosage schedule will be needed, e.g., morning and evening injections of a combination insulin in constant respective dosage (**A**). To avoid hypo- or hyperglycemias, dietary carbohydrate (CH) intake must be synchronized with the time course of insulin absorption from the s.c. depot. Caloric intake is to be distributed (50% CH, 30% fat, 20% protein) in small meals over the day so as to achieve a steady CH supply—snacks, late-night meal. Rapidly absorbable CH (sweets, cakes) must be avoided (hyperglycemic peaks) and replaced with slowly digestible ones. Any change in eating and living habits can upset control of blood sugar: skipping a meal or unusual physical stress lead to hypoglycemia; increased CH intake provokes hyperglycemia.

Hypoglycemia is heralded by warning signs: tachycardia, unrest, tremor, pallor, profuse sweating. Some of these are due to the release of glucose-mobilizing epinephrine. *Countermeasures:* glucose administration, rapidly absorbed CH orally or 10–20 g glucose i.v. in case of unconsciousness; if necessary, injection of glucagon, the pancreatic hyperglycemic hormone.

Even with optimal control of blood sugar, s.c. administration of insulin cannot fully replicate the physiological situation. In healthy subjects, absorbed glucose and insulin released from the pancreas simultaneously reach the liver in high concentration, whereby effective presystemic elimination of both substances is achieved. In the diabetic, s.c. injected insulin is uniformly distributed in the body. Since insulin concentration in blood supplying the liver cannot rise, less glucose is extracted from portal blood. A significant amount of glucose enters extrahepatic tissues, where it has to be utilized.

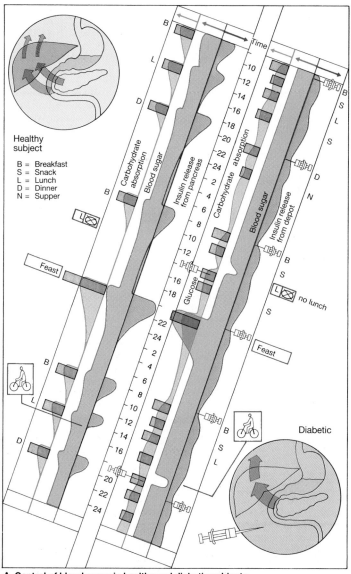

A. Control of blood sugar in healthy and diabetic subjects

Treatment of "Maturity-Onset" Diabetes Mellitus

In overweight adults, a diabetic metabolic condition may develop (type II, or adult diabetes) when there is a relative insulin deficiency—enhanced demand cannot be met by a diminishing insulin secretion. The **cause of increased insulin requirement** is a loss of **insulin receptors** on cell membranes, e.g., of adipocytes. Accordingly, insulin sensitivity of cells declines. This can be illustrated by comparing concentration-binding curves in cells from normal and obese individuals (**A**). In the obese, the maximum binding possible (plateau of curve) is displaced downward, indicative of the reduction in receptor numbers. Also, at low insulin concentrations, there is less binding of insulin, compared with the control condition. For a given metabolic effect (say, utilization of carbohydrates contained in a piece of cake) a certain number of receptors must be occupied. As shown by the binding curves (dashed lines), this can still be achieved with a reduced receptor number; although only at a higher concentration of insulin.

Development of adult diabetes (B). Compared with a normal subject, the obese subject requires a continually elevated output of insulin (orange curves) to avoid an excessive rise of blood glucose levels (green curves) during a glucose load. When the secretory capacity of the pancreas decreases, this is first noted as a rise in blood glucose during glucose loading (latent diabetes). Subsequently, not even the fasting blood glucose level can be maintained (manifest, overt diabetes). A diabetic condition has developed, although insulin release is not lower than that in a healthy person (relative insulin deficiency).

Treatment. Caloric restriction to restore body weight to normal is associated with an increase in insulin receptor number or cellular responsiveness. The releasable amount of insulin is again adequate to maintain a normal metabolic rate.

Therapy of first choice is weight reduction, not administration of drugs! Should the diabetic condition fail to resolve, consideration should first be given to insulin replacement (p. 246). **Oral antidiabetics of the *sulfonylurea type*** increase the sensitivity of B cells towards glucose, enabling them to increase release of insulin. These drugs probably promote depolarization of the B cell membrane by closing off ATP-gated K^+-channels. Normally, these channels are closed when intracellular levels of glucose, hence of ATP, increase. This drug class includes tolbutamide (500–2000 mg/day) and glyburide (glibenclamide) (1.75–10.5 mg/day). In some patients, it is not possible to stimulate insulin secretion from the outset, in others therapy fails later on. Matching dosage of the oral antidiabetic and caloric intake follows the same principles as apply to insulin (p. 246). Hypoglycemia is the most important unwanted effect. Enhancement of the hypoglycemic effect can result from drug interactions: displacement of antidiabetic drug from plasma protein binding sites by sulfonamides, acetylsalicylic acid. Gastrointestinal disturbances, ethanol intolerance, and allergic reactions are possible.

Metformin is a **biguanide derivative** that lowers blood glucose levels by inhibiting absorption and promoting metabolism of glucose. Because there is a danger of flooding the body with lactic acid (lactate acidosis, lethality 50%), it is used only in exceptional circumstances.

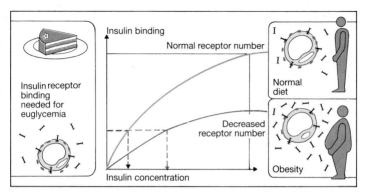

A. Insulin concentration and binding in normal and overweight subjects

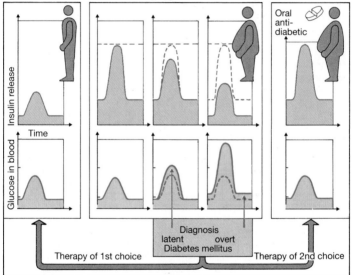

B. Development of maturity-onset diabetes

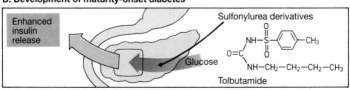

C. Action of oral antidiabetic drugs

Drugs for Maintaining Calcium Homeostasis

At rest, the intracellular concentration of free calcium ions (Ca^{2+}) is kept at 0.1 μM. During excitation, a transient rise of up to 10 μM elicits contraction in muscle cells and secretion in glandular cells. The cellular content of Ca^{2+} is in equilibrium with the extracellular Ca^{2+} concentration (approx. 1000 μM), as is the plasma protein-bound fraction of calcium in blood. Ca^{2+} may crystallize with phosphate to form durapatite (hydroxylapatite), the mineral of bone. Osteoclasts are phagocytes that mobilize Ca^{2+} by resorption of bone. Slight changes in extracellular Ca^{2+} concentration can alter organ function: thus, excitability of skeletal muscle increases markedly as Ca^{2+} is lowered (e.g., in hyperventilation tetany). Three hormones are available to the body for maintaining a constant extracellular Ca^{2+} concentration.

Vitamin D hormone is derived from *vitamin D (cholecalciferol)*. Vitamin D (vit. D) can also be produced in the body; it is formed in the skin from dehydrocholesterol during irradiation with UV light. When there is lack of solar radiation, dietary intake becomes essential, cod liver oil being a rich source. Metabolically active *vit. D hormone* results from two successive hydroxylations: in the liver at position 25 (→ calcifediol) and in the kidney at position 1 (→ calcitriol = vit. D hormone). 1-Hydroxylation depends on the level of calcium homeostasis and is stimulated by parathormone and a fall in plasma levels of Ca^{2+} or phosphate. Vit. D hormone promotes enteral absorption and renal resorption of calcium and phosphate. As a result of the increased concentration of calcium and phosphate in blood, there is an increased tendency

for these ions to be deposited in bone in the form of durapatite crystals. In vit. D deficiency, bone mineralization is inadequate (rickets, osteomalacia). **Therapeutic use** aims at *replacement*. Mostly, vit. D is given; in liver disease calcifediol may be indicated, in renal disease calcitriol. Effectiveness, as well as rate of onset and cessation of action increase in the order vit. D, 25-OH vit.D, 1,25-di-OH vit. D. **Overdosage** may induce hypercalcemia with deposits of calcium salts in tissues (particularly in kidney and blood vessels): calcinosis.

The polypeptide **parathormone** is released from the parathyroid glands when plasma Ca^{2+} level falls. It *stimulates osteoclasts* to increase bone resorption; in the kidneys it promotes calcium resorption, while phosphate excretion is enhanced. As blood phosphate concentration diminishes, the tendency of calcium to precipitate as bone mineral decreases. By stimulating the formation of vit. D hormone, parathormone has an indirect effect on the enteral uptake of Ca^{2+} and phosphate. In **parathormone deficiency**, **vitamin D** can be used as a substitute that, unlike parathormone, is effective orally.

The polypeptide **calcitonin** is secreted by thyroid C-cells during imminent hypercalcemia. It lowers plasma Ca^{2+} concentration by *inhibiting osteoclast activity*. Its uses include hypercalcemia and osteoporosis. Remarkably, calcitonin injection may produce a sustained *analgesic effect* that is not restricted to bone pain.

Hypercalcemia can be treated by administering 0.9% NaCl solution plus furosemide (if necessary), the osteoclast inhibitors calcitonin, plicamycin (mithramycin), or clodronic acid (a biphosphonate), the calcium chelators EDTA sodium or sodium citrate, as well as glucocorticoids.

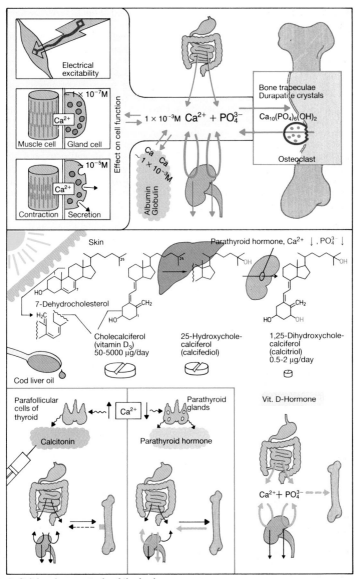

$1 \times 10^{-3}M$ $Ca^{2+} + PO_4^{3-}$

$Ca_{10}(PO_4)_6(OH)_2$

Electrical excitability

Muscle cell   Gland cell $\leftarrow 1 \times 10^{-7}M$

Contraction   Secretion $10^{-5}M$

Effect on cell function

Ca^{2+}

Bone trabeculae
Durapatite crystals

Osteoclast

Albumin Globulin $1 \times 10^{-3}M$ Ca   Ca

Skin   Parathyroid hormone, Ca^{2+} ↓, PO_4^{3-} ↓

7-Dehydrocholesterol

Cholecalciferol (vitamin D$_3$)
50–5000 µg/day

25-Hydroxycholecalciferol (calcifediol)

1,25-Dihydroxycholecalciferol (calcitriol)
0.5–2 µg/day

Cod liver oil

Parafollicular cells of thyroid   Parathyroid glands   Vit. D-Hormone

Calcitonin Ca^{2+} Parathyroid hormone

$Ca^{2+} + PO_4^{3-}$

A. Calcium homeostasis of the body

Drugs for Treating Bacterial Infections

When bacteria overcome the cutaneous or mucosal barriers and penetrate into body tissues, a bacterial *infection* is present. Frequently the body succeeds in removing the invaders, without outward signs of disease, by mounting an immune response. If bacteria multiply faster than the body's defenses can destroy them, *infectious disease* develops with inflammatory signs, e.g., purulent wound infection or urinary tract infection. Appropriate treatment employs substances that injure bacteria and thereby prevent their further multiplication, without harming cells of the host organism (**1**).

Apropos nomenclature: **antibiotics** are produced by microorganisms (fungi, bacteria) and are directed "against life" at any phylogenetic level (prokaryotes, eukaryotes). **Chemotherapeutic agents** originate from chemical synthesis. This distinction has been lost in current usage.

Specific damage to bacteria is particularly practicable when a substance interferes with a metabolic process that occurs in bacterial but not in host cells. Clearly this applies to inhibitors of cell wall synthesis, because human or animal cells lack a cell wall. The **points of attack of antibacterial agents** are schematically illustrated in a grossly simplified bacterial cell, as depicted in **2**.

In the following discussion, polymyxins and tyrothricin are not mentioned further. These polypeptide antibiotics enhance cell membrane permeability. Because of their poor tolerability, they are prescribed in humans only for topical use.

The effect of antibacterial drugs can be observed *in vitro* (**3**). Bacteria multiply in a growth medium under controlled conditions. If the medium contains an antibacterial drug, two results can be discerned: (1) bacteria are killed—**bactericidal effect**; (2) bacteria survive, but do not multiply—**bacteriostatic effect**. Although variations may occur under therapeutic conditions, the different drugs can be classified according to their respective primary mode of action (color tone in **2** and **3**).

When bacterial growth remains unaffected by an antibacterial drug, bacterial **resistance** is present. This may occur because of certain metabolic characteristics that confer a natural insensitivity to the drug on a particular strain of bacteria (*natural resistance*). Depending on whether a drug affects only few or numerous types of bacteria, the terms **narrow-spectrum** (e.g., penicillin G) or **broad-spectrum** (e.g., tetracyclines) **antibiotic** are applied. Naturally susceptible bacterial strains can be transformed under the influence of antibacterial drugs into resistant ones (*acquired resistance*), when a random genetic alteration (mutation) gives rise to a resistant bacterium. Under the influence of the drug, the susceptible bacteria die off, whereas the mutant multiplies unimpeded. The more frequently a given drug is applied, the more probable the emergence of resistant strains (e.g., hospital strains with multiple resistance)!

Resistance can also be acquired when DNA responsible for nonsusceptibility (so-called *resistance plasmid*) is passed on from other resistant bacteria by conjugation or transduction.

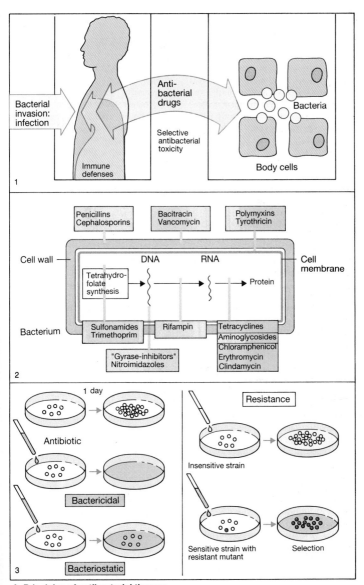

A. Principles of antibacterial therapy

Inhibitors of Cell Wall Synthesis

In most bacteria, a cell wall surrounds the cell like a rigid shell that protects against noxious outside influences and prevents rupture of the plasma membrane from a high internal osmotic pressure. The structural stability of the cell wall is due mainly to the **murein (peptidoglycan) lattice**. This consists of basic building blocks linked together to a large macromolecule. Each basic unit contains the two linked amino sugars N-acetylglucosamine and N-acetylmuramyl acid; the latter bears a peptide chain. The building blocks are synthesized in the bacterium, transported outward through the cell membrane, and assembled as illustrated schematically. The enzyme transpeptidase cross-links the peptide chains of adjacent amino sugar chains.

Inhibitors of cell wall synthesis are suitable antibacterial agents, because animal or human cells lack a cell wall. They exert a **bactericidal** action on growing or multiplying germs. Members of this class include the β-lactam antibiotics *penicillins* and *cephalosporins*, in addition to *bacitracin* and *vancomycin*.

Penicillins (A). The parent substance of this group is **penicillin G (benzylpenicillin)**. It is obtained from cultures of mold fungi, originally from Penicillium notatum. Penicillin G contains the basic structure common to all penicillins, **6-aminopenicillanic acid** (p. 257, 6-APA) comprised of a thiazolidine and a 4-membered β-**lactam ring**. 6-APA itself lacks antibacterial activity. Penicillins disrupt cell wall synthesis by inhibiting **transpeptidase**. When bacteria are in their growth and replication phase, penicillins are bactericidal; due to cell wall defects, the bacteria swell and burst.

Penicillins are generally well tolerated; with penicillin G, the **daily dose** can range from approx. 0.6 g i.m. (= 10^6 international units, 1 mega-I.U.) to 60 g by infusion. The most important **adverse effects** are due to *hypersensitivity* (incidence up to 5%), with manifestations ranging from skin eruptions to anaphylactic shock (in less than 0.05% of patients). Known penicillin allergy is a contraindication for these drugs. Because of an increased risk of sensitization, penicillins must not be used locally. *Neurotoxic effects*, mostly convulsions, may occur if the brain is exposed to extremely high concentrations, e.g., after rapid i.v. injection of a large dose or intrathecal injection.

Penicillin G undergoes rapid renal **elimination** mainly in unchanged form (plasma $t^{1}/_{2}$: 0.5 h). The **duration of effect can be prolonged** by:

1. *Use of higher doses*, enabling plasma levels to remain above the minimally effective antibacterial concentration;

2. *Combination with probenicid*. Renal elimination of penicillin occurs chiefly via the anion (acid)- secretory system of the proximal tubule (–COOH of 6-APA). The acid probenecid (p. 290) competes for this route and thus retards penicillin elimination;

3. *Intramuscular administration in depot form*. In its anionic form (–COO⁻), penicillin G forms poorly water-soluble salts with substances containing a positively charged amino group (procaine, p. 199; clemizole, an antihistaminic; benzathine, dicationic). Depending on the substance, release of penicillin from the depot occurs over a variable interval.

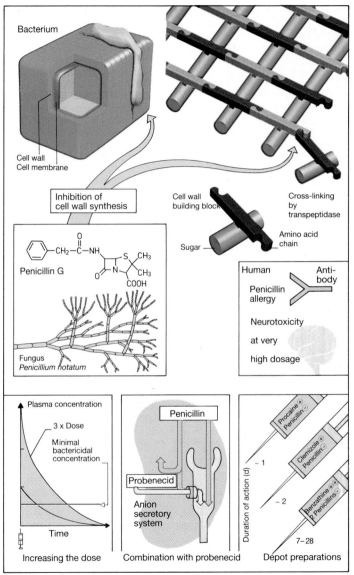

A. Penicillin G: structure and origin; mode of action of penicillins; methods for prolonging duration of action

Although very well tolerated, **penicillin G** has *disadvantages* (**A**) that limit its therapeutic usefulness: (1) It is inactivated by gastric acid, which cleaves the β-lactam ring, necessitating parenteral administration. (2) The β-lactam ring can also be opened by bacterial enzymes (β-lactamases); in particular, penicillinase, which can be produced by staphylococcal strains, renders them resistant to penicillin G. (3) The antibacterial spectrum is narrow; although it encompasses many gram-positive bacteria, gram-negative cocci and spirochetes, many gram-negative pathogens are unaffected.

Derivatives with a different substituent on 6-APA possess **advantages** (**B**): (1) **Acid resistance** permits oral administration, provided that enteral absorption is possible. All derivatives shown in (**B**) can be given orally. *Penicillin V* (phenoxymethylpenicillin) exhibits antibacterial properties similar to those of penicillin G. (2) Due to their **penicillinase-resistance**, *isoxazolylpenicillins* (*oxacillin,* dicloxacillin, floxacillin) are suitable for the (oral) treatment of infections caused by penicillinase-producing staphylococci. (3) **Extended-activity spectrum**: The aminopenicillin *amoxicillin* is active against many gram-negative organisms, e.g., coli bacteria. It can be protected from destruction by penicillinase by combination with *clavulanic acid,* an *inhibitor of penicillinase.*

The structurally close congener *ampicillin* (no 4-hydroxy group) has a similar activity spectrum. However, because it is poorly absorbed (< 50%) and therefore causes more extensive damage to the gut microbial flora, it should be given only by injection.

A still broader spectrum (including Pseudomonas bacteria) is shown by *carboxypenicillins* (carbenicillin,

ticarcillin) and *acylaminopenicillins* (mezlocillin, azlocillin, piperacillin). These substances are neither acid-stable nor penicillinase- resistant.

Cephalosporins (C). These β-**lactam antibiotics** are also fungal products and have bactericidal activity due to **inhibition of transpeptidase.** Their shared basic structure (gray square) is 7-aminocephalosporanic acid, as exemplified by *cephalexin.* Cephalosporins are acid-stable, but many are poorly absorbed. Because they must be given parenterally, most—including those with high activity—are used only in clinical settings. A few, e.g., cephalexin, are suitable for oral use. Cephalosporins are penicillinase-resistant, but cephalosporinase-forming organisms do exist. Some derivatives are, however, also resistant to this β-lactamase. Cephalosporins are broad-spectrum antibacterials. Newer derivatives (e.g. cefotaxime, cefmenoxime, cefoperazone, ceftriaxone, ceftazidime, moxalactam) are also effective against pathogens resistant to various other antibacterials. Cephalosporins are mostly well tolerated. All can cause allergic reactions, some also renal injury, alcohol intolerance, and bleeding (vit. K antagonism).

Other inhibitors of cell wall synthesis. The antibiotics bacitracin and vancomycin interfere with the transport of peptidoglycans through the cytoplasmic membrane and are active only against gram-positive bacteria. **Bacitracin** is a polypeptide mixture, markedly nephrotoxic and used only topically. **Vancomycin** is a glycopeptide and the drug of choice for the (oral) treatment of bowel inflammations occurring as a complication of antibiotic therapy (pseudomembranous enterocolitis caused by *Clostridium difficile*). It is not absorbed.

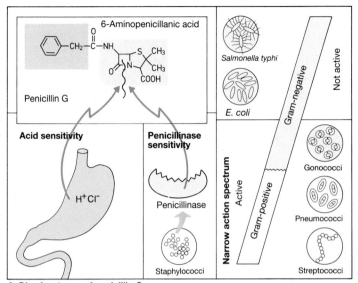

A. Disadvantages of penicillin G

6-Aminopenicillanic acid

Penicillin G

Acid sensitivity

H⁺ Cl⁻

Penicillinase sensitivity

Penicillinase

Staphylococci

Salmonella typhi

E. coli

Gram-negative — Not active

Narrow action spectrum — Active

Gram-positive

Gonococci

Pneumococci

Streptococci

B. Derivatives of penicillin G

	Acid	Penicillinase	Spectrum	Concentration needed to inhibit penicillin G-sensitive bacteria
Penicillin V	Resistant	Sensitive	Narrow	
Oxacillin	Resistant	Resistant	Narrow	
Amoxicillin	Resistant	Sensitive	Broad	

C. Cephalosporin

Cephalexin	Resistant	Resistant, but sensitive to cephalosporinase	Broad	

Inhibitors of Tetrahydrofolate Synthesis

Tetrahydrofolic acid (THF) is a co-enzyme in the synthesis of purine bases and thymidine. These are constituents of DNA and RNA and required for cell growth and replication. Lack of THF leads to inhibition of cell proliferation. Formation of THF from dihydrofolate (DHF) is catalyzed by the enzyme dihydrofolate reductase. DHF is made from folic acid, a vitamin that cannot be synthesized in the body, but must be taken up from exogenous sources. Most bacteria do not have a requirement for folate, because they are capable of synthesizing folate, more precisely DHF, from precursors. Selective interference with bacterial biosynthesis of THF can be achieved with sulfonamides and trimethoprim.

Sulfonamides structurally resemble *p*-aminobenzoic acid (PABA), a precursor in bacterial DHF synthesis. As false substrates, sulfonamides competitively *inhibit* utilization of PABA, hence *DHF synthesis*. Because most bacteria cannot take up exogenous folate, they are depleted of DHF. Sulfonamides thus possess *bacteriostatic activity* against a *broad spectrum* of pathogens. Sulfonamides are produced by chemical synthesis. The basic structure is shown in (**A**). Residue R determines the pharmacokinetic properties of a given sulfonamide. Most sulfonamides are well absorbed via the enteral route. They are metabolized to varying degrees and eliminated through the kidney. Rates of elimination, hence duration of effect, may vary widely. Some members are poorly absorbed from the gut and are thus suitable for the treatment of bacterial bowel infections. Adverse effects may include, among others, allergic reactions, sometimes with severe skin damage, displacement of other plasma protein-bound drugs or bilirubin in neonates (danger of kernicterus, hence contraindication for the last weeks of gestation and in the neonate).

Trimethoprim inhibits bacterial DHF reductase, the human enzyme being significantly less sensitive than the bacterial one (rarely bone marrow depression). The 2,4-diaminopyrimidine, trimethoprim, has bacteriostatic activity against a broad spectrum of pathogens. It is used mostly as a component of co-trimoxazole.

Co-trimoxazole is a combination of *trimethoprim* and the sulfonamide *sulfamethoxazole*. Since THF synthesis is inhibited at two successive steps, the antibacterial effect of co-trimoxazole is better than that of the individual components. Resistant pathogens are infrequent, and a bactericidal effect may occur. Adverse effects correspond to those of the components.

Although initially developed as an antirheumatic agent (p. 292) **sulfasalazine** (salazosulfapyridine) is used mainly in the treatment of inflammatory bowel disease (colitis ulcerativa and terminal ileitis or Crohn's disease). Gut bacteria split this compound into the sulfonamide sulfapyridine and *mesalamine (5-aminosalicylic acid)*. The latter is probably the anti-inflammatory agent (inhibition of leukotriene synthesis?), but must be present on the gut mucosa in high concentrations. Coupling to the sulfonamide prevents premature absorption in upper small bowel segments. The cleaved-off sulfonamide can be absorbed and may produce typical adverse effects (see above).

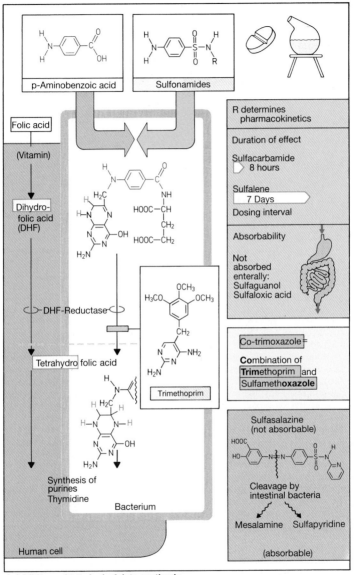

A. Inhibitors of tetrahydrofolate synthesis

Inhibitors of DNA Function

Deoxyribonucleic acid (DNA) serves as a template for the synthesis of nucleic acids. Ribonucleic acid (RNA) executes protein synthesis and thus permits cell growth. Synthesis of new DNA is a prerequisite for cell division. Substances that inhibit reading of genetic information at the DNA template damage the regulatory center of cell metabolism. The substances listed below are useful as antibacterial drugs because they do not affect human cells.

Gyrase inhibitors. The enzyme gyrase (topoisomerase II) permits the orderly accommodation of a ~1000 μm long bacterial chromosome in a bacterial cell of ~1 μm. Within the chromosomal strand, double-stranded DNA has a double helical configuration. The former, in turn, is arranged in loops that are shortened by supercoiling. The gyrase catalyzes this operation, as illustrated, by opening, underwinding, and closing the DNA double strand such that the full loop need not be rotated.

Derivatives of 4-quinolone-3-carboxylic acid (green portion of ofloxacin formula) are inhibitors of bacterial gyrases. They appear to prevent specifically the resealing of opened strands and thereby act bactericidally. These agents are absorbed after oral ingestion. The older drug, *nalidixic acid*, affects exclusively gram-negative bacteria and attains effective concentrations only in urine; it is used as a urinary tract antiseptic. *Norfloxacin* has a broader spectrum. *Ofloxacin, ciprofloxacin*, and *enoxacin* also yield systemically effective concentrations and are used for infections of internal organs.

Besides gastrointestinal problems and allergy, adverse effects particularly involve the CNS (confusion, hallucinations, seizures). Since they can damage epiphyseal chondrocytes and joint cartilages in laboratory animals, gyrase inhibitors should not be used during pregnancy, lactation, and periods of growth.

Azomycin (nitroimidazole) derivatives, such as **metronidazole**, damage DNA by complex formation or strand breakage. This occurs in obligate anaerobes, i.e., bacteria growing under oxygen exclusion. Under these conditions, conversion to reactive metabolites that attack DNA takes place (e.g., the hydroxylamine shown). The effect is bactericidal. A similar mechanism is involved in the antiprotozoal action on *Trichomonas vaginalis* (causative agent of vaginitis and urethritis) and *Entamoeba histolytica* (causative agent of large bowel inflammation, amebic dysentery and hepatic abscesses). Metronidazole is well absorbed via the enteral route; it is also given i.v. or topically. Because metronidazole is considered potentially mutagenic, carcinogenic, and teratogenic in the human, it should not be used longer than 10 days, if possible, and be avoided during pregnancy and lactation. *Tinidazole* may be considered equivalent to metronidazole.

Rifampin inhibits the bacterial enzyme that catalyzes DNA template-directed RNA transcription, i.e., DNA-dependent RNA polymerase. Rifampin acts bactericidally against mycobacteria (*M. tuberculosis, M. leprae*), as well as many gram-positive and gram-negative bacteria. It is well absorbed after oral ingestion. Because resistance may develop with frequent usage, it is restricted to the treatment of tuberculosis and leprosy (p. 266).

Rifampin is contraindicated in the first trimester of gestation and during lactation.

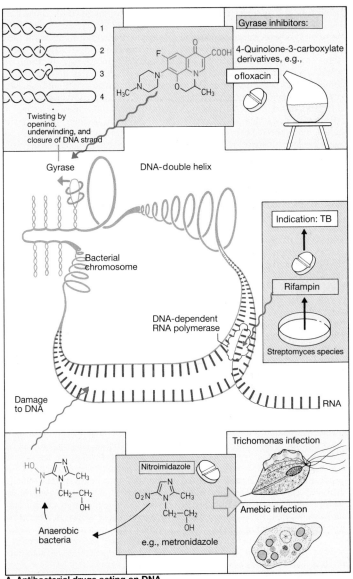

A. Antibacterial drugs acting on DNA

Inhibitors of Protein Synthesis

Protein synthesis means translation into a peptide chain of a genetic message first copied (transcribed) into mRNA (p. 260). Amino acid (AA) assembly occurs at the ribosome. Delivery of amino acids to mRNA involves different transfer RNA molecules (tRNA), each of which binds a specific AA. Each tRNA bears an "anticodon" nucleobase triplet that is complementary to a particular mRNA coding unit (codon, consisting of three nucleobases).

Incorporation of an AA normally involves the following steps (**A**):

1. The ribosome "focuses" two codons on mRNA; one (at the left) has bound its tRNA–AA complex, the AA having already been added to the peptide chain; the other (at the right) is ready to receive the next tRNA–AA complex.

2. After the latter attaches, the AA of the two adjacent complexes are linked by the action of the enzyme peptide synthetase (peptidyltransferase). Concurrently, AA and tRNA of the left complex disengage.

3. The left tRNA dissociates from mRNA. The ribosome can advance along the mRNA strand and focus on the next codon.

4. Consequently, the right tRNA–AA complex shifts to the left, allowing the next complex to be bound at the right.

These individual steps are susceptible to inhibition by **antibiotics** of different groups. The examples shown originate primarily from Streptomyces bacteria, some of the aminoglycosides also being derived from Micromonospora bacteria.

1a. **Tetracyclines** inhibit the binding of tRNA–AA complexes. Their action is bacteriostatic and affects a broad spectrum of pathogens.

1b. **Aminoglycosides** induce the binding of "wrong" tRNA–AA complexes, resulting in synthesis of false proteins. Aminoglycosides are bactericidal. Their activity spectrum encompasses mainly gram-negative organisms. Streptomycin and kanamycin are used predominantly in the treatment of tuberculosis.

Note on spelling: -mycin designates origin from Streptomyces species; -micin (e.g., gentamicin) from Micromonospora species.

2. **Chloramphenicol** inhibits peptide synthetase. It has bacteriostatic activity against a broad spectrum of pathogens. The chemically simple molecule is now produced synthetically.

3. **Erythromycin** suppresses advancement of the ribosome. Its action is predominantly bacteriostatic and directed against gram-positive organisms.

For oral administration, the acid-labile base erythromycin (E) is dispensed as a salt (E. stearate) or an ester (e.g., E. succinate). Erythromycin is well tolerated. It is a suitable substitute in penicillin allergy or resistance. Erythromycin is the most important member of the macrolide antibiotic group, which includes josamycin and spiramycin.

Clindamycin has antibacterial activity similar to that of erythromycin. It exerts a bacteriostatic effect mainly on gram-positive aerobic, as well as on anaerobic pathogens. Clindamycin is a semisynthetic chloroanalogue of lincomycin, which derives from a Streptomyces species. Taken orally, clindamycin is better absorbed than lincomycin, has greater antibacterial efficacy and is thus preferred. Both penetrate well into bone tissue.

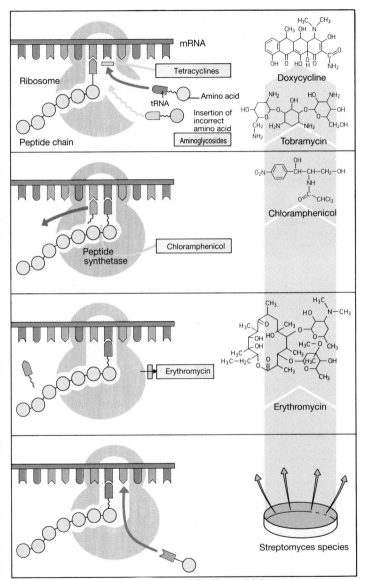

A. Protein synthesis and modes of action of antibacterial drugs

Tetracyclines are absorbed from the gastrointestinal tract to differing degrees, depending on the substance, absorption being nearly complete for *doxycycline* and *minocycline*. Intravenous injection is rarely needed (*rolitetracycline* is available only for i.v. administration). The most common unwanted effect is *gastrointestinal upset* (nausea, vomiting, diarrhea, etc.) due to (1) a direct mucosal irritant action of these substances and (2) damage to the natural bacterial gut flora (broad-spectrum antibiotics) allowing colonization by pathogenic organisms, including candida fungi. Concurrent ingestion of antacids or milk would, however, be inappropriate because tetracyclines form *insoluble complexes* with *plurivalent cations* (e.g., Ca^{2+}, Mg^{2+}, Al^{3+}, $Fe^{2+/3+}$) resulting in their inactivation; that is, absorbability, antibacterial activity, and local irritant action are abolished. The ability, to chelate Ca^{2+} accounts for the propensity of tetracyclines to accumulate in growing teeth and bones. As a result, there occurs an irreversible yellow-brown *discoloration of teeth* and a reversible *inhibition of bone growth*. Because of these adverse effects, tetracycline should not be given after the second month of pregnancy and not prescribed to children aged 8 years and under. Other adverse effects are increased *photosensitivity* of the skin and *hepatic damage*, mainly after i.v. administration.

The broad-spectrum antibiotic **chloramphenicol** is completely absorbed after oral ingestion. It undergoes even distribution in the body and readily crosses diffusion barriers such as the blood–brain barrier. Despite these advantageous properties, use of chloramphenicol is rarely indicated (e.g., in CNS infections) because of the danger of bone marrow damage. *Two types of bone marrow depression*

can occur: (1) a dose-dependent, toxic, reversible form manifested during therapy and (2) a frequently fatal form that may occur after a latency of weeks and is not dose-dependent. Due to high tissue penetrability, the danger of bone marrow depression must also be taken into account after local use (e.g., eye drops).

Aminoglycoside antibiotics consist of glycoside-linked amino-sugars (cf. gentamicin $C_{1\alpha}$, a constituent of the gentamicin mixture). They contain numerous hydroxyl groups and amino groups that can bind protons. Hence, these compounds are highly polar, poorly membrane permeable, and not absorbed enterally. *Neomycin* and *paromomycin* are given orally in order to eradicate intestinal bacteria (prior to bowel surgery or for reducing ammonia formation by gut bacteria in hepatic coma). Aminoglycosides for the treatment of serious infections must be injected (e.g., *gentamicin, tobramycin, amikacin, netilmicin, sisomycin*). In addition, local inlays of a gentamycin-releasing carrier can be used in infections of bone or soft tissues. Aminoglycosides gain access to the bacterial interior by the use of bacterial *transport systems*. In the kidney, they enter the cells of the proximal tubules via an uptake system for oligopeptides. Tubular cells are susceptible to damage (*nephrotoxicity*, mostly reversible). In the inner ear, sensory cells of the vestibular apparatus and Corti's organ may be injured (*ototoxicity*, in part reversible).

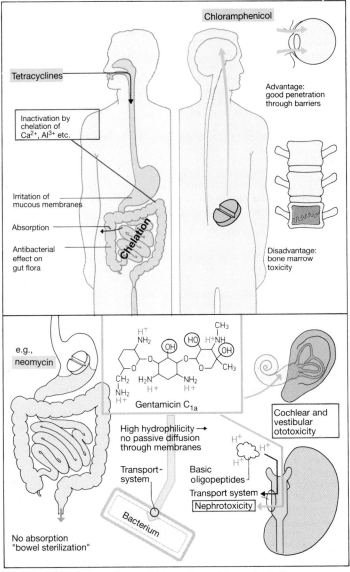

A. Aspects of the therapeutic use of tetracyclines, chloramphenicol, and aminoglycosides

Drugs for Treating Mycobacterial Infections

Mycobacteria are responsible for two diseases: tuberculosis, mostly caused by *M. tuberculosis*, and leprosy due to *M. leprae*. The therapeutic principle applicable to both is combined treatment with two or more drugs. Combination therapy prevents the emergence of resistant mycobacteria. Because the antibacterial effects of the individual substances are additive, correspondingly smaller doses are sufficient. Therefore, the risk of individual adverse effects is lowered. Most drugs are active against only one of the two diseases.

Antitubercular Drugs (1)

Drugs of choice are: isoniazid, rifampin, ethambutol, along with streptomycin and pyrazinamide. Less well tolerated, second-line agents include: *p*-aminosalicylic acid, cycloserine, viomycin, kanamycin, amikacin, capreomycin, ethionamide.

Isoniazid is bactericidal against growing *M. tuberculosis*. Its mechanism of action remains unclear. (In the bacterium it is converted to isonicotinic acid, which is membrane impermeable, hence, likely to accumulate intracellularly.) Isoniazid is rapidly absorbed after oral administration. In the liver, it is inactivated by acetylation, the rate of which is genetically controlled and shows a characteristic distribution in different ethnic groups (fast vs. slow acetylators). Notable adverse effects are: peripheral neuropathy, optic neuritis preventable by administration of vitamin B_6 (pyridoxine); hepatitis, jaundice.

Rifampin. Source, antibacterial activity, and routes of administration are described on p. 260. Albeit mostly well tolerated, this drug may cause several adverse effects including he-

patic damage, hypersensitivity with flu-like symptoms, disconcerting but harmless red/orange discoloration of body fluids, enzyme induction (failure of oral contraceptives).

Ethambutol. The cause of its specific antitubercular action is unknown. Ethambutol is given orally. It is generally well tolerated, but may cause dose-dependent damage to the optic nerve with disturbances of vision (red/green blindness, visual field defects).

Pyrazinamide exerts a bactericidal action by an unknown mechanism. It is given orally. Pyrazinamide may impair liver function; hyperuricemia results from inhibition of renal urate elimination.

Streptomycin must be given i.v. (pp. 262ff) like other aminoglycoside antibiotics. It damages the inner ear and the labyrinth. Its nephrotoxicity is comparatively minor.

Antileprotic Drugs (2)

Rifampin is frequently given in combination with one or both of the two following agents:

Dapsone is a sulfone that, like sulfonamides, inhibits dihydrofolate synthesis (p. 258). It is bactericidal against susceptible strains of M. leprae. Dapsone is given orally. The most frequent adverse effect is methemoglobinemia with accelerated erythrocyte degradation (hemolysis).

Clofazimine is a dye with bactericidal activity against M. leprae and anti-inflammatory properties. It is given orally, but is incompletely absorbed. Because of its high lipophilicity, it accumulates in adipose and other tissues and leaves the body only rather slowly ($t_{1/2}{\sim}70$ days). Red-brown skin pigmentation is an unwanted effect, particularly in fair-skinned patients.

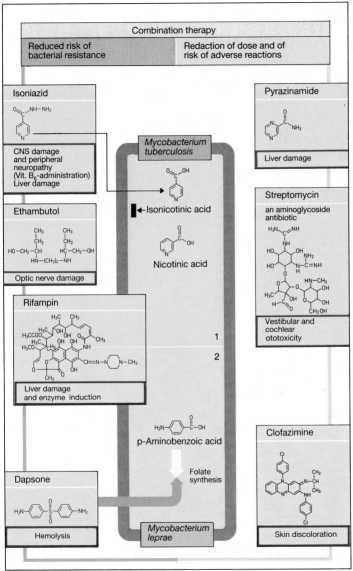

A. Drugs used to treat infections with mycobacteria (1. tuberculosis, 2. leprosy)

Drugs Used in the Treatment of Fungal Infections

Infections due to fungi are usually confined to the skin or mucous membranes: local or superficial mycosis. However, in immune deficiency states, internal organs may also be affected: systemic or deep mycosis.

Mycoses are most commonly due to: *dermatophytes*, which affect the skin, hair, and nails following external infection; *Candida albicans*, a yeast organism normally found on body surfaces, which may cause infections of mucous membranes, less frequently of the skin or internal organs when natural defenses are impaired (immunosuppression, or damage of microflora by broad-spectrum antibiotics).

Imidazole derivatives inhibit ergosterol synthesis. This steroid forms an integral constituent of cytoplasmic membranes of fungal cells, analogous to cholesterol in animal plasma membranes. Fungi exposed to imidazole derivatives stop growing (fungistatic effect) or die (fungicidal effect). The spectrum of affected fungi is very broad. Because they are poorly absorbed and poorly tolerated systemically, most imidazoles are suitable only for topical use (*clotrimazole*, econazole, oxiconazole, isoconazole, bifonazole). Rarely, this use may result in contact dermatitis. *Miconazole* is given locally, or systemically by short-term infusion (despite its poor tolerability). Because it is well absorbed, *ketoconazole* is available for oral administration. Adverse effects are rare; however, the possibility of fatal liver damage should be noted. Remarkably, ketoconazole may inhibit steroidogenesis.

The **polyene antibiotics**, amphotericin B and nystatin, are of bacterial origin. They insert themselves into fungal cell membranes (probably next to ergosterol molecules) and to cause formation of hydrophilic channels. The resultant increase in membrane permeability, e.g., to K$^+$ ions, accounts for the fungicidal effect. *Amphotericin B* is active against most organisms responsible for systemic mycoses. Because of its poor absorbability, it must be given by infusion, which is, however, poorly tolerated (chills, fever, CNS disturbances, impaired renal function, phlebitis at the infusion site). Applied topically to skin or mucous membranes, amphotericin B is useful in the treatment of candidal mycosis. Because of the low rate of enteral absorption, oral administration in intestinal candidiasis can be considered a topical treatment. *Nystatin* is only used for topical therapy.

Flucytosine is converted in Candida fungi to fluorouracil by the action of a specific cytosine deaminase. As an antimetabolite, this compound disrupts DNA and RNA synthesis (p. 280), resulting in a fungicidal effect. Given orally, flucytosine is rapidly absorbed. It is well tolerated in humans and often combined with amphotericin B to allow dose reduction of the latter.

Griseofulvin originates from molds and has activity only against dermatophytes. Presumably, it acts as a spindle poison to inhibit fungal mitosis. Although targeted against local mycoses, griseofulvin must be used systemically. It is incorporated in newly formed keratin. "Impregnated" in this manner, keratin becomes unsuitable as a fungal nutrient. The time required for the eradication of dermatophytes corresponds to the renewal period of skin, hair, or nails. Griseofulvin may cause uncharacteristic adverse effects. In onychomycosis, removal of the infected nail may be preferable to months of pharmacotherapy.

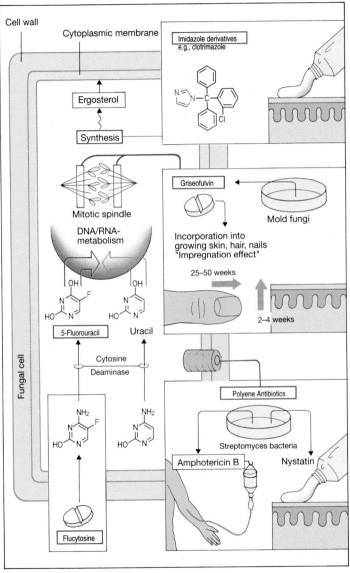

A. Antifungal drugs

Chemotherapy of Viral Infections

Selective interference with the viral life cycle is still difficult to achieve. This restricts the treatment of viral infections. Viruses essentially consist of genetic material (nucleic acids, yellow strand in **A**) and a capsular envelope made up of proteins (blue hexagons). They lack a metabolic system but depend on the infected cell for their growth and replication.

Viral replication (A): (1) The viral particle attaches to the cell membrane (adsorption). (2) It is taken up into the cell interior by endocytosis (penetration). (3) The protein coat opens ("uncoating"). The genetic material of the virus (here DNA, in other viruses RNA) can now act on the cell's metabolic system. (4a) The genetic material is replicated (DNA in this instance) and RNA is produced for the purpose of protein synthesis. (4b) The proteins are used either as capsomers or enzymes catalyzing viral multiplication, e.g., DNA polymerase. (5) Nucleic acids and capsomers are assembled into new virus particles (maturation). (6) Release of new viruses can be associated with host cell destruction. Disease symptoms occur.

Amantadine presumably interferes with "uncoating" or perhaps with "assembly," but only in influenza A viruses (RNA viruses, viral flu). It is also used prophylactically and, if possible, must be taken *before* the outbreak of symptoms. Amantadine is also an antiparkinsonian agent.

Interferons (IFN) are glycoproteins that, among other products, are released from virus-infected cells. In neighboring cells, interferon stimulates the production of "antiviral proteins." These inhibit the synthesis of viral proteins by (preferential) destruction of viral DNA or by suppressing its translation. Interferons are not directed against a specific virus, but have a broad spectrum of antiviral action that is, however, species-specific. Thus, interferon for use in humans must be obtained from cells of human origin, such as leukocytes (IFN-α) or fibroblasts (IFN-β). Interferons are also used to treat certain tumors (e.g., hairy-cell leukemia).

Antimetabolites are "false" DNA building blocks (**B**) or nucleosides. These normally consist of a nucleobase (e.g., thymidine) and the sugar deoxyribose. In antimetabolites, one of the components is defective (rendered in red).

Idoxuridine and congeners are incorporated into DNA with deleterious results. This also applies to the synthesis of human DNA. Therefore, idoxuridine and analogues are suitable only for topical use (e.g., in herpes simplex keratitis).

Vidarabine inhibits virally induced DNA polymerase more strongly than it does the endogenous enzyme. **Acyclovir** (a guanine analogue with an acyclic sugar rudiment) displays the *highest degree of selectivity of action*. Inactive by itself, it must first undergo phosphorylation by a virally induced thymidine kinase. This may occur only in infected cells. Here the active form selectively inhibits viral DNA polymerase. Acyclovir is well tolerated even with systemic administration and used in severe herpes simplex or herpes zoster infections. **Zidovudine** (**azidothymidine** = AZT) selectively inhibits "reverse transcriptase," a virus-specific enzyme present in HIV that first transcribes viral RNA into host cell single-stranded DNA. These drugs are used in AIDS to slow progression of the disease. Eradication of the virus (i.e., a cure) is not possible. They are not well tolerated.

Ganciclovir is an antimetabolite active against cytomegaly virus, e.g., responsible for retinitis in AIDS patients.

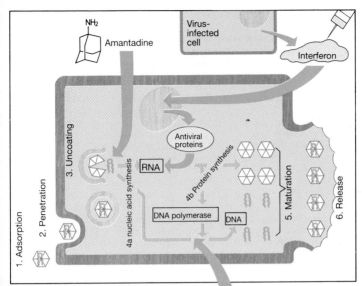

A. Virus multiplication and modes of action of antiviral agents

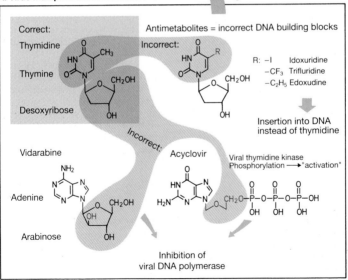

B. Chemical structure of virustatic antimetabolites

Disinfectants

Disinfection denotes the inactivation or killing of *pathogens* (protozoa, bacteria, fungi, viruses) in the human environment. This can be achieved by chemical or physical means; the latter will not be discussed here. **Sterilization** refers to the killing of *all* germs, whether pathogenic, dormant, or non-pathogenic; **antisepsis** to the *reduction* in the number of germs.

Agents for chemical disinfection ideally should cause *rapid, complete,* and *persistent* inactivation of all germs, but at the same time exhibit low toxicity (systemic toxicity, tissue irritancy, antigenicity) and be nondeleterious to inanimate materials. These requirements call for chemical properties that may exclude each other, therefore compromises guided by the intended use have to be made.

Disinfectants come from various chemical classes, including oxidants, halogens, alcohols, aldehydes, organic acids, phenols, cationic surfactants (detergents), and heavy metals. The **basic mechanisms of action** involve denaturation of proteins, inhibition of enzymes, or a reaction with nucleic acids. Effect and speed of action are concentration-dependent.

Activity spectrum. Disinfectants inactivate bacteria (gram-positive > gram-negative > mycobacteria), less effectively their sporal forms, and few (e.g., formaldehyde) are virucidal.

Applications

Room disinfection and *surface (floor) disinfection.* Mixtures of phenols, halogen-releasing substances (sodium hypochlorite), and detergents can be employed in relatively high concentrations, because direct contact with the human body does not occur and the materials to be disinfected are durable. Phenols lose their activity at alkaline pH. Combined with sodium hypochlorite, they are suitable for the disinfection of organic matter (excrements, sputum) since they are not inactivated by the latter, unlike aldehydes.

Disinfection of instruments. Instruments that cannot be heat- or steam-sterilized can be precleaned (to decrease amount of organic matter) and then disinfected with aldehydes and detergents. Chemical disinfection procedures are indispensable for diagnostic instruments containing heat-sensitive synthetic materials (endoscopic probes, catheters).

Skin "disinfection." Antiseptic skin preparation is desirable prior to surgical procedures to reduce the risk of wound infection. Swabbing with iodine tincture (2% iodine) or chlorhexidine solution (0.02%) is more effective than rubbing with alcohol. Regular use of disinfectants by medical personnel (surgical "scrub") reduces the risk of germ transmission. Mixtures of alcohols, aldehydes, phenols, and cationic surfactants are available for this purpose. In such mixtures, rapid action is achieved by use of ethanol 80%, isopropyl alcohol 70%, or formaldehyde and a persistent effect by use of poorly volatile substances, such as benzyl alcohol or glutaraldehyde. Frequency of use places high demands on compatibility.

This also applies to *wound disinfection*, e.g., with hydrogen peroxide (0.2–1% solution, short action) or potassium permanganate (0.001% solution, slightly astringent).

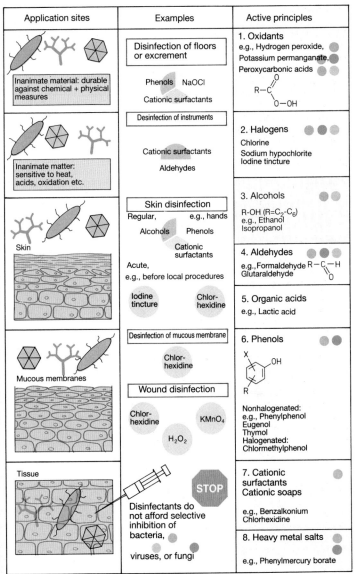

Application sites	Examples	Active principles
Inanimate material: durable against chemical + physical measures	Disinfection of floors or excrement Phenols NaOCl Cationic surfactants	1. Oxidants e.g., Hydrogen peroxide, Potassium permanganate, Peroxycarbonic acids $$R-\overset{\displaystyle O}{\underset{\displaystyle O-OH}{C}}$$
Inanimate matter: sensitive to heat, acids, oxidation etc.	Desinfection of instruments Cationic surfactants Aldehydes	2. Halogens Chlorine Sodium hypochlorite Iodine tincture
Skin	Skin disinfection Regular, e.g., hands Alcohols Phenols Cationic surfactants Acute, e.g., before local procedures Iodine tincture Chlor-hexidine	3. Alcohols R-OH (R=C_2-C_6) e.g., Ethanol Isopropanol
		4. Aldehydes e.g., Formaldehyde $R-\overset{\displaystyle C}{\underset{\displaystyle O}{}}-H$ Glutaraldehyde
		5. Organic acids e.g., Lactic acid
Mucous membranes	Desinfection of mucous membrane Chlor-hexidine Wound disinfection Chlor-hexidine KMnO$_4$ H_2O_2	6. Phenols Nonhalogenated: e.g., Phenylphenol Eugenol Thymol Halogenated: Chlormethylphenol
Tissue	STOP Disinfectants do not afford selective inhibition of bacteria, viruses, or fungi	7. Cationic surfactants Cationic soaps e.g., Benzalkonium Chlorhexidine
		8. Heavy metal salts e.g., Phenylmercury borate

A. Disinfectants

Drugs for Treating Endo- and Ectoparasitic Infestations

Adverse hygienic conditions favor human infestation with multicellular organisms (referred to here as parasites). Skin and hair are colonization sites for arthropod ectoparasites, such as insects (lice, fleas) and arachnids (mites). Against these, insecticidal or arachnicidal agents, respectively, can be used. Endoparasites invade the intestines or even internal organs, and are mostly members of the phyla of flatworms and roundworms. They are combated with anthelmintics.

Anthelmintics. As shown in the table, the newer agents *praziquantel* and *mebendazole* are adequate for the treatment of diverse worm diseases. They are generally well tolerated, as are the other agents listed.

Insecticides. Whereas fleas can be effectively dealt with by disinfection of clothes and living quarters, lice and mites require the topical application of insecticides to the infested subject.

DDT (chlorphenothane) kills insects after absorption of a very low amount, e.g., via foot contact with sprayed surfaces (contact insecticide). The cause of death is nervous system damage and seizures. In humans DDT causes acute neurotoxicity only after absorption of very large amounts. DDT is chemically stabile and degraded in the environment and body at extremely slow rates. As a highly lipophilic substance, it accumulates in fat tissues. Widespread use of DDT in pest control has led to its accumulation in food chains to alarming levels. For this reason its use has now been banned in many countries.

Lindane is the active γ-isomer of hexachlorocyclohexane. It also exerts a neurotoxic action on insects (as well as humans). Irritation of skin or mucous membranes may occur after topical use. Lindane is active also against intradermal mites (*Sarcoptes scabiei*, causative agent of scabies), besides lice and fleas. It is more readily degraded than DDT.

Permethrin, a synthetic pyrethroid, exhibits similar antiparasitic activity and may be the drug of choice due to its slower cutaneous absorption, fast hydrolytic inactivation, and rapid renal elimination.

Worms (helminths)	Anthelmintic drug of choice
Flatworms (platyhelminths) Tape worms (cestodes) Flukes (trematodes) e.g., *Schistosoma* species (bilharziasis)	Praziquantel* Niclosamide Praziquantel
Roundworms (nematodes) Pinworm (*Enterobius vermicularis*) Whipworm (*Trichuris trichiura*) Roundworm (*Ascaris lumbricoides*) *Trichinella spiralis*** *Strongyloides stercoralis* Hookworm (*Necator americanus a.,* *Ancylostoma duodenale*)	Mebendazole or pyrantel pamoate Mebendazole Mebendazole or pyrantel pamoate Mebendazole and thiabendazole Thiabendazole Mebendazole or pyrantel pamoate

*   Not for ocular or spinal cord cysticercosis
** Thiabendazole: intestinal phase; mebendazole: tissue phase

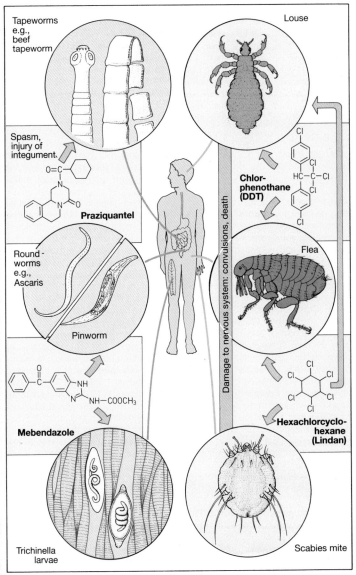

A. Endo- and ectoparasites: therapeutic agents

Antimalarials

The causative agents of malaria are plasmodia. The infective form, the sporozoite, is inoculated into skin capillaries when infected female *Anopheles* mosquitoes (**A**) suck blood from humans. The sporozoites invade liver parenchymal cells where they develop into primary tissue schizonts. After multiple fission, these schizonts produce numerous merozoites that enter the blood. The preerythrocytic stage is symptom-free. In blood, the parasite enters erythrocytes (erythrocytic stage) where it again multiplies by schizogony, resulting in the formation of more merozoites. Rupture of the infected erythrocytes releases the merozoites and pyrogens. A fever attack ensues and more erythrocytes are infected. The generation period for the next crop of merozoites determines the interval between fever attacks. With *Plasmodium vivax* and *P. ovale*, there can be a parallel multiplication in the liver (paraerythrocytic stage). Moreover, some sporozoites may become dormant in the liver as "hypnozoites" before entering schizogony. When the sexual forms (gametocytes) are ingested by a feeding mosquito, they can initiate the sexual reproductive stage of the cycle that results in a new generation of transmittable sporozoites.

Different antimalarials selectively kill different developmental forms of the parasite. The mechanism of action is known for some of them: pyrimethamine inhibits dihydrofolate reductase (p. 258), as does chlorguanide (proguanil) via its active metabolite. The sulfonamide sulfadoxine inhibits synthesis of dihydrofolic acid (p. 258). Chloroquine accumulates within the acidic vacuoles of blood schizonts and inhibits polymerization of heme, the latter being toxic for the schizonts.

Antimalarial drug choice takes into account tolerability and plasmodial resistance.

Tolerability. The first available antimalarial, quinine, has the smallest therapeutic margin. All newer agents are rather well tolerated.

P. falciparum, responsible for the most dangerous form of malaria, is particularly prone to develop **drug resistance**. The incidence of resistant strains rises with increasing frequency of drug use. Resistance has been reported for chloroquine and also the combination pyrimethamine/ sulfadoxine.

Drug choice for antimalarial chemoprophylaxis. In areas with a risk of malaria, continuous intake of antimalarials affords the best protection against the disease, although not against infection. *The drug of choice is chloroquine.* Because of its slow excretion (plasma $t^1/_2 \sim 3$ days and longer), a single weekly dose is sufficient. In areas with resistant *P. falciparum*, alternative regimens are chloroquine plus pyrimethamine/ sulfadoxine (or chlorguanide, or doxycycline), the chloroquine analogue amodiaquin, as well as quinine or the better tolerated derivative mefloquine (blood-schizonticidal). Agents active against blood schizonts do not prevent the (symptom-free) hepatic infection, only the disease-causing infection of erythrocytes ("suppression therapy"). On return from an endemic malaria region, a 2-week course of primaquine is adequate for eradication of the late hepatic stages (*P. vivax* and *P. ovale*).

Antimalarial therapy employs the same agents and is based on the same principles. The blood-schizonticidal halofantrine is reserved for therapy only.

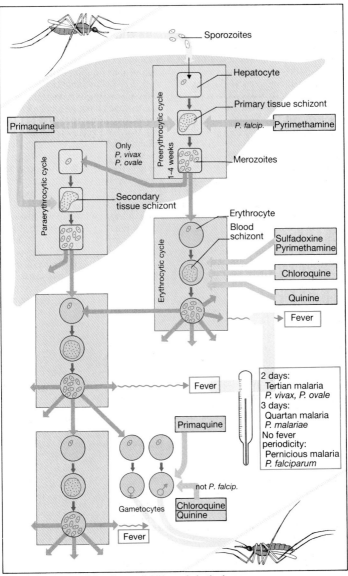

Sporozoites

Hepatocyte

Preerythrocytic cycle
1–4 weeks

Primary tissue schizont

P. falcip.   Pyrimethamine

Primaquine

Paraerythrocytic cycle

Only
P. vivax
P. ovale

Secondary
tissue schizont

Merozoites

Erythrocyte
Blood
schizont

Erythrocytic cycle

Sulfadoxine
Pyrimethamine

Chloroquine

Quinine

Fever

Fever

2 days:
  Tertian malaria
  P. vivax, P. ovale
3 days:
  Quartan malaria
  P. malariae
No fever
periodicity:
  Pernicious malaria
  P. falciparum

Primaquine

not *P. falcip.*

Gametocytes

Chloroquine
Quinine

Fever

**A. Malaria: stages of the plasmodial life cycle in the human;
therapeutic approaches**

Chemotherapy of Malignant Tumors

A tumor (neoplasm) consists of cells that proliferate independently of the body's inherent "building plan." A malignant tumor (cancer) is present when the tumor tissue destructively invades healthy surrounding tissue or when dislodged tumor cells form secondary tumors (metastases) in other organs. A cure requires the elimination of all malignant cells (curative therapy). When this is not possible, attempts can be made to slow tumor growth and thereby prolong the patient's life or improve quality of life (palliative therapy). Chemotherapy is faced with the problem that the malignant cells are endogenous and are not endowed with special metabolic properties.

Cytostatics (A) are cytotoxic substances that particularly affect proliferating or dividing cells. Rapidly dividing malignant cells are preferentially injured. Tissues with a low mitosis rate are largely unaffected; likewise, most healthy tissues. This, however, also applies to malignant tumors consisting of slowly dividing differentiated cells. Tissues that have a physiologically high mitotic rate are bound to be affected by cytostatic therapy. Thus, **typical adverse effects** occur:

Loss of hair results from injury to hair follicles; *gastrointestinal disturbances*, such as diarrhea, from inadequate replacement of enterocytes whose life span is limited to a few days; *nausea and vomiting* from stimulation of area postrema chemoreceptors (p. 300); and *lowered resistance to infection* from weakening of the immune system. A normal immune response to a pathogen requires rapid multiplication of T- and B-lymphocytes. In addition, increased numbers of phagocytes (e.g., neutrophil granulocytes) are released from the bone marrow. This reaction is also inhibited because cytostatics cause a *bone marrow depression*. Resupply of blood cells depends on the mitotic activity of bone marrow stem and daughter cells. When myeloid proliferation is arrested, the short-lived granulocytes are the first to be affected (neutropenia), then blood platelets (thrombopenia) and, finally, the more long-lived erythrocytes (anemia). *Infertility* is caused by suppression of spermatogenesis or follicle maturation. Most cytostatics disrupt DNA metabolism. This entails the risk of a potential genomic alteration in healthy cells (*mutagenic* effect). Conceivably, the latter accounts for the occurrence of leukemias several years after cytostatic therapy (*carcinogenic* effect). Furthermore, congenital malformations are to be expected when cytostatics must be used during pregnancy (*teratogenic* effect).

Cytostatics possess different **mechanisms of action**. Frequently, a combination of cytostatics permits an improved therapeutic effect with fewer adverse reactions. Initial success can be followed by loss of effect because of the emergence of resistant tumor cells.

Damage to the mitotic spindle (B). The contractile proteins of the spindle apparatus must draw apart the replicated chromosomes before the cell can divide. This process is prevented by the so-called *spindle poisons* (see also colchicine, p. 290) that arrest mitosis at metaphase. The cytostatics *vincristine* and *vinblastine* exert a cell-cycle–specific effect. They originate from the periwinkle plant, *Vinca rosea*, and are, therefore, referred to as *vinca alkaloids*. Damage to the nervous system is a distinct adverse effect.

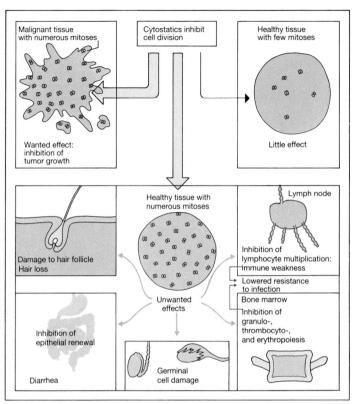

A. Chemotherapy of tumors: principal and adverse effects

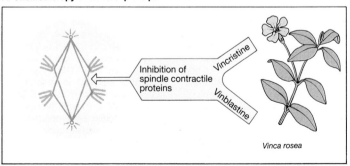

B. Cytostatics: inhibition of mitosis by vinca alkaloids

Inhibition of DNA and RNA synthesis (A). Mitosis is preceded by replication of chromosomes (DNA synthesis) and increased protein synthesis (RNA synthesis). Existing DNA (gray) serves as a template for the synthesis of new (blue) DNA or RNA. *De novo* synthesis may be inhibited by:

Damage to the template (1). Alkylating cytostatics are reactive compounds that transfer alkyl residues into a covalent bond with DNA. For instance, mechlorethamine (*nitrogen mustard*) is able to cross-link double-stranded DNA on giving off its chlorine atoms. Correct reading of genetic information is thereby rendered impossible. Other alkylating agents are *chlorambucil, melphalan, thiotepa, cyclophosphamide* (p. 293), *ifosfamide, lomustine*, and *busulfan*. Specific adverse reactions include irreversible pulmonary fibrosis due to busulfan and hemorrhagic cystitis caused by cyclophosphamide metabolites (preventable by the uro-protective mesna). *Cisplatin* binds to (but does not alkylate) DNA strands. **Cytostatic antibiotics** insert themselves into the DNA double-strand. This may lead to strand breakage (e.g., with *bleomycin*). The *anthracycline antibiotics daunorubicin* and *doxorubicin (adriamycin)* may induce cardiomyopathy. Bleomycin can also cause pulmonary fibrosis.

Inhibition of nucleobase synthesis (2). Tetrahydrofolic acid (THF) is required for the synthesis of both purine bases and thymidine. Formation of THF from folic acid involves dihydrofolate reductase (p. 258). The *folate analogues aminopterin* and *methotrexate (amethopterin)* inhibit enzyme activity as false substrates. As cellular stores of THF are depleted, synthesis of DNA and RNA building blocks ceases. The effect of these antimetabolites can be reversed by administration of folinic acid (5-formyl-THF, leucovorin, citrovorum factor).

Incorporation of false building blocks (3). Unnatural nucleobases (6-*mercaptopurine; fluorouracil*) or nucleosides with incorrect sugars (*cytarabine*) act as antimetabolites. They inhibit DNA/RNA synthesis or lead to synthesis of incorrect nucleic acids.

6-Mercaptopurine results from biotransformation of the inactive precursor *azathioprine* (p. 37). The urostatic allopurinol inhibits the degradation of 6-mercaptopurine such that coadministration of the two drugs permits dose reduction of the latter.

Immunosuppressants. Suppression of immune responses is desirable in the prevention of transplant rejection or the management of autoimmune disorders. Immune suppression can be achieved with the *cytostatics cyclophosphamide* and *azathioprine*, the *glucocorticoid prednisolone*, as well as the polypeptid antibiotic *cyclosporin A*.

Cyclosporin *A* is produced by fungi and consists of 11 partly atypical aminoacids. It is absorbed enterally, albeit incompletely. Cyclosporin A exerts a more selective action than do other immunosuppressants. It inhibits the production of cytotoxic T lymphocytes, presumably by inhibiting the transcription in T-helper cells of genes coding for interleukins and other lymphokines. The successes of modern transplantation medicine are in large measure attributable to the introduction of this agent. Its utility in autoimmune diseases is under investigation. Renal damage is prominent among its adverse effects.

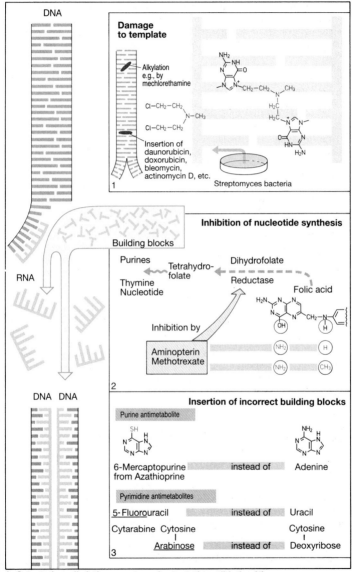

Damage to template

Alkylation e.g., by mechlorethamine

Cl−CH₂−CH₂
          N−CH₃
Cl−CH₂−CH₂

Insertion of daunorubicin, doxorubicin, bleomycin, actinomycin D, etc.

1

Streptomyces bacteria

DNA

RNA

Inhibition of nucleotide synthesis

Building blocks

Purines   Tetrahydro-   Dihydrofolate
Thymine   folate
Nucleotide   Reductase   Folic acid

Inhibition by

Aminopterin
Methotrexate

2

DNA DNA

Insertion of incorrect building blocks

Purine antimetabolite

6-Mercaptopurine   instead of   Adenine
from Azathioprine

Pyrimidine antimetabolites

5- Fluorouracil   instead of   Uracil

Cytarabine Cytosine   Cytosine
       Arabinose   instead of   Deoxyribose

3

A. Cytostatics: alkylating agents and cytostatic antibiotics (1), inhibitors of tetrahydrofolate synthesis (2), antimetabolites (3)

Angina Pectoris

An anginal pain attack signals a transient hypoxia of the myocardium. As a rule, the *oxygen deficit* results from inadequate myocardial blood flow due to narrowing of larger coronary arteries. The underlying causes are: most commonly, an atherosclerotic change of the vascular wall (*coronary sclerosis* with exertional angina); very infrequently, a spasmodic constriction of a morphologically healthy coronary artery (*coronary spasm* with angina at rest; variant angina); or more often, a coronary spasm occurring in an atherosclerotic vascular segment.

The *goal of treatment* is to prevent myocardial hypoxia either by raising blood flow (*oxygen supply*) or by lowering myocardial blood demand (*oxygen demand*) (**A**).

Factors determining oxygen supply. The force driving myocardial blood flow is the *pressure difference* between the coronary ostia (*aortic pressure*) and the opening of the coronary sinus (*right atrial pressure*). Blood flow is opposed by *coronary flow resistance,* which includes three components. (1) Due to their large caliber, the *proximal coronary segments* do not normally contribute significantly to flow resistance. However, in coronary sclerosis or spasm, pathological obstruction of flow occurs here. Whereas the more common coronary sclerosis cannot be overcome pharmacologically, the less common coronary spasm can be relieved by appropriate vasodilators (nitrates, nifedipine). (2) The caliber of *arteriolar resistance vessels* controls blood flow through the coronary bed. Arteriolar caliber is determined by myocardial O_2 tension and local concentrations of metabolic products, and is "automatically" adjusted to the required blood flow (**B**, healthy subject). This *metabolic autoregulation* explains why anginal attacks in coronary sclerosis occur only during exercise (**B**, patient). At rest, the pathologically elevated flow resistance is compensated by a corresponding decrease in arteriolar resistance, ensuring adequate myocardial perfusion. During exercise, further dilation of arterioles is impossible. As a result, there is ischemia associated with pain. Pharmacological agents that act to dilate arterioles would thus be inappropriate because at rest they may divert blood from underperfused into healthy vascular regions on account of redundant arteriolar dilatation. The resulting "steal effect" could provoke an anginal attack. (3) The intramyocardial pressure, i.e., systolic squeeze, compresses the capillary bed. Myocardial blood flow is halted during systole and occurs almost entirely during diastole. *Diastolic wall tension* ("*preload*") depends on ventricular volume and filling pressure. The organic nitrates reduce preload by decreasing venous return to the heart.

Factors determining oxygen demand. The heart muscle cell consumes the most energy to generate contractile force. Oxygen demand rises with an increase in (1) *heart rate*, (2) *contraction velocity*, (3) *systolic wall tension* ("afterload"). The latter depends on ventricular volume and the systolic pressure needed to empty the ventricle. As peripheral resistance increases, aortic pressure rises, hence the resistance against which ventricular blood is ejected. Oxygen demand is lowered by β-blockers and calcium antagonists, as well as by nitrates (p. 284).

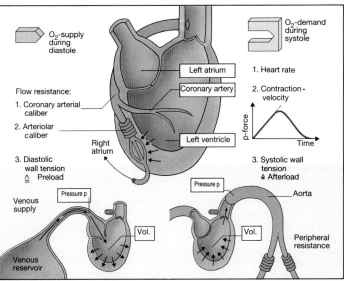

A. O$_2$-supply and demand of the myocardium

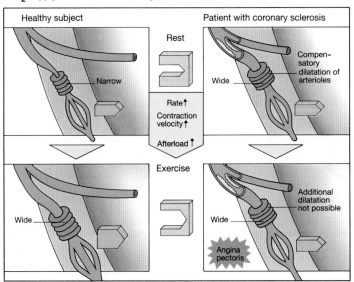

B. Pathogenesis of exertion angina in coronary sclerosis

Antianginal Drugs

Antianginal agents derive from three drug groups, the pharmacological properties of which have already been presented in more detail, viz., the organic nitrates (p. 120), the calcium antagonists (p. 122), and the β-blockers (pp. 92ff).

Organic nitrates (A) increase blood flow, hence oxygen supply, because diastolic wall tension (preload) declines as venous return to the heart is diminished. Thus, the nitrates enable myocardial flow resistance to be reduced even in the presence of coronary sclerosis with angina pectoris. In angina due to coronary spasm, arterial dilatation overcomes the vasospasm and restores myocardial perfusion to normal. Oxygen demand falls because of the ensuing decrease in the two variables that determine systolic wall tension (afterload): ventricular filling volume and aortic blood pressure.

Calcium antagonists (B) decrease oxygen demand by lowering aortic pressure, one of the components contributing to afterload. The dihydropyridine *nifedipine* is devoid of a cardiodepressant effect, but may give rise to reflex tachycardia and an associated increase in oxygen demand. The catamphiphilic drugs *verapamil* and *diltiazem* are cardiodepressant. Reduced beat frequency and contractility contribute to a reduction in oxygen demand; however, AV-block and mechanical insufficiency can dangerously jeopardize heart function. In coronary spasm, calcium antagonists can induce spasmolysis and improve blood flow.

β-Blockers (C) protect the heart against the oxygen-wasting effect of sympathetic drive by inhibiting β-receptor–mediated increases in cardiac rate and speed of contraction.

Uses of antianginal drugs (D). For relief of acute anginal attack, rapidly absorbed drugs devoid of cardiodepressant activity are preferred. The drug of choice is *nitroglycerin* (NTG, 0.8–2.4 mg sublingually; onset of action within 1–2 min; duration of effect approx. 30 min). Isosorbide dinitrate (ISDN) can also be used (5–10 mg sublingually); compared with NTG, its action is somewhat delayed in onset, but of longer duration. Finally, nifedipine may be useful (5 to 20 mg, capsule to be bitten and the contents swallowed).

For sustained daytime **angina prophylaxis**, *nitrates* are of limited value because "nitrate pauses" of about 12 h are appropriate if nitrate tolerance is to be avoided. If attacks occur during the day, *ISDN*, or its metabolite *isosorbide mononitrate*, may be given in the morning and at noon (e.g., ISDN 40 mg in extended-release capsules). Because of hepatic presystemic elimination, NTG is not suitable for oral administration. Continuous delivery via a transdermal patch would also not seem advisable because of the potential development of tolerance.

The choice between *calcium antagonists* must take into account the differential effect of nifedipine versus verapamil or diltiazem on cardiac performance (see above). When *β-blockers* are given, the potential consequences of reducing cardiac contractility (withdrawal of sympathetic drive) must be kept in mind. Since vasodilating β_2-receptors are blocked, an increased risk of vasospasm cannot be ruled out. Therefore, monotherapy with β-blockers is recommended only in angina due to coronary sclerosis, but not in variant angina.

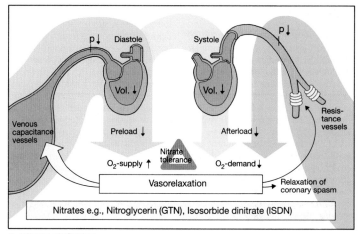

A. Effects of nitrates

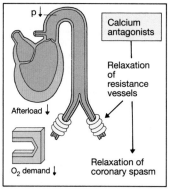

B. Effects of Ca-antagonists

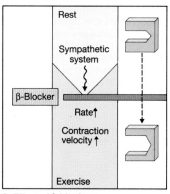

C. Effect of β-blockers

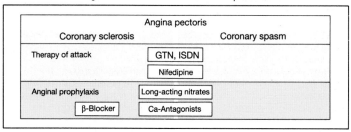

D. Clinical uses of anti-anginal drugs

Hypertension

Arterial hypertension (high blood pressure) generally does not impair the well-being of the affected individual; however, in the long term it leads to vascular damage and secondary complications (A). The aim of antihypertensive therapy is to prevent the latter and, thus, to prolong life expectancy.

Hypertension infrequently results from another disease, such as a catecholamine-secreting tumor (pheochromocytoma); in most cases the cause cannot be determined: **essential (primary) hypertension**. Antihypertensive drugs are indicated when blood pressure cannot be sufficiently controlled by means of **weight reduction** or a **low-salt diet**. In principle, lowering of either cardiac output or peripheral resistance may decrease blood pressure (cf. p. 288, blood pressure determinants). The available drugs influence one or both of these determinants.

The therapeutic utility of antihypertensives is determined by their efficacy and tolerability. The choice of a specific drug is determined on the basis of a benefit : risk assessment of the relevant drugs, in keeping with the patient's individual needs. Accordingly, there are first-line agents for initiating therapy (A).

Initially, an attempt is made to normalize blood pressure by instituting **single-drug therapy** (monotherapy). The choice of drug may be based on considerations such as the following: β-blockers (p. 92) are particularly useful for the treatment of juvenile hypertension with tachycardia and high cardiac output; however, in patients disposed to bronchospasm, even β-selective blockers are contraindicated. Thiazide diuretics (p. 158) are potentially well suited in hypertension associated with congestive heart failure; however, they would be unsuitable in hypokalemic states. When hypertension is accompanied by angina pectoris, the preferred choice would be a β-blocker or calcium antagonist rather than a diuretic (p. 122). As for the calcium antagonists, it should be noted that verapamil, unlike nifedipine, possesses cardiodepressant activity. ACE inhibitors (p. 124) have recently gained acceptance as first-line antihypertensive drugs.

In **multidrug therapy**, it is necessary to consider which agents rationally complement each other. A β-blocker (bradycardia, cardiodepression due to sympathetic blockade) can be effectively combined with nifedipine (reflex tachycardia), but obviously not with verapamil (bradycardia, cardiodepression). Where vasodilators such as dihydralazine or minoxidil (p. 118) are given, β-blockers would serve to prevent reflex tachycardia, and diuretics to counteract fluid retention.

Abrupt termination of continuous treatment can be followed by rebound hypertension (particularly with short $t^{1/2}$ β-blockers).

Drugs for the control of hypertensive crises include nifedipine (capsule, to be chewed and swallowed), clonidine (p.o. or i.v., p. 96), dihydralazine (i.v.), and sodium nitroprusside (p. 120, by infusion). The nonselective α-blocker phentolamine (p. 90) is indicated only in pheochromocytoma.

Antihypertensives for hypertension **in pregnancy** are β_1-selective adrenoceptor-blockers, methyldopa (p. 96), and dihydralazine (i.v. infusion) for eclampsia (massive rise in blood pressure with CNS symptoms).

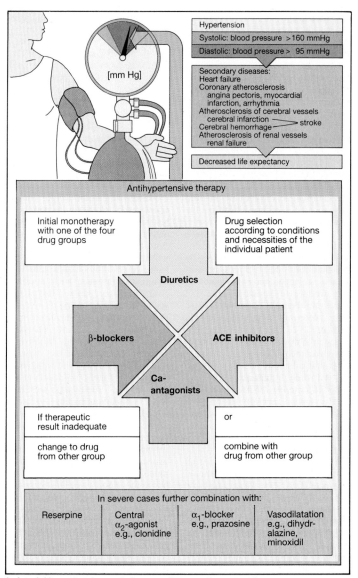

Hypertension

Systolic: blood pressure >160 mmHg

Diastolic: blood pressure > 95 mmHg

Secondary diseases:
Heart failure
Coronary atherosclerosis
    angina pectoris, myocardial
    infarction, arrhythmia
Atherosclerosis of cerebral vessels
    cerebral infarction
    Cerebral hemorrhage ──→ stroke
Atherosclerosis of renal vessels
    renal failure

Decreased life expectancy

Antihypertensive therapy

Initial monotherapy with one of the four drug groups

Drug selection according to conditions and necessities of the individual patient

Diuretics

β-blockers

ACE inhibitors

Ca-antagonists

If therapeutic result inadequate

change to drug from other group

or

combine with drug from other group

In severe cases further combination with:

| Reserpine | Central α₂-agonist e.g., clonidine | α₁-blocker e.g., prazosine | Vasodilatation e.g., dihydralazine, minoxidil |

A. Arterial hypertension and pharmacotherapeutic approaches

Hypotension

The venous side of the circulation, excluding the pulmonary circulation, accommodates ~60% of the total blood volume; because of the low venous pressure (mean approx. 15 mmHg), it is part of the *low-pressure system*. The arterial vascular beds, representing the *high-pressure system* (mean pressure approx. 100 mmHg), contain ~10%. The arterial pressure generates the driving force for perfusion of tissues and organs. Blood draining from the latter collects in the low-pressure system and is pumped back by the heart into the high-pressure system.

The arterial blood pressure (ABP) depends on: (1) the volume of blood per unit of time that is forced by the heart into the high-pressure system—cardiac output corresponds to the product of stroke volume and heart rate (beats/min), stroke volume being determined by venous filling pressure; (2) the counterforce opposing the flow of blood, i.e., peripheral resistance, which is a function of arteriolar caliber.

Chronic hypotension (systolic BP <105 mmHg). *Primary idiopathic hypotension* generally has no clinical importance. If symptoms such as lassitude and dizziness occur, a program of physical exercise instead of drugs is advisable.

Secondary hypotension is a sign of an underlying disease that should be treated first. If stroke volume is too low, as in heart failure, a cardiac glycoside can be given to increase myocardial contractility and stroke volume. When stroke volume is decreased due to insufficient blood volume, plasma substitutes will be helpful in treating blood loss, whereas aldosterone deficiency requires administration of a mineralocorticoid. A parasympatholytic (or electrical pacemaker) can restore cardiac rate in bradycardia.

Acute hypotension. *Failure of orthostatic regulation.* A change from the recumbent to the erect position (orthostasis) will cause blood within the low-pressure system to sink towards the feet because the veins in body parts below the heart will be distended, despite a reflex venoconstriction, by the weight of the column of blood in the blood vessels. The fall in stroke volume is partly compensated by a rise in heart rate. The remaining reduction of cardiac output can be countered by elevating the peripheral resistance, enabling blood pressure and organ perfusion to be maintained. An orthostatic malfunction is present when counter-regulation fails and hence cerebral blood flow falls with resultant symptoms, such as dizziness, "black-out," or even loss of consciousness. In the *sympatheticotonic form*, sympathetically mediated circulatory reflexes are intensified (more pronounced tachycardia and rise in peripheral resistance, i.e. diastolic pressure); however, there is failure to compensate for the reduction in venous return. Prophylactic treatment with sympathomimetics therefore would hold little promise. Instead, cardiovascular fitness training would appear more important. An increase in venous return may be achieved in two ways. Increasing NaCl intake augments salt and fluid reserves and hence the blood volume (contraindications: hypertension, heart failure). Constriction of venous capacitance vessels might be produced by dihydroergotamine. Whether this effect could also be achieved by an α-sympathomimetic remains debatable. In the very rare *asympatheticotonic form*, use of sympathomimetics would certainly be reasonable.

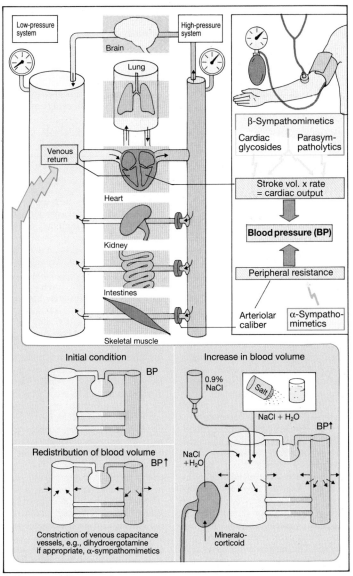

A. Treatment of hypotension

Gout

Gout is an inherited metabolic disease that results from **hyperuricemia**, an elevation in the blood of uric acid, the end-product of purine degradation. The typical **gout attack** consists of a highly painful inflammation of the first metatarsophalangeal joint ("podagra"). Gout attacks are triggered by precipitation of sodium urate crystals in the synovial fluid of joints.

During the early stage of inflammation, urate crystals are phagocytosed by polymorphonuclear leukocytes (1) that engulf the crystals by their ameboid cytoplasmic movements (2). The phagocytic vacuole fuses with a lysosome (3). The lysosomal enzymes are, however, unable to degrade the sodium urate. Further ameboid movement dislodges the crystals and causes rupture of the phagolysosome. Lysosomal enzymes are liberated into the granulocyte, resulting in its destruction by self-digestion and damage to the adjacent tissue. Inflammatory mediators, such as prostaglandins and chemotactic factors, are released (4). More granulocytes are attracted and suffer similar destruction; the inflammation intensifies—the gout attack flares up.

Treatment of the gout attack aims to interrupt the inflammatory response. The drug of choice is **colchicine**, an alkaloid from the autumn crocus (*Colchicum autumnale*). It is known as a "spindle poison" because it arrests mitosis at metaphase by inhibiting contractile spindle proteins. Its antigout activity is due to inhibition of contractile proteins in the neutrophils, whereby ameboid mobility and phagocytotic activity are prevented. The most common *adverse effects* of colchicine are abdominal pain, vomiting, and diarrhea, probably due to inhibition of mitoses in the rapidly dividing gastrointestinal epithelial cells. Colchicine is usually given orally (e.g., 0.5 mg hourly until pain subsides or gastrointestinal disturbances occur).

Nonsteroidal anti-inflammatory drugs, such as **indomethacin** and **phenylbutazone,** are also effective. In severe cases, **glucocorticoids** may be indicated.

Effective **prophylaxis of gout attacks** requires that urate blood levels be lowered to 6 mg/100 ml.

Diet. Purine (cell nuclei)-rich foods should be avoided, e.g., organ meats. Milk, dairy products, and eggs are low in purines and are recommended. Coffee and tea are permitted, since the methylxanthine caffeine does not enter purine metabolism.

Uricostatics decrease urate production. **Allopurinol,** as well as its accumulating metabolite alloxanthine (oxypurinol), inhibit xanthine oxidase, which catalyzes urate formation from hypoxanthine via xanthine. These precursors are readily eliminated via the urine. Allopurinol is given orally (300–800 mg/day). Except for infrequent allergic reactions, it is well tolerated and the drug of choice for gout prophylaxis. At the start of therapy, gout attacks may occur, but they can be prevented by concurrent administration of colchicine (0.5–1.5 mg/day). **Uricosurics,** such as **probenecid, benzbromarone** (100 mg/day), or **sulfinpyrazone** promote renal excretion of uric acid. They saturate the organic acid transport system in the proximal renal tubules, making it unavailable for urate reabsorption. When underdosed, they inhibit only the acid secretory system, which has a smaller transport capacity. Urate elimination is then inhibited and a gout attack is possible. In patients with urate stones in the urinary tract, uricosurics are contraindicated.

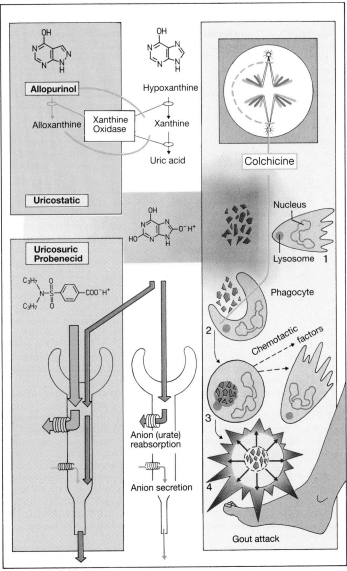

Allopurinol

Hypoxanthine

Alloxanthine — Xanthine Oxidase → Xanthine

Uric acid

Uricostatic

Colchicine

Nucleus

Lysosome 1

Uricosuric Probenecid

Phagocyte

2

Chemotactic factors

Anion (urate) reabsorption

3

Anion secretion

4

Gout attack

A. Gout and its therapy

Rheumatoid Arthritis

Rheumatoid arthritis or **chronic polyarthritis** is a progressive inflammatory joint disease that intermittently attacks more and more joints, predominantly those of the fingers and toes. The probable cause of rheumatoid arthritis is a pathological reaction of the immune system. This malfunction can be promoted or triggered by various conditions, including genetic disposition, age-related wear and tear, hypothermia, and infection. An initial noxious stimulus elicits an **inflammation of synovial membranes**, that, in turn, leads to release of antigens through which the inflammatory process is maintained. Inflammation of the synovial membrane is associated with liberation of inflammatory mediator substances that, among other actions, chemotactically stimulate migration of phagocytic blood cells (granulocytes, macrophages) into the synovial tissue. The phagocytes produce destructive enzymes that promote tissue damage. Due to the production of prostaglandins and leukotrienes (p. 188) and other factors, the inflammation spreads to the entire joint. As a result, joint cartilage is damaged and the joint is ultimately immobilized or fused.

Pharmacotherapy. Acute relief of inflammatory symptoms can be achieved by **prostaglandin synthesis inhibitors**; nonsteroidal anti-inflammatory drugs, (NSAIDs), such as diclofenac, indomethacin, piroxicam, p. 190) and **glucocorticoids** (p. 234). The inevitably **chronic** use of *NSAIDs* is likely to cause *adverse effects*, in particular gastric and duodenal ulceration, impaired renal function with sodium and water retention, bone marrow depression (aplastic anemia, leukopenia), allergic skin rash, and bronchial asthma. Patients on indomethacin may experience CNS disturbances (headache, confusion, depression). Neither NSAIDs nor glucocorticoids can halt the progressive destruction of joints. Long-term treatment with **gold salts** (i.m. aurothioglucose, aurothiomalate; p.o. auranofin), **hydroxychloroquine** or **penicillamine** can help reduce the need for NSAIDs and glucocorticoids. Since acute symptomatic relief cannot be achieved, these drugs are designated **disease-modifying agents**. Among possible mechanisms of action, inhibition of macrophage activity and inhibition of release or activity of lysosomal enzymes are being discussed. Frequent adverse reactions are: damage to skin and mucous membranes, renal toxicity, and blood dyscrasias. These necessitate withdrawal of medication in more than one-third of patients. **Sulfasalazine** is currently enjoying a revival as a disease-modifying agent.

In very severe cases, attempts are made to **suppress the autoimmune reaction** by means of glucocorticoids and cytostatic drugs (azathioprine, methotrexate, cyclophosphamide, p. 280). Among the latter, methotrexate is presently preferred.

Phenylbutazone and **apazone** exert potent anti-inflammatory effects that are useful in the treatment of rheumatoid disease, gout, superficial thrombophlebitis, and musculoskeletal disorders. The high toxicity of phenylbutazone (agranulocytosis, aplastic anemia, nephrotic syndrome, hepatic and renal necrosis, allergic reactions, exfoliative dermatitis) has resulted in its complete ban in some countries or its withdrawal from general availability on prescription.

Surgical removal of the inflamed synovial membrane (**synovectomy**) frequently provides long-term relief.

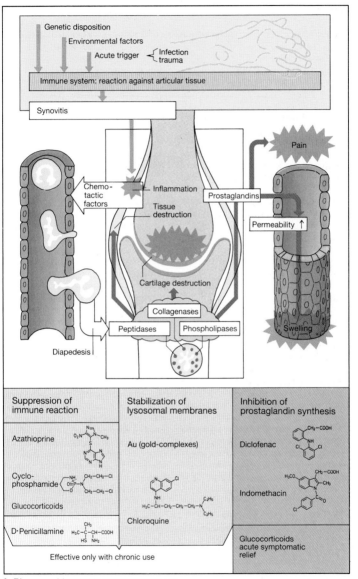

A. Rheumatoid arthritis and its treatment

Migraine

Migraine is a syndrome characterized by recurrent attacks of intense headache and nausea that occur at irregular intervals and last for several hours. In classical migraine, the attack is typically heralded by an "aura" accompanied by spreading homonymous visual field defects with colored sharp edges ("fortification" spectra). In addition, the patient cannot focus on certain objects, has a ravenous appetite for particular foods, and is hypersensitive to odors (hyperosmia) or light (photophobia). The exact cause of these complaints is unknown; however, a disturbance in cranial blood flow is the likely underlying pathogenetic mechanism. In addition to an often inherited predisposition, precipitating factors are required to provoke an attack, e.g., psychic stress, lack of sleep, certain foods. Pharmacotherapy of migraine has two aims: stopping the acute attack and preventing subsequent ones.

Treatment of the attack. For symptomatic relief, headaches are treated with analgesics (acetaminophen, acetylsalicylic acid) and nausea is treated with metoclopramide (pp. 114, 300). Since there is delayed gastric emptying during the attack, drug absorption can be markedly retarded and hence effective plasma levels are not obtained. Because metoclopramide stimulates gastric emptying, it promotes absorption of ingested analgesic drugs and thus facilitates pain relief.

If acetylsalicylic acid is administered i.v., its bioavailability is complete. Therefore, i.v. injection may be advisable in acute attacks.

Should analgesics prove insufficiently effective, ergotamine and the 5-HT$_1$ agonist sumatriptan may help control the acute attack in most cases or prevent an imminent attack. Unlike sumatriptan, ergotamine causes vasoconstriction or vasodilatation (p. 126) depending on the existing vascular tone. As a dopamine agonist, ergotamine activates receptors in the area postrema controlling the excitability of the emetic center (pp. 114, 300). Ergotamine can thus enhance or prolong nausea.

With frequent intake ($>$ once per week), ergotamine-containing remedies themselves may paradoxically provoke headaches. The latter then change in character from intermittent to continuous chronic headache. Following ingestion of drug, headaches transiently abate, prompting further consumption of migraine remedies. A vicious circle ensues. As a result of chronic drug use, typical adverse effects may develop: impaired peripheral blood flow (gangrene) with ergotamine (ergotism); gastrointestinal bleeding or renal toxicity with analgesics. Drugs for acute relief are thus not suitable for migraine prophylaxis.

Prophylaxis. Taken regularly over a longer period, a heterogeneous group of drugs comprising propranolol and metoprolol (β-blockers), flunarizine (antihistaminic, dopamine and calcium antagonist), pizotyline = pizotifen, and methysergide (5-HT antagonists) may decrease the frequency, intensity, and duration of migraine attacks. Because of a low incidence of adverse reactions, β-blockers (p. 92) and flunarizine are drugs of first choice. Adverse effects of flunarizine include sedation and extrapyramidal motor disturbances.

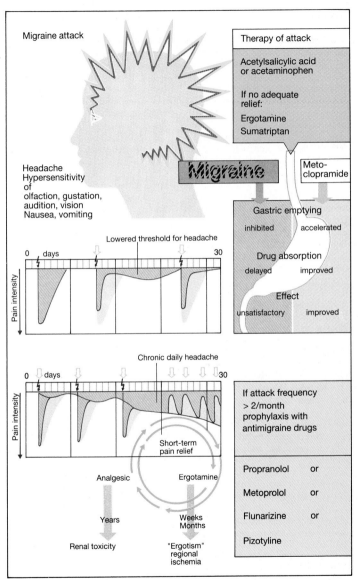

Migraine attack

Therapy of attack

Acetylsalicylic acid
or acetaminophen

If no adequate
relief:

Ergotamine
Sumatriptan

Metoclopramide

Migraine

Headache
Hypersensitivity
of
olfaction, gustation,
audition, vision
Nausea, vomiting

Gastric emptying

inhibited   accelerated

Drug absorption

delayed   improved

Effect

unsatisfactory   improved

Lowered threshold for headache

0   days   30

Pain intensity

Chronic daily headache

0   days   30

Pain intensity

Short-term
pain relief

Analgesic   Ergotamine

Years   Weeks
Months

Renal toxicity   "Ergotism"
regional
ischemia

If attack frequency
> 2/month
prophylaxis with
antimigraine drugs

Propranolol   or

Metoprolol   or

Flunarizine   or

Pizotyline

A. Migraine and its treatment

Common Cold

The common cold—colloquially, the flu, catarrh, or grippe (strictly speaking, the rarer infection with influenza viruses)—is an acute infectious inflammation of the upper respiratory tract. Its symptoms, sneezing, running nose (due to rhinitis), hoarseness (laryngitis), difficulty in swallowing and sore throat (pharyngitis and tonsillitis), cough associated with first serous then mucous sputum (tracheitis, bronchitis), sore muscles, and general malaise can be present sequentially or concurrently in varying combination or sequence. The term stems from an old popular belief that these complaints are caused by exposure to chilling or dampness. The causative pathogens are different viruses (rhino-, adeno-, parainfluenza v.) that are transmitted by aerosol droplets produced by coughing and sneezing.

Therapeutic measures. Causal treatment with a *virustatic* is not possible at present. Since cold symptoms abate spontaneously, there is no compelling need to use drugs. However, conventional remedies are intended for *symptomatic relief.*

Rhinitis. Nasal discharge could be prevented by *parasympatholytics*; however, other atropine-like effects (p. 104) would have to be accepted. Therefore, parasympatholytics are hardly ever used, although a corresponding action is probably exploited in the case of H_1-*antihistaminics*, an ingredient of many cold remedies. Locally applied (nasal drops) vasoconstricting α-*sympathomimetics* (p. 84) decongest the nasal mucosa and dry up secretions, clearing the nasal passage. Long-term use may cause damage to nasal mucous membranes (p. 90).

Sore throat, swallowing problems. Demulcent lozenges containing *surface anesthetics* such as ethylaminobenzoate (benzocaine) or tetracaine (p. 198) may provide relief; however, the risk of allergic reactions should be borne in mind.

Cough. Since coughing serves to expel excess tracheobronchial secretions, suppression of this physiological reflex is justified only when coughing is dangerous (after surgery) or unproductive because of absent secretions. *Codeine* and *noscapine* (p. 202) suppress cough by a central action.

Mucous airway obstruction. *Mucolytics,* such as acetylcysteine, split disulfide bonds in mucus, hence reduce its viscosity and promote clearing of bronchial mucus. Other expectorants (e.g., hot beverages, potassium iodide, and ipecac) stimulate production of watery mucus. Acetylcysteine is indicated in cystic fibrosis patients and inhaled as an aerosol. Whether mucolytics are indicated in the common cold and whether expectorants like bromohexine effectively lower viscosity of bronchial secretions may be questioned.

Fever. *Antipyretic analgesics* (acetylsalicylic acid, acetaminophen, p. 190) are indicated only when there is high fever. Fever is a natural response and useful in monitoring the clinical course of an infection.

Muscle aches and pains, headache. *Antipyretic analgesics* are effective in relieving these symptoms.

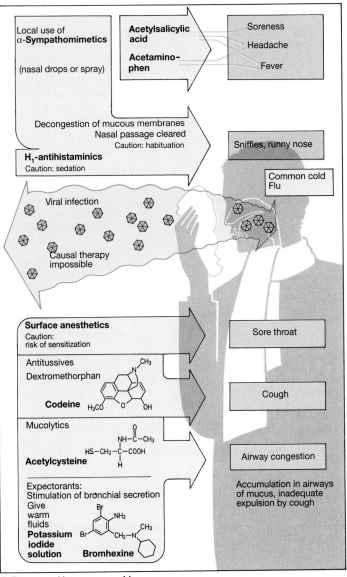

A. Drugs used in common cold

Allergic Disorders

IgE-mediated allergic reactions (p. 72) involve mast cell release of *histamine* (p. 114) and production of *other mediators* (such as leukotrienes, p. 188). Resultant responses include: *relaxation of vascular smooth muscle,* as evidenced locally by vasodilation (e.g., conjunctival congestion) or systemically by hypotension (as in anaphylactic shock); *enhanced capillary permeability* with transudation of fluid into tissues—swelling of conjunctiva and mucous membranes of the upper airways ("hay fever"), cutaneous wheal formation; *contraction of bronchial smooth muscle*—bronchial asthma; *stimulation of intestinal smooth muscle*—diarrhea.

1. Stabilization of mast cells. *Cromolyn* prevents IgE-mediated release of mediators, although only after *chronic treatment.* It is applied *locally*: conjunctiva, nasal mucosa, bronchial tree (inhalation), intestinal mucosa (absorption almost nil with oral intake). Indications: *prophylaxis of hay fever, allergic asthma,* and *food allergies.*

2. Blockade of histamine receptors. Allergic reactions are predominantly mediated by H_1 receptors. H_1 *antihistaminics* (p. 114) are mostly used orally. Their therapeutic effect is often disappointing. Indications: allergic rhinitis (*hay fever*).

3. Functional antagonists of mediators of allergy.

a) **α-Sympathomimetics**, such as naphazoline, oxymetazoline, and tetrahydrozoline, are applied topically to the conjunctival and nasal mucosa to produce local vasoconstriction and decongestion and to dry up secretions (p. 90). Because they may cause mucosal damage, their use should be short-term.

b) **Epinephrine**, given i.v., is the *most important drug in the management of anaphylactic shock;* it constricts vessels, reduces capillary permeability, and dilates bronchi.

c) **β2-Sympathomimetics**, such as terbutaline, fenoterol, and albuterol are employed in *bronchial asthma,* mostly by inhalation, and parenterally in emergencies. Even after inhalation, effective amounts can reach the systemic circulation and cause enough stimulation of cardiac β-receptors to produce tachycardia or arrhythmias. During chronic administration, the sensitivity of bronchial musculature is likely to decline.

d) **Theophylline** belongs to the methylxanthines. Whereas caffeine (1,3,7-trimethylxanthine) predominantly stimulates the CNS and constricts cerebral blood vessels, theophylline (1,3-dimethylxanthine) possesses additional marked bronchodilator, cardiostimulant, vasorelaxant, and diuretic actions. These effects are attributed to both inhibition of phosphodiesterase (→ cAMP elevation, p. 66) and antagonism at adenosine receptors. In *bronchial asthma,* theophylline can be given orally for prophylaxis or parenterally to control the attack. Manifestations of overdosage include tonic-clonic seizures and cardiac arrhythmias as early signs.

e) **Ipratropium** (p. 104) can be inhaled to induce bronchodilation; however, it often lacks sufficient effectiveness in allergic bronchospasm.

f) **Glucocorticoids** (p. 234) display significant antiallergic activity and probably interfere with different stages of the allergic response. Indications: *hay fever, bronchial asthma* (preferably local application of analogues with high presystemic elimination, e.g., beclomethasone, budesonide), *anaphylactic shock* (i.v. in high dosage).

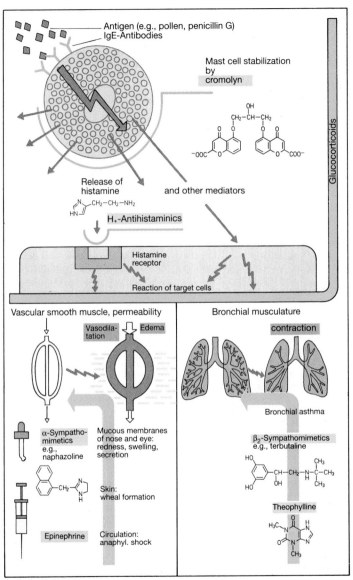

A. Anti-allergic therapy

Emesis

In emesis the stomach empties retrogradely. The pyloric sphincter is closed while cardia and esophagus relax to allow gastric contents to be propelled orad by a forceful synchronous contraction of abdominal wall muscles and diaphragm. Glottal closure prevents entry of vomitus into the trachea. As a rule there is prodromal salivation or yawning. Coordination between these different stages depends on the **medullary center for emesis**, which can be activated by diverse stimuli. These are conveyed via the **vestibular apparatus, visual, olfactory,** and **gustatory inputs** as well as **viscerosensory afferents** from the upper alimentary tract. Furthermore, **psychic experiences** may also activate the emetic center. The mechanisms underlying **motion sickness** (kinetosis, sea sickness) and **vomiting during pregnancy** are still unclear.

The emetic center itself cannot be reached by polar substances because it is protected by the blood–brain barrier. However, these can indirectly excite the center by activating **chemoreceptors** in the **area postrema**.

Antiemetic therapy. Vomiting can be a useful reaction enabling the body to eliminate an orally ingested poison. Antiemetic drugs are used to prevent kinetosis, pregnancy vomiting, cytotoxic drug-induced or postoperative vomiting, as well as vomiting due to radiation therapy.

Kinetoses (motion sicknesses). Effective prophylaxis can be achieved with the parasympatholytic scopolamine (p. 106) and H_1 antihistaminics (p. 114) of the diphenylmethane type (e.g., diphenhydramine, meclizine). Antiemetic activity is not a property shared by all parasympatholytics or antihistaminics. The efficacy of the drugs mentioned depends on the actual situation of the individual (gastric filling, ethanol consumption), environmental conditions (e.g., the behavior of fellow travellers), and the type of motion experienced. The drugs should be taken 30 min before the start of travel and repeated every 4–6 h. Scopolamine applied transdermally through an adhesive patch can provide effective protection for up to 3 days.

Pregnancy vomiting is prone to occur in the first trimester; thus pharmacotherapy would coincide with the period of maximal fetal vulnerability with respect to chemical injury. Accordingly, antiemetics (antihistaminics, or neuroleptics if required) should be used only when continuous vomiting threatens to disturb electrolyte and water balance to a degree that places the fetus at risk.

Drug-induced vomiting. Numerous drugs elicit vomiting via stimulation of chemoreceptors in the area postrema. This reaction can be attenuated or suppressed by drugs that possess blocking activity at dopamine receptors (phenothiazines: prochlorperazine, methotrimeprazine; butyrophenones: haloperidol, p. 114), 5-HT_3 receptors (ondansetron), or both (metoclopramide, in high dosage). Synthetic cannabinoids (nabilone, dronabinol) and corticosteroids (methylprednisolone, dexamethasone) are also effective in controlling emesis and can be combined with other antiemetics. This regimen is particularly important as an adjunct to cytostatic therapy because most antineoplastic drugs exert an emetic effect.

Vomiting subsequent to **surgery**, during **radiation therapy** and **uremia,** or due to diseases accompanied by **elevated intracranial pressure** is also treated with neuroleptics or metoclopramide.

Anticipatory nausea and vomiting can be attenuated by a benzodiazepine such as lorazepam.

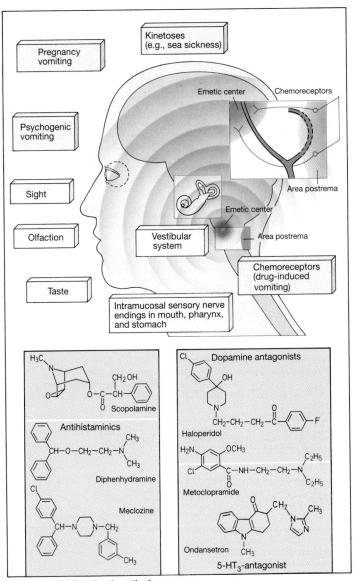

A. Emetic stimuli and antiemetic drugs

Further Reading

Berkowitz RL, Couston DR, Mochiezuki TK. Handbook of prescribing medications during pregnancy. Boston: Little, Brown, 1981.

Bowman WC, Rand MJ. Textbook of pharmacology. 2nd ed. Oxford: Blackwell, 1980.

D'Arcey PF, Griffin JP. Iatrogenic diseases. Oxford: Oxford University Press, 1986.

Davies DM, ed. Textbook of adverse drug reactions. 4th ed. Oxford: Oxford University Press, 1991.

Folb PI, Dukes MNG. Drug safety in pregnancy. Amsterdam: Elsevier, 1990.

Gibaldi M. Biopharmaceutics and clinical pharmacokinetics. 3rd ed. Philadelphia: Lea & Febiger, 1984.

Gilman AG, Rall TW, Nies AS, Taylor P. Goodman & Gilman's the pharmacological basis of therapeutics. 8th ed. New York: Pergamon Press, 1990.

Griffin JP, D'Arcey PF, Speirs CJ. Adverse drug interactions. 4th ed. London: Wright (Butterworth), 1988.

Hansten PD, Horn JR. Drug interactions and updates. Philadelphia: Lea & Febiger, 1990.

Katzung BG. Basic and clinical pharmacology. 5th ed. Norwalk, CT: Appleton & Lange, 1992.

Klaassen CD, Amdur MO, Doull J. Casarett and Doull's toxicology: The basic sience of poisons. 3rd ed. New York: Macmillan, 1986.

Koda-Kimble MA, Young LY. Applied therapeutics: the clinical use of drugs. 5th ed. Vancouver: Applied Therapeutics, 1992.

Laurence DR, Bennett PN. Clinical pharmacology. 6th ed. Edinburgh: Churchill Livingstone, 1987.

Levine RL. Pharmacology: drug actions and reactions. 4th ed. Boston: Little, Brown, 1990.

Rang HP, Dale MM: Pharmacology. 2nd ed. Edinburgh: Churchill Livingstone, 1991.

Rowland M, Tozer TN. Clinical pharmacokinetics: concepts and applications. Philadelphia: Lea & Febiger, 1980.

Rubin PC. Prescribing in pregnancy. London: British Medical Journal, 1987.

Stryer L. Biochemistry. New York: WH Freeman, 1988.

Wingard LB, Brody TM, Larner J, Schwartz A. Human pharmacology: molecular to clinical. St. Louis: Mosby-Year Book, 1991.

Drug Indexes

Nomenclature. The terms *active agent* and *pharmacon* designate substances that are capable of modifying life processes irrespective of whether the effects elicited may benefit or harm the organisms concerned. By this definition, a toxin is also a pharmacon. Taken in a narrower sense, a pharmacon means a substance that is used for therapeutic purposes. An unequivocal term for such a substance is *medicinal drug.*

A drug can be identified by different designations:
– the chemical name
– the generic (nonproprietary) name
– a trade or brand name

The drug diazepam may serve as an illustrative example. Chemically, this compound is called 7-chloro-1,3-dihydro-1-methyl-5-phenyl-2H-1,4-benzo-diazepin-2-one, a term too unwieldy for everyday use. A simpler name is diazepam. This is not a legally protected name but a *generic (nonproprietary) name.* An INN (= international nonproprietary name) is a generic name that has been agreed upon by an international commission.

Preparations containing diazepam were first marketed under the *trade name* Valium by its manufacturer, Hoffmann–La Roche, Inc. This name is a registered trademark. After patent protection for the manufacture of diazepam-containing drug preparations expired, other companies were free to produce preparations containing this drug. Each invented a proprietary name for its "own" preparation. As a result, there now exists a plethora of proprietary labels for diazepam preparations (as of 1991, more than 50). Some of these easily reveal the active ingredient, because the company name is simply added to the generic name, e.g., Diazepam-(company's name). Other designations are new creations, as for example, Vivol.

Similarly, some other commercially successful drugs are sold under more than 20 different brand labels. The number of proprietary names, therefore, greatly exceeds the number of available drugs.

For the sake of clarity, only INNs or generic (nonproprietary) names are used in this atlas to designate drugs, such as the name "diazepam" in the above example.

Use of Indexes

The indexes are meant to help the reader:

1. identify a commercial preparation for a given drug. This information is found in the index "Generic Name → Proprietary Name."

2. obtain information about the pharmacological properties of the active ingredient in a commercial preparation. In order to find the generic (nonproprietary) name, the second index "Proprietary Name → Generic Name" can be consulted. Page references pertaining to the drug can then be looked up in the Index. The list of proprietary names given below will necessarily be incomplete due to their multitude. For drugs that are marketed under several brand names, the trade name of the original manufacturer will be listed; in the case of some frequently prescribed generics, some proprietary names of other manufacturers will also be listed. Brand names that clearly reveal the drug's identity have been omitted. Combination preparations have not been included, barring a few exceptions.

Many a brand name is not listed in the index "Proprietary Name → Generic Name." In these cases, it will be useful to consult the packaging information, which should list the generic (nonproprietary) name or INN.

Generic Name	Proprietary Name
A	
Acebutolol	Monitan, Sectral
Acenocoumarol	Sinthrome, Sintrom
Acetaminophen	Acephen, Anacin-3, Calpol, Datril, Panadol, Tempra, Tylenol, Valadol
Acetazolamide	Diamox, Glaupax
Acetylcysteine	Airbron, Fabrol, Mucomyst, Parvolex
Acetyldigoxin	Acylanid
Acetylsalicylic acid (aspirin)	Angettes, Arthrisin, Asadrine, Ecotrin, Entrophen, Platet, Pyronoval, Solprin, Supasa
Acyclovir	Zovirax
ACTH	See corticotropin
Actinomycin D	See dactinomycin
ADH	See vasopressin
Adrenaline	See epinephrine
Adriamycin	See doxorubicin
Ajmaline	Cardiorhythmine, Gilurytmal
Albuterol (salbutamol)	Novosalmol, Proventil, Salbulin, Ventolin
Alcuronium	Alloferin
Aldosterone	Aldocorten
Allopurinol	Alloprin, Caplenal, Hamarin, Novopurol, Urosin, Zyloprim, Zyloric
Alprazolam	Xanax
Alprenolol	Aptine, Gubernal
Alprostadil	Minprog, Prostin VR
Aluminum hydroxide	Aldrox, Alu-Cap, Alu-Tab, Amphojel, Fluagel
Amantadine	Ambaxine, Solu-Contenton, Symmetrel, Virofral
Ambroxol	Ambril, Bronchopront, Mucosolvan
Amikacin	Amikin, Briclin, Novamin
Amiloride	Arumil, Colectril, Cordarex, Midamor
Amiloride + Hydrochlorothiazide	Moduret
Aminocaproic acid	Amicar, Epsicapron
Aminomethylbenzoic acid	Gumbix
5-Aminosalicylic acid	see Mesalamine
Amiodarone	Cordarex, Cordarone
Amitriptyline	Amitril, Domical, Elavil, Endep, Enovil, Lentizol, Levate, Mevaril, Tryptizol
Amodiaquine	Camoquin, Flavoquine
Amoxicillin	Almodan, Amoxil, Clamoxyl, Moxacin, Novamoxin
Amphotericin B	Amphozone, Fungilin, Fungizone, Moronal
Ampicillin	Amcill, Amfipen, Omnipen, Penbritin, Polycillin, Principen, Totacillin, Vidopen
Amrinone	Inocor, Wincoram
Ancrod	Arvin
Angiotensinamide	Hypertensin
Aprindine	Amidonal, Fibocil
Aspirin	see acetylsalicylic acid

Amphetamine	see dextroamphetamine
Atenolol	Antipressan, Premormine, Tenormin, Totamol
Atracurium	Tracrium
Atropine	Atropisol, Borotropin
Auranofin	Ridaura
Aurothioglucose	Aureotan, Auromyose, Solganal
Azathioprine	Azanin, Berkaprine, Imuran, Imurek
Azidothymidine (AZT)	see Zidovudine
Azlocillin	Azlin, Securopen
Aztreonam	Azactam

B

Bacitracin	Altracin, Baciguent, Topitracin
Baclofen	Lioresal
Beclomethasone	Aldecin, Becloforte, Becodisks, Beconase, Becotide, Propaderm
Benzbromarone	Desuric, Nacaricin, Normurat, Uricovac
Benzocaine	Anaesthesin
Benztropine	Cogentin
Betaxolol	Betoptic, Kerlone
Bezafibrate	Befizal, Bezalip
Bifonazole	Amycor, Mycospor, Mycosporan
Biperiden	Akeniton, Akinophyl
Bisacodyl	Bicol, Broxalax, Dulcolax, Durolax, Laxabene, Laxanin, Nigalax, Pyrilax, Telemin, Ulcolax
Bismuth subsalicylate	Pepto-Bismol
Bisoprolol	Concor, Detensiel, Emcor, Monocor
Bleomycin	Blenoxane
Bromazepam	Durazanil, Lectopam, Lexotan
Bromhexine	Auxit, Bisolvon, Ophthosol
Bromocriptine	Parlodel, Pravidel, Serono-Bagren
Brotizolam	Lendorm(A), Lendormin
Budesonide	Preferid, Pulmicort, Rhinocort, Spirocort
Bumetanide	Bumex, Burinex, Fontego, Fordiuran, Lixil
Bunitrolol	Stresson
Bupranolol	Betadran, Betadrenol, Looser, Panimit
Buprenorphine	Buprene, Temgesic
Buserelin	Suprefact
Busulfan	Mielucin, Mitosan, Myleran, Sulfabutin

C

Calcifediol	Calderol, Dedrogyl, Hidroferol
Calcitonin	Calcimer, Calcitare, Calsynar, Cibacalcin, Karil
Calcitriol	Rocaltrol
Calcium carbonate	Cacit, Calchichew, Calcidrink, Calsan, Caltrate, Nu-Cal
Camazepam	Albego
Canrenone	Kanrenol, Soldactone, Venactone
Capreomycin	Capastat, Caprolin
Captopril	Acediur, Acepril, Capoten, Cesplon, Hypertil, Lopirin, Tensobon
Carazolol	Conducton, Suacron
Carbachol	Doryl, Miostat, Sirtal

Carbamazepine	Epitol, Tegretol, Timonil
Carbenicillin	Anabactyl(A), Carindapen, Geopen, Pyopen
Carbenoxolone	Biogastrone, Bioplex, Neogel, Sanodin
Carbidopa + Levodopa	Isicom, Nacom, Sinemet
Carbimazole	Neo-Mercazole, Neo-Thyreostat
Carteolol	Arteoptic, Caltidren, Carteol, Cartrol, Endak, Tenalin, Teoptic
Cefmenoxime	Bestcall, Cemix, Tacef
Cefoperazone	Cefobid, Cefobis, Tomabef
Cefotaxime	Claforan
Cefoxitin	Mefoxin
Ceftazidime	Fortaz, Fortum, Tacicef
Ceftriaxone	Acantex, Rocephin
Cellulose	Avicel
Cephalexin	Cepexin(A), Ceporex, Keflex, Losporal
Chloralhydrate	Lorinal, Noctec, Somnos, Welldorm, Elixir
Chlorambucil	Leukeran
Chloramphenicol	Chloromycetin, Chloroptic, Kemicetine, Leukomycin, Paraxin, Sno Phenicol, Sopamycetin, Spersanicol
Chlorhexidine	Baxedin, Chlor-hex, Chlorhexitulle, Corsodyl, Hibidil, Hibiscrub, Hibisol, Hibitane, Plak-out
Chloroquine	Aralen, Avloclor, Nivaquine, Quinachlor
Chlorpromazine	Hibanil, Largactil, Megaphen, Thorazine
Chlorthalidone	Hygroton
Cholecalciferol	D-Tabs, Vigantol, Vigorsan
Cholestyramine	Cuemid, Questran
Chorionic gonadotropin (HCG)	Entromone, Follutein, Pregnesin, Pregnyl, Profasi
Cimetidine	Dyspamet, Peptol, Tagamet
Ciprofloxacin	Cipro, Ciprobay, Ciproxin
Cisplatin	Platinex, Platinol
Clavulanic acid + Amoxicillin	Augmentin
Clemastine	Tavegil, Tavist
Clindamycin	Cleocin, Dalacin, Sobelin
Clodronic acid	Clasteon, Ossiten, Ostac
Clofazimine	Lamprene
Clofibrate	Atromid-S, Claripex, Skleromexe
Clomethiazole	Distraneurin, Hemineurin
Clomiphene	Clomid, Dyneric, Omifin, Pergotime, Serophene
Clonazepam	Clonopin, Iktorivil, Rivotril
Clonidine	Catapres, Dixarit
Clorazepate	Novoclopate, Tranxene
Clostebol	Steranobol
Clotiazepam	Clozan, Rize, Tienor, Trecalmo, Veratran
Clotrimazole	Canesten, Clotrimaderm, Gyne-Lotrimin, Mycelex, Trimysten
Codeine	Codicept, Paveral
Colestipol	Cholestabyl, Cholestid
Corticotropin	Acthar, Cortigel, Cortrophin
Cortisol	see hydrocortisone

Cortisone	Cortelan, Cortistab, Cortogen, Cortone
Cotrimoxazole	Bactrim, Protrin, Septra
Cromolyn	Intal, Nalcron, Opticrom, Rynacrom, Vistacrom
Cyanocobalamine	Anacobin, Bedoz, Cytacon, Cytamen, Rubion, Rubramin, Sytobex
Cyclofenil	Fertodur, Ondogyne, Ondonid, Rehibin, Sexovid
Cyclopenthiazide	Navidrix
Cyclophosphamide	Cytoxan, Endoxan, Procytox
Cyclosporine	Sandimmune
Cyproheptadine	Anarexol, Nuran, Periactin, Peritol, Vimicon
Cyproterone acetate	Androcur, Cyprostat
Cytarabine	Alexan, Cytosar, Udicil

D

Dactinomycin (actinomycin D)	Cosmegen
Dantrolene	Dantrium
Dapsone	Avlosulfone, Diphenasone, Eporal, Udolac
Daunorubicin	Cerubidine, Daunoblastin, Ondena
Desipramine	Norpramin, Pertofran
Desmopressin	DDAVP, Desmospray, Minirin, Stimate
Desogestrel + Ethinylestradiol	Marvelon
Dexamethasone	Decadron, Deronil, Hexadrol, Maxidex, Spersadex
Dexetimide	Tremblex
Dextroamphetamine	Dexedrine, Synatan
Diazepam	Apaurin, Atensine, Diazemuls, Eridan, Lembrol, Meval, Noan, Stesolid, Tensium, Valium Roche, Valium, Vatran, Vivol
Diazoxide	Eudemine, Hyperstat, Mutabase, Proglicem
Diclofenac	Allvoran, Diclophlogont, Rhumalgan, Voltaren, Voltarol
Dicloxacillin	Diclocil, Dynapen, Pathocil
Diethylstilbestrol	Honvol
Digitoxin	Crystodigin, Digicor, Digimerck, Digitaline, Purodigin, Tardigal
Digoxin	Digacin, Lanicor, Lanoxin, Lenoxin, Novodigoxin
Digoxin immune FAB	Digibind
Dihydralazine	Dihyzin, Nepresol
Dihydroergotamine	Angionorm, D.E.H.45, Dihydergot, Divegal, Endophleban
Diltiazem	Cardizem, Tildiem
Dinoprost	Minprostin F2 Alpha, Prostin F2 Alpha
Dinoprostone	Prepidil, Prostin E2
Diphenhydramine	Allerdryl, Benadryl, Insommal, Nautamine
Diphenoxylate	Diarsed, Lomotil, Retardin
Dipyrone	Metilon, Novalgin
Disopyramide	Dirythmin, Norpace, Rythmodan
Dobutamine	Dobutrex
Domperidone	Evoxin, Motilium, Nauzelin, Peridon
Doxorubicin	Adriamycin, Adriblastin

Doxycycline	C-Pak, Doxicin, Nordox, Vibramycin
Doxylamine	Decapryn
Droperidol	Droleptan, Inapsine

E

Econazole	Ecostatin, Gyno-Pevaryl, Pevaryl
Ecothiopate	Phospholine Iodide
Enalapril	Innovace, Vasotec, Xanef
Enflurane	Ethrane
Enoxacin	Bactidan, Comprecin, Enoram
Ephedrine	Bofedrol, C.A.M., Efedron, Va-tro-nol
Epinephrine (adrenaline)	Epifrin, EpiPen, Eppy, Ganda E, Lyophrin, Simplene, Suprarenin Vaponefrine
Ergonovine (ergometrine)	Ergotrate Maleate, Ermalate
Ergotamine	Ergomar, Gynergen, Lingraine, Medihaler Ergotamine, Migril
Erythromycin	E-mycin, Eryc, Erymax, Erythromid, Erythroped, Ilosone
Erythromycin estolate	Dowmycin, Ilosone, Novorythro
Erythromycin ethylsuccinate	EES, Erythrocin, Wyamycin
Erythromycin propionate	Cimetrin
Erythromycin stearate	Erymycin, Erythrocin
Erythromycin succinate	Monomycin
Erythropoietin (epoetin alfa)	Epogen
Esmolol	Brevibloc
Estradiol	Estrace
Estradiol benzoate	Progynon
Estradiol valerate	Delestrogen, Dioval
Estriol	Theelol
Ethacrynic acid	Edecrin, Hydromedin, Reomax
Ethambutol	Etibi, Myambutol
Ethinyl estradiol	Estinyl, Lynoral
Ethionamide	Trecator
Ethosuximide	Petinimid, Suxinutin, Zarontin
Etretinate	Tegison, Tigason

F

Famotidine	Pepcid, Pepdul
Felypressin	Octapressin
Fenfluramine	Ganal, Ponderal, Ponderax, Pondimin
Fenoprofen	Fenopron, Nalfon, Nalgesic, Progesic
Fenoterol	Berotec, Partusisten
Fentanyl	Sublimaze
Fentanyl + Droperidol	Innovar
Flecainide	Tambocor
Flucloxacillin (floxacillin)	Floxapen, Ladropen, Stafoxil
Flucytosine	Alcoban, Ancotil
Fludrocortisone	Alflorone, F-Cortef, Florinef
Flumazenil	Anexate
Flunarizine	Flugeral, Sibelium
Flunitrazepam	Narcozep, Rohypnol
Fluorouracil	Adrucil, Efudex, Efudix

Fluoxetine	Prozac
Folic acid	Foldine, Folvite
Furosemide	Dryptal, Fusid, Lasix, Seguril, Uritol

G

Gallamine	Flaxedil
Gallopamil	Algocor, Corgal, Procorum, Wingom
Ganciclovir	Cymevene, Cytovene
Gelatin colloids	Gelafundin, Haemaccel
Gemfibrozil	Lopid
Gentamicin	Cidomycin, Garamycin, Genticin, Refobacin, Sulmycin
Glyburide (glibenclamide)	Calabren, Daonil, DiaBeta, Euglucon, Micronase
Glyceryltrinitrate	See nitroglycerin
Gonadorelin	Factrel, Relefact
Goserelin	Zoladex
Griseofulvin	Fulcin, Fulvicin, Grisovin, Likuden
Guanethidine	Ismelin, Visutensil

H

Haloperidol	Haldol, Serenace
Halothane	Fluothane, Narkotan
HCG	See chorionic gonadotropin
Heparin	Calciparin, Hepalean, Hepsal, Liquemin, Uniparin
Heparin low molecular	Fragmin, Fraxiparin
Hetastarch (HES)	Hespan
Hexachlorophane	See lindane
Hexobarbital	Evipan
Hydralazine	Alazine, Apresoline
Hydrochlorothiazide	Aprozide, Diaqua, Diuchlor, Esidrix, Hydromal, Hydrosaluric, Neo-Codema
Hydrocortisone (cortisol)	Alocort, Cortate, Cortef, Cortenema, Hyderm, Hyocort, Rectocort, Unicort
Hydromorphone	Dilaudid, Hymorphan
Hydroxocobalamin	Acti-B12, Alpha-redisol, Cobalin-H, Droxomin, Hybalamine, Vibal L. A.
Hydroxychloroquine	Plaquenil
Hydroxyethyl starch	Hespan
Hydroxyprogesterone caproate	Duralutin, Gesterol L.A., Hylutin, Hyroxon, Primolut Depot, Pro-Depo
Hyoscine butylbromide	Buscopan

I

Ibuprofen	Actiprophen, Advil, Brufen, Fenbid, Lidifen, Motrin, Nuprin, Trendar
Idoxuridine	Dendrid, Herpid, Herplex, Kerecid, Stoxil
Ifosfamide	Ifex, Mitoxana
Imipramine	Dynaprin, Impril, Janimine, Melipramin, Tofranil, Typramine

Indomethacin	Ammuno, Imbrilon, Indocid, Indocin, Indomee, Indomod, Metacen
Interferon	Fiblaferon 3
Interferon-alpha2	Berofor alpha 2
Interferon-alpha2a	Roferon A3
Interferon-alpha2b	Intron A
Ipratropium	Atrovent, Itrop, Rinatec
Isoconazole	Gyno-Travogen, Travogen, Travogyn
Isoflurane	Forane
Isoniazid	Armazid, Isotamine, Lamiazid, Nydrazid, Rimifon, Teebaconin
Isoproterenol (isoprenaline)	Aludrin, Isuprel, Medihaler-Iso, Saventrine
Isosorbide dinitrate	Cedocard, Coradus, Coronex, Isoket, Isordil, Sorbitrate, Vascardin
Isosorbide mononitrate	Coleb, Elantan, Imdur, Ismo, Isotrate
Isotretinoin	Acutane Roche, Roaccutane

K

Kanamycin	Anamid, Kannasyn, Kantrex, Klebcil
Kaolin + pectin (attapulgite)	Donnagel-MB, Kaopectate, Pectokay
Ketamine	Ketalar
Ketoconazole	Nizoral

L

Lactulose	Cephulac, Chronulac, Duphalac
Leuprolide (leuprorelin)	Lupron
Levodopa	Dopaidan, Dopar, Larodopa
Levodopa + Benserazide	Madopar, Prolopa
Levodopa + Carbidopa	Sinemet
Levomepromazine	See methotrimeprazine
Lidocaine	Dalcaine, Lidopen, Nulicaine, Xylocain, Xylocard
Lincomycin	Albiotic, Cillimycin, Lincocin
Lindane	Hexit, Kwell, Kwilldane, Quellada, Scabene
Liothyronine	Cytomel
Lisinopril	Carace, Prinivil, Zestril
Lisuride	Cuvalit, Dopergin, Lysenyl
Lithium carbonate	Camcolit, Carbolite, Duoralith, Eskalith, Liskonum, Lithane, Lithobid, Lithotabs, Priadel
Lomustine	CCNU, CeeNu
Loperamide	Imodium
Lorazepam	Alzapam, Ativan, Loraz
Lorcainide	Lopantrol, Lorivox, Remivox,
Lormetazepam	Loramet, Noctamid
Lovastatin	Mevacor, Mevinacor
Lypressin	Diapid, Syntopressin, Vasopressin

M

Mannitol	Isotol, Osmitrol,
Mebendazole	Vermox

Mechlorethamine	Mustargen
Meclizine (meclozine)	Antivert, Antrizine, Bonamine, Whevert
Meclofenamate	Meclomen
Medroxyprogesterone acetate	Amen, Depo-Provera, Farlutal, Oragest, Provera
Mefloquine	Lariam
Melphalan	Alkeran
Meperidine (pethidine)	Demerol, Dolantin, Pethidine Roche
Mepivacaine	Carbocaine, Isocaine
Mercaptopurine	Purinethol
Mesalamine	Asocol, Mesacal, Pentasa, Propasa, Rezipas
Mesna	Mesnex, Uromitexan
Mesterolone	Androviron, Proviron
Metamizol	See dipyrone
Metaproterenol (orciprenaline)	Alupent, Metaprel
Metformin	Diabex, Glucophage
Methadone	Dolophine, Methadose, Physeptone
Methamphetamine	Desoxyn, Methampex
Methimazole (thiamazole)	Tapazole
Methohexital	Brevital
Methotrimeprazine	Levoprome, Nozinan
Methotrexate	Folex, Maxtrex, Mexate
Methoxyflurane	Methofane, Penthrane
Methylcellulose	Celevac, Citrucel, Cologel, Lacril, Murocel
Methyldopa	Aldomet, Amodopa, Dopamet, Novomedopa, Presinol, Sembrina
Methylergonovine	Methergin
Methylphenidate	Ritalin
Methyltestosterone	Android, Metandren, Testred, Virilon
Methysergide	Deseril, Sansert
Metoclopramide	Clopra, Emex, Maxeran, Maxolan, Primperan, Reclomide, Reglan
Metoprolol	Betaloc, Lopressor
Metronidazole	Clont, Femazole, Flagyl, Metronid, Protostat, Satric, Zadstat
Mexiletine	Mexitil
Mezlocillin	Mezlin
Miconazole	Daktarin, Dermonistat, Micatin, Monistat
Midazolam	Hypnovel, Versed
Mifepristone (RU-486)	Mifegyne
Minocycline	Minocin, Vectrin
Minoxidil	Loniten, Regaine, Rogaine
Misoprostol	Cytotec
Mithramycin	See plicamycin
Molsidomine	Corvaton, Duracoron, Molsidolat
Morphine	MST Continus, Oramorph
Morphine hydrochloride	Morphitec
Morphine sulfate	Duramorph, Epimorph, Roxanol, Statex

N

Nabilone	Cesamet
Nadolol	Corgard

Nalbuphine	Nubain
Nalidixic acid	Negram, Nogram
Naloxone	Narcan
Nandrolone	Anabolin, Androlone, Deca-Durabolin, Hybolin Decanoate, Hybolin, Kabolin
Naphazoline	Albalon, Degest-2, Privine, Vasocon
Naproxen	Naprosyn, Naxen, Synflex
Neomycin	Mycifradin, Myciguent, Nivemycin
Neostigmine	Prostigmin
Netilmicin	Netillin, Netromycin
Niclosamide	Niclocide, Yomesan
Nifedipine	Adalat Retard, Adalat, Coracten, Procardia
Nimodipine	Nimotop
Nitrazepam	Mogadon, Somnite
Nitrendipine	Bayotensin, Baypress
Nitroglycerin	Ang-O-Span, Deponit, Nitrocap, Nitrogard, Nitronal, Sustac, Tridil
Nitroprusside sodium	Nipride, Nitropress
Nizatidine	Axid
Nordazepam	Tranxillium N, Vegesan
Norepinephrine (noradrenaline)	Arterenol, Levophed
Norethindrone (norethisterone)	Micronor, Noriday, Nor-Q D, Norlutin, Primolut N
Norfloxacin	Noroxin, Utinor
Noscapine	Coscopin, Coscotab
Nystatin	Korostatin, Mycostatin, Mykinac, Nilstat, Nystan, Nystex, O-V Statin

O

Ofloxacin	Tarivid
Omeprazole	Losec
Opium tincture (laudanum)	Paregoric
Orciprenaline	See metaproterenol
Ornipressin	POR 8
Oxacillin	Bactocill, Prostaphlin
Oxazepam	Oxpam, Serax, Zapex
Oxiconazole	Oxistat
Oxprenolol	Apsolox, Trasicor
Oxymetazoline	Afrin, Allerest, Coricidin, Dristan, Neo-Synephrine, Sinarest
Oxytocin	Pitocin, Syntocinon

P

Pancuronium	Pavulon
Papaverine	Cerebid, Cerespan, Delapav, Myobid, Papacon, Pavabid, Pavadur, Vasal
Paracetamol	See acetaminophen
Paromomycin	Humatin
Penicillamine	Cuprimine, Depen, Distamine, Pendramine
Penicillin G	Bicillin, Cryspen, Crystapen, Deltapen, Lanacillin, Megacillin, Parcillin, Pensorb, Pentids, Permapen, Pfizerpin
Penicillin G, Benzathine	Bicillin, Megacillin, Penidural, Tardocillin

Penicillin V	Apsin VK, Betapen-VK, Bopen-VK, Calvepen, Cocillin-VK, Distaquaine V-K, Lanacillin-VK, Ledercillin-VK, Nadopen-V, Novopen-VK, Pen-Vee K, Penapar-VK, Penbec-V, Pfizerpen VK, Robicillin-VK, Stabillin V-K, Uticillin-VK, V-Cil-K, V-Cillin K, Veetids
Pentazocine	Fortal, Talwin
Pentobarbital	Butylone, Nembutal, Novarectal, Pentanca
Pentoxifylline	Trental
Pergolide	Celance, Permax
Perindopril	Coversum, Coversyl
Permethrin	Elimite, Lyclear, Nix, Permanone
Pethidine	See meperidine
Phencyclidine	Sernyl
Phenobarbital	Barbita, Gardenal, Solfoton
Phenolphthalein	Alophen, Correctol, Espotabs, Evac-U-gen, Evac-U-lax, Ex-Lax, Modane, Prulet
Phenoxybenzamine	Dibenyline, Dibenzyline
Phenprocoumon	Liquamar, Marcumar
Phentolamine	Regitin, Rogitin
Phenylbutazone	Algoverine, Azolid, Butacote, Butagen, Butazolidin, Malgesic
Phenytoin	Dilantin, Epanutin
Physostigmine	Antilirium
Phytomenadione	Konakion
Pilocarpine	Akarpine, Almocarpine, I-Pilopine, Isopto Carpine, Miocarpine, Ocusert, Pilokair
Pindolol	Visken
Pipecuronium	Arduan
Piperacillin	Pipracil, Pipril
Pirenzepine	Gastrozepin
Piroxicam	Felden
Pizotyline (pizotifen)	Litec, Mosegor, Sandomigran
Plicamycin	Mithracin
Pravastatin	Lipostat, Pravachol
Prazepam	Centrax
Praziquantel	Biltricide
Prazosin	Hypovase, Minipress
Prednisolone	Ak Pred, Articulose, Codelsol, Cortalone, Delta-Cortef, Deltastab, Hydeltrasol, Inflamase, Key-Pred, Metalone, Metreton, Pediapred, Predate, Predcor, Predenema, Predfoam, Prednesol, Prelone
Prednisone	Meticorten, Orasone, Panasol, Winpred
Prilocaine	Citanest, Xylonest
Primaquine	Primaquine
Primidone	Myidone, Mysoline, Sertan
Probenecid	Benemid, Probalan
Procainamide	Procan SR, Promine, Pronestyl, Rhythmin
Progesterone	Cyclogest, Femotrone, Gestone, Progestasert

Promethazine	Anergan, Avomine, Ganphen, Mallergan, Pentazine, Phenazine, Phenergan, Prometh, Prorex, Provigan, Remsed
Propafenone	Arythmol, Rhythmol
Propranolol	Berkolol, Cardinol, Detensol, Inderal
Propylthiouracil	Propyl-Thyracil
Pyrantel Pamoate	Antiminth, Combantrin
Pyrazinamide	Aldinamide, Tebrazid, Zinamide
Pyridostigmine	Mestinon, Regonol
Pyridoxine	Bee-six, Comploment Continus, Hexa-Betalin, Pyroxine
Pyrimethamine	Daraprim
Pyrimethamine + Sulfadoxine	Fansidar

Q

Quinidine	Cardioqin, Cin-Quin, Kiditard, Kinidin, Quinalan, Quinidex, Quinora
Quinine	Quinaminoph, Quinamm, Quine, Quinite

R

Ranitidine	Zantac
Reserpine	Sandril, Serpalan, Serpasil, Zepine
Rifampin (rifampicin)	Rifadin, Rimactan
Ritodrine	Yutopar
Rolitetracycline	Reverin, Transcycline

S

Salazosulfapyridine	see sulfasalazine
Salbutamol	see albuterol
Salicylic acid	Acnex, Sebcur, Soluver, Trans-Ver-Sal
Scopolamine	Scopoderm TTS, Transderm Scop, Triptone
Selegiline	Deprenyl, Eldepryl
Senna	Black Draught, Fletcher's Castoria, Genna, Gentle Nature, Nytilax, Senolax, Senokot
Simvastatin	Zocor
Sitosterol	Sito-Lande
Sotalol	Sotacor
Spectinomycin	Trobicin
Spiramycin	Rovamycin, Selectomycin
Spironolactone	Aldactone, Spiroctan
Streptokinase	Kabikinase, Streptase
Streptomycin	Strepolin, Streptosol
Succinylcholine	Anectine, Quelicin, Succostrin
Sucralfate	Antepsin, Carafate, Sulcrate
Sulfadoxine + Pyrimethamine	Fansidar
Sulfamethoxazole	Gantanol
Sulfapyridine	Dagenan
Sulfasalazine (salazosulfapyridine)	Azulfidine, Salazopyrin
Sulfinpyrazone	Anturan, Aprazone
Sulfisoxazole	Gantrisin, Gulfasin
Sulprostone	Nalador
Sulthiame	Ospolot

T

t-PA (alteplase)	Activase
Temazepam	Euhypnos, Normison, Restoril
Terbutaline	Brethine, Bricanyl
Terfenadine	Seldane, Triludan
Testerone undecanoate	Andriol
Testosterone	Restandol, Sustanon
Testosterone cypionate	Androcyp, Andronate, Duratest, Testoject
Testosterone enanthate	Andro, Delatestryl, Everone, Testone
Testosterone propionate	Testex
Tetracaine	Anethaine, Pontocaine
Tetrahydrozoline (tetryzoline)	Collyrium, Murine, Tyzine, Visine
Thalidomide	Contergan
Theophylline	Aerolate, Bronkodyl, Constant-T, Elixophyllin, Lasma, Nuelin, Pro-Vent, Quibron-T, Slo-bid, Slo-Phylli, Somophyllin-T, Sustaire, Theolair, Uniphyl
Thiabendazole	Mintezol
Thiamazole	See methimazole
Thiopental	Pentothal, Trapanal
Thiotepa	Thiotepa Lederle
Thrombin	Thrombinar, Thrombostat
Thyroxine	Choloxin, Eltroxin
Ticarcillin	Ticar, Timentin
Timolol	Betim, Blocadren, Timoptic, Timoptol
Tinidazol	Fasigyn CH, Simplotan, Sorquetan
Tobramycin	Nebcin, Tobralex, Tobrex
Tocainide	Tonocard
Tolbutamide	Mobenol, Oramide, Orinase, Rastinon
Tramadol	Tramal
Tranexamic acid	Cyklocapron
Tranylcypromine	Parnate
Triamcinolone	Adcortyl, Aristocort, Kenacort, Ledercort, Volon
Triamcinolone acetonide	Adicort, Azmacort, Kenalog, Kenalone, Triam-A
Triamterene	Dyrenium, Dytac
Triazolam	Halcion
Trifluridine	Viroptic
Trihexiphenidyl	Aparkane, Artane, Tremin, Trihexane
Trimethaphan	Arfonad
Trimethoprim	Ipral, Monotrim, Proloprim, Trimpex
Tubocurarine	Jexin, Tubarine
Tyrothricin	Hydrotricine, Tyrozets

U

Urokinase	Abbokinase, Ukidan

V

Valproic acid	Depakene

Vancomycin	Vancocin, Vancomycin CP Lilly
Vasopressin	Pitressin
Vecuronium	Norcuron
Verapamil	Berkatens, Calan, Cordilox, Isoptin, Securon, Univer, Verelan
Vidarabine	Vira-A
Vinblastine	Velban, Velbe
Vincristine	Oncovin
Vit. B12	Bay-Bee, Berubigen, Betalin 12, Cabadon, Cobex, Cyanoject, Cyomin, Pemavit, Redisol, Rubesol, Sytobex, Vibal
Vit. B6	Bee Six, Hexa-Betalin, Pyroxine
Vit. D	Drisdol, D-Vi-sol

W

Warfarin	Coumadin, Marevan, Panwarfin, Sofarin

X

Xanthinol nicotinate (Xanthinol niacinate)	Complamin
Xylometazoline	Chlorohist, Neosynephrine II, Otrivin, Sinutab

Z

Zidovudine (AZT)	Retrovir

Proprietary Name	Generic Name
A	
Abbokinase CAN	Urokinase
Acantex	Ceftriaxone
Acediur	Captopril
Acephen	Acetaminophen
Acepril	Captopril
Acnex	Salicylic acid
Acthar	Corticotropin
Acti-B12	Hydroxocobalamin
Actiprophen	Ibuprofen
Activase	t-PA (alteplase)
Acutane Roche	Isotretinoin
Acylanid	Acetyldigoxin
Adalat Retard	Nifedipine
Adalat	Nifedipine
Adcortyl	Triamcinolone
Adicort	Triamcinolone acetonide
Adriblastin	Doxorubicin
Adrucil	Fluorouracil
Advil	Ibuprofen
Aerolate	Theophylline
Afrin	Oxymetazoline
Airbron	Acetylcysteine
Ak Pred	Prednisolone
Akarpine	Pilocarpine
Akeniton	Biperiden
Akinophyl	Biperiden
Alazine	Hydralazine
Albalon	Naphazoline
Albego	Camazepam
Albiotic	Lincomycin
Alcoban	Flucytosine
Aldactone	Spironolactone
Aldecin	Beclomethasone
Aldinamide	Pyrazinamide
Aldocorten	Aldosterone
Aldomet	Methyldopa
Aldrox	Aluminum hydroxide
Alexan	Cytarabine
Alflorone	Fludrocortisone
Algocor	Gallopamil
Algoverine	Phenylbutazone
Alkeran	Melphalan
Allerdryl	Diphenhydramine
Allerest	Oxymetazoline
Alloferin	Alcuronium
Alloprin	Allopurinol
Allvoran	Diclofenac
Almocarpine	Pilocarpine
Almodan	Amoxicillin

Alocort	Hydrocortisone (cortisol)
Alophen	Phenolphthalein
Alpha-redisol	Hydroxocobalamin
Altracin	Bacitracin
Alu-Cap	Aluminum hydroxide
Alu-Tab	Aluminum hydroxide
Aludrin	Isoproterenol (Isoprenaline)
Alupent	Metaproterenol
Alzapam	Lorazepam
Ambaxine	Amantadine
Ambril	Ambroxol
Amcill	Ampicillin
Amen	Medroxyprogesterone acetate
Amfipen	Ampicillin
Amicar	Aminocaproic acid
Amidonal	Aprindine
Amikin	Amikacin
Amitril	Amitriptyline
Ammuno	Indomethacin
Amodopa	Methyldopa
Amoxil	Amoxicillin
Amphojel	Aluminum hydroxide
Amphozone	Amphotericin B
Amycor	Bifonazole
Anabactyl(A)	Carbenicillin
Anabolin	Nandrolone
Anacin-3	Acetaminophen
Anacobin	Cyanocobalamine
Anaesthesin	Benzocaine
Anamid	Kanamycin
Anarexol	Cyproheptadine
Ancotil	Flucytosine
Andriol	Testerone undecanoate
Andro	Testosterone enanthate
Androcur	Cyproterone acetate
Androcyp	Testosterone cypionate
Android	Methyltestosterone
Androlone	Nandrolone
Andronate	Testosterone cypionate
Androviron	Mesterolone
Anectine	Succinylcholine
Anergan	Promethazine
Anethaine	Tetracaine
Anexate	Flumazenil
Ang-O-Span	Nitroglycerin
Angettes	Acetylsalicylic acid
Angionorm	Dihydroergotamine
Antepsin	Sucralfate
Antilirium	Physostigmine
Antiminth	Pyrantel Pamoate
Antipressan	Atenolol
Antivert	Meclizine (meclozine)

Antrizine	Meclizine (meclozine)
Anturan	Sulfinpyrazone
Apaurin	Diazepam
Aprazone	Sulfinpyrazone
Apresoline	Hydralazine
Aprozide	Hydrochlorothiazide
Apsin VK	Penicillin V
Apsolox	Oxprenolol
Aptine	Alprenolol
Aralen	Chloroquine
Arduan	Pipecuronium
Arfonad	Trimethaphan
Aristocort	Triamcinolone
Armazid	Isoniazid
Arteoptic	Carteolol
Arterenol	Norepinephrine (noradrenaline)
Arthrisin	Acetylsalicylic acid
Articulose	Prednisolone
Arumil	Amiloride
Arvin	Ancrod
Arythmol	Propafenone
Asacol	Mesalamine
Asadrine	Acetylsalicylic acid
Atensine	Diazepam
Ativan	Lorazepam
Atromid-S	Clofibrate
Atropisol	Atropine
Atrovent	Ipratropium
Augmentin	Clavulanic acid + Amoxicillin
Aureotan	Aurothioglucose
Auromyose	Aurothioglucose
Auxit	Bromhexine
Avicel	Cellulose
Avloclor	Chloroquine
Avlosulfone	Dapsone
Avomine	Promethazine
Axid	Nizatidine
Azactam	Aztreonam
Azanin	Azathioprine
Azlin	Azlocillin
Azmacort	Triamcinolone acetonide
Azolid	Phenylbutazone
Azulfidine	Sulfasalazine

B

Baciguent	Bacitracin
Bactidan	Enoxacin
Bactocill	Oxacillin
Bactrim	Cotrimoxazole
Barbita	Phenobarbital
Baxedin	Chlorhexidine
Bay-Bee	Vit. B12

Bayotensin	Nitrendipine
Baypress	Nitrendipine
Becloforte	Beclomethasone
Becodisks	Beclomethasone
Beconase	Beclomethasone
Becotide	Beclomethasone
Bedoz	Cyanocobalamine
Bee Six	Vit. B6
Bee-six	Pyridoxine
Befizal	Bezafibrate
Benadryl	Diphenhydramine
Benemid	Probenecid
Berkaprine	Azathioprine
Berkatens	Verapamil
Berkolol	Propranolol
Berofor alpha 2	Interferon-alpha2
Berotec	Fenoterol
Berubigen	Vit. B12
Bestcall	Cefmenoxime
Betadran	Bupranolol
Betadrenol	Bupranolol
Betalin	Vit. B12
Betaloc	Metoprolol
Betapen-VK	Penicillin V
Betim	Timolol
Betoptic	Betaxolol
Bezalip	Bezafibrate
Bicillin	Penicillin G
Bicillin	Penicillin G Benzathine
Bicol	Bisacodyl
Biltricide	Praziquantel
Biogastrone	Carbenoxolone
Bioplex	Carbenoxolone
Bisolvon	Bromhexine
Black Draught	Senna
Blenoxane	Bleomycin
Blocadren	Timolol
Bofedrol	Ephedrine
Bonamine	Meclizine (meclozine)
Bopen-VK	Penicillin V
Borotropin	Atropine
Brethine	Terbutaline
Brevibloc	Esmolol
Brevital	Methohexital
Bricanyl	Terbutaline
Briclin	Amikacin
Bronchopront	Ambroxol
Bronkodyl	Theophylline
Broxalax	Bisacodyl
Brufen	Ibuprofen
Bumex	Bumetanide
Buprene	Buprenorphine

Burinex	Bumetanide
Buscopan	Hyoscine butylbromide
Butacote	Phenylbutazone
Butagen	Phenylbutazone
Butazolidin	Phenylbutazone
Butylone	Pentobarbital

C

C-Pak	Doxycycline
C.A.M.	Ephedrine
Cabadon	Vit. B12
Cacit	Calcium carbonate
Calabren	Glyburide (glibenclamide)
Calan	Verapamil
Calchichew	Calcium carbonate
Calcidrink	Calcium carbonate
Calciferol	Vit. D
Calcimer	Calcitonin
Calciparin	Heparin
Calcitare	Calcitonin
Calderol	Calcifediol
Calpol	Acetaminophen
Calsan	Calcium carbonate
Calsynar	Calcitonin
Caltidren	Carteolol
Caltrate	Calcium carbonate
Calvepen E	Penicillin V
Camcolit	Lithium carbonate
Camoquin	Amodiaquine
Canesten	Clotrimazole
Capastat	Capreomycin
Caplenal	Allopurinol
Capoten	Captopril
Caprolin	Capreomycin
Carace	Lisinopril
Carafate	Sucralfate
Carbocaine	Mepivacaine
Carbolite	Lithium carbonate
Cardinol	Propranolol
Cardioqin	Quinidine
Cardiorhythmine	Ajmaline
Cardizem	Diltiazem
Carindapen	Carbenicillin
Carteol	Carteolol
Cartrol	Carteolol
Catapres	Clonidine
CCNU	Lomustine
Cedocard	Isosorbide dinitrate
CeeNu	Lomustine
Cefobid	Cefoperazone
Cefobis	Cefoperazone
Celance	Pergolide

Celevac	Methylcellulose
Cemix	Cefmenoxime
Centrax	Prazepam
Cepexin(A)	Cephalexin
Cephulac	Lactulose
Ceporex	Cephalexin
Cerebid	Papaverine
Cerespan	Papaverine
Cerubidine	Daunorubicin
Cesamet	Nabilone
Cesplon	Captopril
Chlor-hex	Chlorhexidine
Chlorhexitulle	Chlorhexidine
Chlorohist	Xylometazoline
Chloromycetin	Cloramphenicol
Chloroptic	Cloramphenicol
Cholestabyl	Colestipol
Cholestid	Colestipol
Choloxin	Thyroxine
Chronulac	Lactulose
Cibacalcin	Calcitonin
Cidomycin	Gentamicin
Cillimycin	Lincomycin
Cimetrin	Erythromycin propionate
Cin-Quin	Quinidine
Cipro	Ciprofloxacin
Ciprobay	Ciprofloxacin
Ciproxin	Ciprofloxacin
Citanest	Prilocaine
Citrucel	Methylcellulose
Claforan	Cefotaxime
Clamoxyl	Amoxicillin
Claripex	Clofibrate
Clasteon	Clodronic acid
Cleocin	Clindamycin
Clomid	Clomiphene
Clonopin	Clonazepam
Clont	Metronidazole
Clopra	Metoclopramide
Clotrimaderm	Clotrimazole
Clozan	Clotiazepam
Cobalin-H	Hydroxocobalamin
Cobex	Vit. B12
Cocillin-VK	Penicillin V
Codelsol	Prednisolone
Codicept	Codeine
Cogentin	Benztropine
Coleb	Isosorbide mononitrate
Colectril	Amiloride
Collyrium	Tetrahydrozoline (tetryzoline)
Cologel	Methylcellulose
Combantrin	Pyrantel Pamoate

Complamin	Xanthinol nicotinate
Complement Continus	Pyridoxine
Comprecin	Enoxacin
Concor	Bisoprolol
Conducton	Carazolol
Constant-T	Theophylline
Contergan	Thalidomide
Coracten	Nifedipine
Coradus	Isosorbide dinitrate
Cordarex	Amiloride
Cordarex	Amiodarone
Cordarone	Amiodarone
Cordilox	Verapamil
Corgal	Gallopamil
Corgard	Nadolol
Coricidin	Oxymetazoline
Coronex	Isosorbide dinitrate
Correctol	Phenolphthalein
Corsodyl	Chlorhexidine
Cortalone	Prednisolone
Cortate	Hydrocortisone (cortisol)
Cortef	Hydrocortisone (cortisol)
Cortelan	Cortisone
Cortenema	Hydrocortisone (cortisol)
Cortigel	Corticotropin
Cortistab	Cortisone
Cortogen	Cortisone
Cortone	Cortisone
Cortrophin	Corticotropin
Corvaton	Molsidomine
Coscopin	Noscapine
Coscotab	Noscapine
Cosmegen	Dactinomycin
Coumadin	Warfarin
Coversum	Perindopril
Coversyl	Perindopril
Cryspen	Penicillin G
Crystapen	Penicillin G
Crystodigin	Digitoxin
Cuemid	Cholestyramine
Cuprimine	Penicillamine
Cuvalit	Lisuride
Cyanoject	Vit. B12
Cyclogest	Progesterone
Cyklocapron	Tranexamic acid
Cymevene	Ganciclovir
Cyomin	Vit. B12
Cyprostat	Cyproterone acetate
Cytacon	Cyanocobalamine
Cytamen	Cyanocobalamine
Cytomel	Liothyronine
Cytosar	Cytarabine

Cytotec	Misoprostol
Cytovene	Ganciclovir
Cytoxan	Cyclophosphamide

D

D-Tabs	Cholecalciferol
D.E.H.45	Dihydroergotamine
Dagenan	Sulfapyridine
Daktarin	Miconazole
Dalcaine	Lidocaine
Dantrium	Dantrolene
Daonil	Glyburide (glibenclamide)
Daraprim	Pyrimethamine
Datril	Acetaminophen
Daunoblastin	Daunorubicin
DDAVP	Desmopressin
Deca-Durabolin	Nandrolone
Decadron	Dexamethasone
Decapryn	Doxylamine
Dedrogyl	Calcifediol
Degest-2	Naphazoline
Delapav	Papaverine
Delatestryl	Testosterone enanthate
Delestrogen	Estradiol valerate
Delta-Cortef	Prednisolone
Deltapen	Penicillin G
Deltastab	Prednisolone
Demerol	Meperidine (pethidine)
Dendrid	Idoxuridine
Depakene	Valproic Acid
Depen	Penicillamine
Depo-Provera	Medroxyprogesterone acetate
Deponit	Nitroglycerin
Deprenyl	Selegiline
Dermonistat	Miconazole
Deronil	Dexamethasone
Deseril	Methysergide
Desmospray	Desmopressin
Desoxyn	Methamphetamine
Desuric	Benzbromarone
Detensiel	Bisoprolol
Detensol	Propranolol
Dexedrine	Dextroamphetamine
DiaBeta	Glyburide (glibenclamide)
Diabex	Metformin
Diamox	Acetazolamide
Diapid	Lypressin
Diaqua	Hydrochlorothiazide
Diarsed	Diphenoxylate
Diazemuls	Diazepam
Dibenyline	Phenoxybenzamine
Dibenzyline	Phenoxybenzamine

Diclocil	Dicloxacillin
Diclophlogont	Diclofenac
Digacin	Digoxin
Digibind	Digoxin immune FAB
Digicor	Digitoxin
Digimerck	Digitoxin
Digitaline	Digitoxin
Dihydergot	Dihydroergotamine
Dihyzin	Dihydralazine
Dilantin	Phenytoin
Dilaudid	Hydromorphone
Diodronel	Etidronate
Dioval	Estradiol valerate
Diphenasone	Dapsone
Dirythmin	Disopyramide
Distamine	Penicillamine
Distaquaine V-K	Penicillin V
Distraneurin	Clomethiazole
Diuchlor	Hydrochlorothiazide
Divegal	Dihydroergotamine
Dixarit	Clonidine
Dobutrex	Dobutamine
Dolantin	Meperidine (pethidine)
Dolophine	Methadone
Dominal	Amitriptyline
Donnagel-MB	Kaolin + pectin (attapulgite)
Dopaidan	Levodopa
Dopamet	Methyldopa
Dopar	Levodopa
Dopergin	Lisuride
Doryl	Carbachol
Dowmycin	Erythromycin estolate
Doxicin	Doxycycline
Drisdol	Vit. D
Dristan	Oxymetazoline
Droleptan	Droperidol
Droxomine	Hydroxycobalamine
Dryptal	Furosemide
Dulcolax	Bisacodyl
Duoralith	Lithium carbonate
Duphalac	Lactulose
Duracoron	Molsidomine
Duralutin	Hydroxyprogesterone caproate
Duramorph	Morphine sulfate
Duratest	Testosterone cypionate
Durazanil	Bromazepam
Durolax	Bisacodyl
D-Vi-Sol	Vit. D
Dynapen	Dicloxacillin
Dynaprin	Imipramine
Dyneric	Clomiphene
Dyrenium	Triamterene

Dyspamet	Cimetidine
Dytac	
E	Triamterene
E-mycin	Erythromycin
Ecostatin	Econazole
Ecotrin	Acetylsalicylic acid
Edecrin	Ethacrynic acid
EES	Erythromycin ethylsuccinate
Efedron	Ephedrine
Efudex	Fluorouracil
Efudix	Fluorouracil
Elantan	Isosorbide mononitrate
Elavil	Amitriptyline
Eldepryl	Selegiline
Elimite	Permethrin
Elixophyllin	Theophylline
Eltroxin	Thyroxine
Emcor	Bisoprolol
Emex	Metoclopramide
Endak	Carteolol
Endep	Amitriptyline
Endophleban	Dihydroergotamine
Endoxan	Cyclophosphamide
Enoram	Enoxacin
Enovil	Amitriptyline
Entromone	Chorionic gonadotropin
Entrophen	Acetylsalicylic acid
Epanutin	Phenytoin
Epifrin	Epinephrine
Epimorph	Morphine sulfate
EpiPen	Epinephrine
Epitol	Carbamazepine
Epogen	Erythropoietin (epoetin alfa)
Eporal	Dapsone
Eppy	Epinephrine
Epsicapron	Aminocaproic acid
Ergomar	Ergotamine
Ergotrate Maleate	Ergonovine (ergometrine)
Eridan	Diazepam
Ermalate	Ergonovine (ergometrine)
Eryc	Erythromycin
Erymax	Erythromycin
Erymycin	Erythromycin stearate
Erythrocin	Erythromycin ethylsuccinate
Erythrocin	Erythromycin stearate
Erythroped	Erythromycin
Esidrix	Hydrochlorothiazide
Eskalith	Lithium carbonate
Espotabs	Phenolphthalein
Estinyl	Ethinyl estradiol
Estrace	Estradiol

Ethrane	Enflurane
Etibi	Ethambutol
Eudemine	Diazoxide
Euglucon	Glyburide (glibenclamide)
Euhypnos	Temazepam
Evac-U-gen	Phenolphthalein
Evac-U-lax	Phenolphthalein
Everone	Testosterone enanthate
Evipan	Hexobarbital
Evoxin	Domperidone
Ex-Lax	Phenolphthalein

F

F-Cortef	Fludrocortisone
Fabrol	Acetylcysteine
Fansidar	Pyrimethamine + Sulfadoxine
Farlutal	Medroxyprogesterone acetate
Fasigyn CH	Tinidazol
Felden	Piroxicam
Femazole	Metronidazole
Femotrone	Progesterone
Fenbid	Ibuprofen
Fenopron	Fenoprofen
Fertodur	Cyclofenil
Fiblaferon 3	Interferon
Fibocil	Aprindine
Flagyl	Metronidazole
Flavoquine	Amodiaquine
Flaxedil	Gallamine
Fletchers Castoria	Senna
Florinef	Fludrocortisone
Floxapen	Flucloxacillin (floxacillin)
Fluagel	Aluminum hydroxide
Flugeral	Flunarizine
Fluothane	Halothane
Foldine	Folic acid
Folex	Methotrexate
Follutein	Chorionic gonadotropin
Folvite	Folic acid
Fontego	Bumetanide
Forane	Isoflurane
Fordiuran	Bumetanide
Fortal	Pentazocine
Fortaz	Ceftazidime
Fortum	Ceftazidime
Fragmin	Heparin low molecular
Fraxiparin	Heparin low molecular
Fulcin	Griseofulvin
Fulvicin	Griseofulvin
Fungilin	Amphotericin B
Fungizone	Amphotericin B
Fusid	Furosemide

G

Ganal	Fenfluramine
Ganda E	Epinephrine
Ganphen	Promethazine
Gantanol	Sulfamethoxazole
Gantrisin	Sulfisoxazole
Garamycin	Gentamicin
Gardenal	Phenobarbital
Gastrozepin	Pirenzepine
Gelafundin	Gelatin colloids
Genna	Senna
Genticin	Gentamicin
Gentle Nature	Senna
Geopen	Carbenicillin
Gesterol L.A.	Hydroxyprogesterone caproate
Gestone	Progesterone
Gilurytmal	Ajmaline
Glaupax	Acetazolamide
Glucophage	Metformin
Grisovin	Griseofulvin
Gubernal	Alprenolol
Gulfasin	Sulfisoxazole
Gumbix	Aminomethylbenzoic acid
Gyne-Lotrimin	Clotrimazole
Gynergen	Ergotamine
Gyno-Pevaryl	Econazole
Gyno-Travogen	Isoconazole

H

Haemaccel	Gelatin colloids
Halcion	Triazolam
Haldol	Haloperidol
Hamarin	Allopurinol
Hemineurin	Clomethiazole
Hepalean	Heparin
Hepsal	Heparin
Herpid	Idoxuridine
Herplex	Idoxuridine
Hespan	Hetastarch (HES)
Hespan	Hydroxyethyl starch
Hexa-Betalin	Pyridoxine
Hexa-Betalin	Vit. B6
Hexadrol	Dexamethasone
Hexit	Lindane
Hibanil	Chlorpromazine
Hibidil	Chlorhexidine
Hibiscrub	Chlorhexidine
Hibisol	Chlorhexidine
Hibitane	Chlorhexidine
Hidroferol	Calcifediol
Honvol	Diethylstilbestrol
Humatin	Paromomycin

Hybalamine	Hydroxycobalamine
Hybolin Decanoate	Nandrolone
Hybolin	Nandrolone
Hydeltrasol	Prednisolone
Hyderm	Hydrocortisone (cortisol)
Hydromal	Hydrochlorothiazide
Hydromedin	Ethacrynic acid
Hydrosaluric	Hydrochlorothiazide
Hydrotricine	Tyrothricin
Hygroton	Chlorthalidone
Hylutin	Hydroxyprogesterone caproate
Hymorphan	Hydromorphone
Hyocort	Hydrocortisone (cortisol)
Hyperstat	Diazoxide
Hypertensin	Angiotensinamide
Hypertil	Captopril
Hypnovel	Midazolam
Hypovase	Prazosin
Hyroxon	Hydroxyprogesterone caproate

I

I-Pilopine	Pilocarpine
Ifex	Ifosfamide
Iktorivil	Clonazepam
Ilosone	Erythromycin estolate
Ilosone	Erythromycin
Imbrilon	Indomethacin
Imdur	Isosorbide mononitrate
Imodium	Loperamide
Impril	Imipramine
Imuran	Azathioprine
Imurek	Azathioprine
Inapsine	Droperidol
Inderal	Propranolol
Indocid	Indomethacin
Indocin	Indomethacin
Indomee	Indomethacin
Indomod	Indomethacin
Inflamase	Prednisolone
Innovace	Enalapril
Innovar	Fentanyl + Droperidol
Inocor	Amrinone
Insommal	Diphenhydramine
Intal	Cromolyn
Intron A	Interferon-alpha2b
Ipral	Trimethoprim
Isicom	Carbidopa + Levodopa
Ismelin	Guanethidine
Ismo	Isosorbide mononitrate
Isocaine	Mepivacaine
Isoket	Isosorbide dinitrate
Isoptin	Verapamil

Isopto Carpine	Pilocarpine
Isordil	Isosorbide dinitrate
Isotamine	Isoniazid
Isotol	Mannitol
Isotrate	Isosorbide mononitrate
Isuprel	Isoproterenol (isoprenaline)
Itrop	Ipratropium

J

Janimine	Imipramine
Jexin	Tubocurarine

K

Kabikinase	Streptokinase
Kabolin	Nandrolone
Kannasyn	Kanamycin
Kanrenol	Canrenone
Kantrex	Kanamycin
Kaopectate	Kaolin + pectin (attapulgite)
Karil	Calcitonin
Kefalar	Ketamine
Keflex	Cephalexin
Kemicetine	Cloramphenicol
Kenacort	Triamcinolone
Kenalog	Triamcinolone acetonide
Kenalone	Triamcinolone acetonide
Kerecid	Idoxuridine
Kerlone	Betaxolol
Key-Pred	Prednisolone
Kiditard	Quinidine
Kinidin	Quinidine
Klebcil	Kanamycin
Konakion	Phytomenadione
Korostatin	Nystatin
Kwell	Lindane
Kwilldane	Lindane

L

Lacril	Methylcellulose
Ladropen	Flucloxacillin (floxacillin)
Lamiazid	Isoniazid
Lamprene	Clofazimine
Lanacillin	Penicillin G
Lanacillin-VK	Penicillin V
Lanicor	Digoxin
Lanoxin	Digoxin
Largactil	Chlorpromazine
Lariam	Mefloquine
Larodopa	Levodopa
Lasix	Furosemide
Lasma	Theophylline
Laxabene	Bisacodyl

Laxanin	Bisacodyl
Lectopam	Bromazepam
Ledercillin-VK	Penicillin V
Ledercort	Triamcinolone
Lembrol	Diazepam
Lendorm(A)	Brotizolam
Lendormin	Brotizolam
Lenoxin	Digoxin
Lentizol	Amitriptyline
Leukeran	Chlorambucil
Leukomycin	Cloramphenicol
Levate	Amitriptyline
Levophed	Norepinephrine (noradrenaline)
Levoprome	Methotrimeprazine
Lexotan	Bromazepam
Lidifen	Ibuprofen
Lidopen	Lidocaine
Likuden	Griseofulvin
Lincocin	Lincomycin
Lingraine	Ergotamine
Lioresal	Baclofen
Lipostat	Pravastatin
Liquamar	Phenprocoumon
Liquemin	Heparin
Liskonum	Lithium carbonate
Litec	Pizotyline (pizotifen)
Lithane	Lithium carbonate
Lithobid	Lithium carbonate
Lithotabs	Lithium carbonate
Lixil	Bumetanide
Lomotil	Diphenoxylate
Loniten	Minoxidil
Looser	Bupranolol
Lopantrol	Lorcainide
Lopid	Gemfibrozil
Lopirin	Captopril
Lopressor	Metoprolol
Loramet	Lormetazepam
Loraz	Lorazepam
Lorinal	Chloralhydrate
Lorivox	Lorcainide
Losec	Omeprazole
Losporal	Cephalexin
Lupron	Leuprolide
Lyclear	Permethrin
Lynoral	Ethinyl estradiol
Lyophrin	Epinephrine
Lysenyl	Lisuride

M

Madopar	Levodopa + Benserazide
Malgesic	Phenylbutazone

Mallergan	Promethazine
Marcumar	Phenprocoumon
Marevan	Warfarin
Marvelon	Desogestrel+Ethinylestradiol
Maxeran	Metoclopramide
Maxidex	Dexamethasone
Maxolan	Metoclopramide
Maxtrex	Methotrexate
Meclomen	Meclofenamate
Medihaler-Iso	Isoproterenol (isoprenaline)
Mefoxin	Cefoxitin
Megacillin	Penicillin G
Megacillin	Penicillin G Benzathine
Megaphen	Chlorpromazine
Melipramin	Imipramine
Mesasal	Mesalamine
Mesnex	Mesna
Mestinon	Pyridostigmine
Metacen	Indomethacin
Metalone	Prednisolone
Metandren	Methyltestosterone
Metaprel	Metaproterenol
Methadose	Methadone
Methampex	Methamphetamine
Methergin	Methylergonovine
Methofane	Methoxyflurane
Meticorten	Prednisone
Metilon	Dipyrone
Metreton	Prednisolone
Metronid	Metronidazole
Mevacor	Lovastatin
Meval	Diazepam
Mevaril	Amitriptyline
Mevinacor	Lovastatin
Mexate	Methotrexate
Mexitil	Mexiletine
Mezlin	Mezlocillin
Micatin	Miconazole
Micronase	Glyburide (glibenclamide)
Micronor	Norethisterone
Midamor	Amiloride
Mielucin	Busulfan
Mifegyne	Mifepristone (RU-486)
Migril	Ergotamine
Minipress	Prazosin
Minirin	Desmopressin
Minocin	Minocycline
Minprog	Alprostadil
Minprostin F2 Alpha	Dinoprost
Mintezol	Thiabendazole
Miocarpine	Pilocarpine
Miostat	Carbachol

Mithracin	Plicamycin
Mitosan	Busulfan
Mitoxana	Ifosfamide
Mobenol	Tolbutamide
Modane	Phenolphthalein
Moduret	Amiloride+Hydrochlorothiazide
Mogadon	Nitrazepam
Molsidolat	Molsidomine
Monistat	Miconazole
Monitan	Acebutolol
Monocor	Bisoprolol
Monomycin	Erythromycin succinate
Monotrim	Trimethoprim
Moronal	Amphotericin B
Morphitec	Morphine hydrochloride
Motrin	Ibuprofen
Mosegor	Pizotyline (pizotifen)
Motilium	Domperidone
Moxacin	Amoxicillin
MST Continus	Morphine
Mucomyst	Acetylcysteine
Mucosolvan	Ambroxol
Murine	Tetrahydrozoline (tetryzoline)
Murocel	Methylcellulose
Mustargen	Mechlorethamine
Mutabase	Diazoxide
Myambutol	Ethambutol
Mycelex	Clotrimazole
Mycifradin	Neomycin
Myciguent	Neomycin
Mycospor	Bifonazole
Mycosporan	Bifonazole
Mycostatin	Nystatin
Myidone	Primidone
Mykinac	Nystatin
Myleran	Busulfan
Myobid	Papaverine
Mysoline	Primidone

N

Nacaricin	Benzbromarone
Nacom	Carbidopa + Levodopa
Nadopen-V	Penicillin V
Nalador	Sulprostone
Nalcron	Cromolyn
Nalfon	Fenoprofen
Nalgesic	Fenoprofen
Naprosyn	Naproxen
Narcan	Naloxone
Narcozep	Flunitrazepam
Narkotan	Halothane
Nautamine	Diphenhydramine

Nauzelin	Domperidone
Navidrix	Cyclopenthiazide
Naxen	Naproxen
Nebcin	Tobramycin
Negram	Nalidixic acid
Nembutal	Pentobarbital
Neo-Codema	Hydrochlorothiazide
Neo-Cytamen	Hydroxocobalamin
Neo-Mercazole	Carbimazole
Neo-Synephrine	Oxymetazoline
Neo-Thyreostat	Carbimazole
Neogel	Carbenoxolone
Neosynephrine II	Xylometazoline
Nepresol	Dihydralazine
Netillin	Netilmicin
Netromycin	Netilmicin
Niclocide	Niclosamide
Nigalax	Bisacodyl
Nilstat	Nystatin
Nimotop	Nimodipine
Nipride	Sodium nitroprusside
Nitrocap	Nitroglycerin
Nitrogard	Nitroglycerin
Nitroglyn	Nitroglycerin
Nitrolingual	Nitroglycerin
Nitronal	Nitroglycerin
Nitrong	Nitroglycerin
Nitropress	Nitroprusside sodium
Nitrostat	Nitroglycerin
Nivaquine	Chloroquine
Nivemycin	Neomycin
Nix	Permethrin
Nizoral	Ketoconazole
Noan	Diazepam
Noctamid	Lormetazepam
Noctec	Chloralhydrate
Nogram	Nalidixic acid
Nor-Q D	Norethisterone
Norcuron	Vecuronium
Nordox	Doxycycline
Noriday	Norethisterone
Norlutin	Norethisterone
Normison	Temazepam
Normurat	Benzbromarone
Noroxin	Norfloxacin
Norpace	Disopyramide
Norpramin	Desipramine
Novalgin	Dipyrone
Novamin	Amikacin
Novamoxin	Amoxicillin
Novarectal	Pentobarbital
Novocaine	Procaine

Novoclopate	Clorazepate
Novodigoxin	Digoxin
Novomedopa	Methyldopa
Novopen-VK	Penicillin V
Novopurol	Allopurinol
Novorythro	Erythromycin estolate
Novosalmol	Albuterol
Nozinan	Methotrimeprazine
Nu-Cal	Calcium carbonate
Nubain	Nalbuphine
Nuelin	Theophylline
Nulicaine	Lidocaine
Nuprin	Ibuprofen
Nuran	Cyproheptadine
Nydrazid	Isoniazid
Nystan	Nystatin
Nystex	Nystatin
Nytilax	Senna

O

O-V Statin	Nystatin
Octapressin	Felypressin
Ocusert	Pilocarpine
Omifin	Clomiphene
Omnipen	Ampicillin
Oncovin	Vincristine
Ondena	Daunorubicin
Ondogyne	Cyclofenil
Ondonid	Cyclofenil
Ophthosol	Bromhexine
Opticrom	Cromolyn
Oragest	Medroxyprogesterone acetate
Oramide	Tolbutamide
Oramorph	Morphine
Orasone	Prednisone
Orinase	Tolbutamide
Osmitrol	Mannitol
Ospolot	Sulthiame
Ossiten	Clodronic acid
Ostac	Clodronic acid
Otrivine	Xylometazoline
Oxistat	Oxiconazole
Oxpam	Oxazepam

P

Panadol	Acetaminophen
Panasol	Prednisone
Panimit	Bupranolol
Panwarfin	Warfarin
Papacon	Papaverine
Paralgin	Dipyrone
Paraxin	Chloramphenicol

Parcillin	Penicillin G
Paregoric	Opium Tincture (laudanum)
Parlodel	Bromocriptine
Parnate	Tranylcypromine
Partusisten	Fenoterol
Parvolex	Acetylcysteine
Pathocil	Dicloxacillin
Pavabid	Papaverine
Pavadur	Papaverine
Paveral	Codeine
Pavulon	Pancuronium
Pectokay	Kaolin + pectin (attapulgite)
Pediapred	Prednisolone
Pemavit	Vit. B12
Pen-Vee K	Penicillin V
Penapar-VK	Penicillin V
Penbec-V	Penicillin V
Penbritin	Ampicillin
Pendramine	Penicillamine
Penidural	Penicillin G Benzathine
Pensorb	Penicillin G
Pentanca	Pentobarbital
Pentasa	Mesalamine
Pentazine	Promethazine
Penthrane	Methoxyflurane
Pentids	Penicillin G
Pentothal	Thiopental
Pepcid	Famotidine
Pepdul	Famotidine
Pepto-Bismol	Bismuth subsalicylate
Peptol	Cimetidine
Pergotime	Clomiphene
Periactin	Cyproheptadine
Peridon	Domperidone
Peritol	Cyproheptadine
Permanone	Permethrin
Permapen	Penicillin G
Permax	Pergolide
Pethidine Roche	Meperidine (pethidine)
Petinimid	Ethosuximide
Pertofran	Desipramine
Pevaryl	Econazole
Pfizerpen VK	Penicillin V
Pfizerpin	Penicillin G
Phenazine	Promethazine
Phenergan	Promethazine
Phospholine Iodide	Ecothiopate
Physeptone	Methadone
Pilokair	Pilocarpine
Pipracil	Piperacillin
Pipril	Piperacillin
Pitocin	Oxytocin

Pitressin	Vasopressin
Plak-out	Chlorhexedine
Plaquenil	Hydroxychloroquine
Platet	Acetylsalicylic acid
Platinex	Cisplatin
Platinol	Cisplatin
Polycillin	Ampicillin
Ponderal	Fenfluramine
Ponderax	Fenfluramine
Pondimin	Fenfluramine
Pontocaine	Tetracaine
POR 8	Ornipressin
Pravachol	Pravastatin
Pravidel	Bromocriptine
Predate	Prednisolone
Predcor	Prednisolone
Predenema	Prednisolone
Predfoam	Prednisolone
Prednesol	Prednisolone
Preferid	Budesonide
Pregnesin	Chorionic gonadotropin
Pregnyl	Chorionic gonadotropin
Prelone	Prednisolone
Premormine	Atenolol
Prepidil	Dinoprostone
Presinol	Methyldopa
Priadel	Lithium carbonate
Primaquine	Primaquine
Primolut Depot	Hydroxyprogesterone caproate
Primolut N	Norethisterone
Primperan	Metoclopramide
Principen	Ampicillin
Prinivil	Lisinopril
Privine	Naphazoline
Pro-Depo	Hydroxyprogesterone caproate
Pro-Vent	Theophylline
Probalan	Probenecid
Procan SR	Procainamide
Procardia	Nifedipine
Procorum	Gallopamil
Procytox	Cyclophosphamide
Profasi	Chorionic gonadotropin
Progesic	Fenoprofen
Progestasert	Progesterone
Proglicem	Diazoxide
Progynon	Estradiol benzoate
Prolopa	Levodopa + Benserazide
Proloprim	Trimethoprim
Prometh	Promethazine
Promine	Procainamide
Pronestyl	Procainamide
Propaderm	Beclomethasone

Propasa	Mesalamine
Propyl-Thyracil	Propylthiouracil
Prorex	Promethazine
Prostaphlin	Oxacillin
Prostigmin	Neostigmine
Prostin E2	Dinoprostone
Prostin F2 Alpha	Dinoprost
Prostin VR	Alprostadil
Protostat	Metronidazole
Protrin	Cotrimoxazole
Proventil	Albuterol
Provera	Medroxyprogesterone acetate
Provigan	Promethazine
Proviron	Mesterolone
Prozac	Fluoxetine
Prulet	Phenolphthalein
Pulmicort	Budesonide
Purinethol	Mercaptopurine
Purodigin	Digitoxin
Pyopen	Carbenicillin
Pyrilax	Bisacodyl
Pyronoval	Acetylsalicylic acid
Pyroxine	Pyridoxine, Vit. B6

Q

Quelicin	Succinylcholine
Quellada	Lindane
Questran	Cholestyramine
Quibron-T	Theophylline
Quinachlor	Chloroquine
Quinalan	Quinidine
Quinaminoph	Quinine
Quinamm	Quinine
Quine	Quinine
Quinidex	Quinidine
Quinite	Quinine
Quinora	Quinidine

R

Rastinon	Tolbutamide
Reclomide	Metoclopramide
Rectocort	Hydrocortisone (cortisol)
Redisol	Vit. B12
Refobacin	Gentamicin
Regaine	Minoxidil
Regitin	Phentolamine
Reglan	Metoclopramide
Regonol	Pyridostigmine
Rehibin	Cyclofenil
Relefact	Gonadorelin
Remivox	Lorcainide
Remsed	Promethazine

Reomax	Ethacrynic acid
Restandol	Testosterone
Restoril	Temazepam
Retardin	Diphenoxylate
Retrovir	Zidovudine (AZT)
Reverin	Rolitetracycline
Rezipas	Mesalamine
Rhinocort	Budesonide
Rhumalgan	Diclofenac
Rhythmin	Procainamide
Rhythmol	Propafenone
Ridaura	Auranofin
Rifadin	Rifampin + Rifampicin
Rimactan	Rifampin + Rifampicin
Rimifon	Isoniazid
Rinatec	Ipratropium
Ritalin	Methylphenidate
Rivotril	Clonazepam
Rize	Clotiazepam
Roaccutane	Isotretinoin
Robicillin-VK	Penicillin V
Rocaltrol	Calcitriol
Rocephin	Ceftriaxone
Roferon A3	Interferon-alpha2a
Rogaine	Minoxidil
Rogitin	Phentolamine
Rohypnol	Flunitrazepam
Rovamycin	Spiramycin
Roxanol	Morphine sulfate
Rubesol	Vit. B12
Rubion	Cyanocobalamine
Rubramin	Cyanocobalamine
Rynacrom	Cromolyn
Rythmodan	Disopyramide

S

Salazopyrin	Sulfasalazine
Salbulin	Albuterol
Sandimmune	Cyclosporine
Sandomigran	Pizotyline (pizotifen)
Sandril	Reserpine
Sanodin	Carbenoxolone
Sanomigran	Pizotyline (pizotifen)
Sansert	Methysergide
Satric	Metronidazole
Saventrine	Isoproterenol(isoprenaline)
Scabene	Lindane
Scopoderm TTS	Scopolamine
Sebcur	Salicylic acid
Sectral	Acebutolol
Securon	Verapamil
Securopen	Azlocillin

Seguril	Furosemide
Seldane	Terfenadine
Selectomycin	Spiramycin
Sembrina	Methyldopa
Senokot	Senna
Senolax	Senna
Septra	Cotrimoxazole
Septrin	(sulfamethoxazole/trimethoprim)
Serax	Oxazepam
Serenace	Haloperidol
Sernyl	Phencyclidine
Serono-Bagren	Bromocriptine
Serophene	Clomiphene
Serpalan	Reserpine
Serpasil	Reserpine
Sertan	Primidone
Sexovid	Cyclofenil
Sibelium	Flunarizine
Simplene	Epinephrine
Simplotan	Tinidazol
Sinarest	Oxymetazoline
Sinemet	Carbidopa + Levodopa
Sinthrome	Acenocoumarol
Sintrom	Acenocoumarol
Sinutab	Xylometazoline
Sirtal	Carbachol
Sito-Lande	Sitosterol
Skleromexe	Clofibrate
Slo-bid	Theophylline
Slo-Phyllin	Theophylline
Sno Phenicol	Chloramphenicol
Sobelin	Clindamycin
Sofarin	Warfarin
Soldactone	canrenone
Solfoton	Phenobarbital
Solganal	Aurothioglucose
Solprin	Acetylsalicylic acid
Solu-Contenton	Amantadine
Soluver	Salicylic acid
Somnite	Nitrazepam
Somnos	Chloralhydrate
Somophyllin-T	Theophylline
Sopamycetin	Chloramphenicol
Sorbitrate	Isosorbide dinitrate
Sorquetan	Tinidazol
Sotacor	Sotalol
Spersadex	Dexamethasone
Spersanicol	Chloramphenicol
Spirocort	Budesonide
Spiroctan	Spironolactone
Stabillin V-K	Penicillin V
Stafoxil	Flucloxacillin (floxacillin)

Statex	Morphine sulfate
Steranobol	Clostebol
Stesolid	Diazepam
Stimate	Desmopressin
Stoxil	Idoxuridine
Strepolin	Streptomycin
Streptase	Streptokinase
Streptosol	Streptomycin
Stresson	Bunitrolol
Suacron	Carazolol
Sublimaze	Fentanyl
Succostrin	Succinylcholine
Sulcrate	Sucralfate
Sulfabutin	Busulfan
Sulmycin	Gentamicin
Supasa	Acetylsalicylic acid
Suprarenin	Epinephrine
Suprefact	Buserelin
Sustac	Nitroglycerin
Sustaire	Theophylline
Sustanon	Testosterone
Suxinutin	Ethosuximide
Symmetrel	Amantadine
Synatan	Dextroamphetamine
Synflex	Naproxen
Syntocinon	Oxytocin
Syntopressin	Lypressin
Sytobex	cyanocobalamin Vit. B 12

T

Tacef	Cefmenoxime
Tacicef	Ceftazidime
Tagamet	Cimetidine
Talwin	Pentazocine
Tambocor	Flecainide
Tapazole	Methimazole
Tardigal	Digitoxin
Tardocillin	Penicillin G Benzathine
Tarivid	Ofloxacin
Tavegil	Clemastine
Tavist	Clemastine
Tebrazid	Pyrazinamide
Teebaconin	Isoniazid
Tegison	Etretinate
Tegretol	Carbamazepine
Telemin	Bisacodyl
Temgesic	Buprenorphine
Tempra	Acetaminophen
Tenalin	Carteolol
Tenormin	Atenolol
Tensium	Diazepam
Tensobon	Captopril

Teoptic	Carteolol
Testex	Testosterone propionate
Testoject	Testosterone cypionate
Testone	Testosterone enanthate
Testred	Methyltestosterone
Theelol	Estriol
Theolair	Theophylline
Thiotepa Lederle	Thiotepa
Thorazine	Chlorpromazine
Thrombinar	Thrombin
Thrombostat	Thrombin
Ticar	Ticarcillin
Tienor	Clotiazepam
Tigason	Etretinate
Tildiem	Diltiazem
Timentin	Ticarcillin
Timonil	Carbamazepine
Timoptic	Timolol
Timoptol	Timolol
Tobralex	Tobramycin
Tobrex	Tobramycin
Tofranil	Imipramine
Tomabef	Cefoperazone
Tonocard	Tocainide
Topitracin	Bacitracin
Totacillin	Ampicillin
Totamol	Atenolol
Tracrium	Atracurium
Tramal	Tramadol
Trans-Ver-Sal	Salicylic acid
Transcycline	Rolitetracycline
Transderm Scop	Scopolamine
Tranxene	Clorazepate
Tranxillium N	Nordazepam
Trapanal	Thiopental
Trasicor	Oxprenolol
Travogen	Isoconazole
Travogyn	Isoconazole
Trecalmo	Clotiazepam
Trecator	Ethionamide
Tremblex	Dexetimide
Trendar	Ibuprofen
Trental	Pentoxifylline
Triam-A	Triamcinolone acetonide
Tridil	Nitroglycerin
Triludan	Terfenadine
Trimpex	Trimethoprim
Trimysten	Clotrimazole
Triptone	Scopolamine
Trobicin	Spectinomycin
Tryptizol	Amitriptyline
Tubarine	Tubocurarine

Tylenol	Acetaminophen
Typramine	Imipramine
Tyrozets	Tyrothricin
Tyzine	Tetrahydrozoline (Tetryzoline)

U

Udicil	Cytarabine
Udolac	Dapsone
Ukidan	Urokinase
Ulcolax	Bisacodyl
Unicort	Hydrocortisone (Cortisol)
Uniparin	Heparin
Uniphyl	Theophylline
Univer	Verapamil
Uricovac	Benzbromarone
Uritol	Furosemide
Uromitexan	Mesna
Urosin	Allopurinol
Uticillin-VK	Penicillin V
Utinor	Norfloxacin

V

V-Cil-K	Penicillin V
V-Cillin K	Penicillin V
Va-tro-nol	Ephedrine
Valadol	Acetaminophen
Valium Roche	Diazepam
Valium	Diazepam
Vancocin	Vancomycin
Vancomycin CP Lilly	Vancomycin
Vaponefrine	Epinephrine
Vasal	Papaverine
Vascardin	Isosorbide dinitrate
Vasocon	Naphazoline
Vasopressin	Lypressin
Vasotec	Enalapril
Vatran	Diazepam
Vectrin	Minocycline
Veetids	Penicillin V
Vegesan	Nordazepam
Velban	Vinblastine
Velbe	Vinblastine
Venactone	Canrenone
Ventolin	Albuterol
Veratran	Clotiazepam
Verelan	Verapamil
Vermox	Mebendazole
Versed	Midazolam
Vibal	Vit. B12
Vibal L. A.	Hydroxycobalamine
Vibramycin	Doxycycline
Vidopen Uk	Ampicillin

Vigantol	Cholecalciferol
Vigorsan	Cholecalciferol
Vimicon	Cyproheptadine
Vira-A	Vidarabine
Virilon	Methyltestosterone
Virofral	Amantadine
Viroptic	Trifluridine
Visine	Tetrahydrozoline (tetryzoline)
Visken	Pindolol
Vistacrom	Cromolyn
Visutensil	Guanethidine
Vivol	Diazepam
Volon	Triamcinolone
Voltaren	Diclofenac
Voltarol	Diclofenac

W

Welldorm Elixir	Chloralhydrate
Whevert	Meclizine (meclozine)
Wincoram	Amrinone
Wingom	Gallopamil
Winpred	Prednisone
Wyamycin	Erythomycin-ethylsuccinate

X

Xanax	Alprazolam
Xanef	Enalapril
Xylocain	Lidocaine
Xylocard	Lidocaine
Xylonest	Prilocaine

Y

Yomesan	Niclosamide
Yutopar	Ritodrine

Z

Zadstat	Metronidazole
Zantac	Ranitidine
Zapex	Oxazepam
Zarontin	Ethosuximide
Zepine	Reserpine
Zestril	Lisinopril
Zinamide	Pyrazinamide
Zocor	Simvastatin
Zoladex	Goserelin
Zovirax	Acyclovir
Zyloprim	Allopurinol
Zyloric U	Allopurinol

Index